The Anatomical Foundations of Regional Anesthesia and Acute Pain Medicine

Macroanatomy
Microanatomy
Sonoanatomy
Functional anatomy

Editor

André P. Boezaart

Departments of Anesthesiology and Orthopaedic Surgery and Rehabilitation
Division of Acute and Perioperative Pain Medicine
University of Florida College of Medicine
Gainesville, Florida
USA

The Anatomical Foundations of Regional

Anesthesia and Acute Pain Medicine

Editor : **André P. Boezaart**

ISBN (eBook): 978-1-68108-191-5

ISBN (Print): 978-1-68108-192-2

Published by Bentham Science Publishers –
Sharjah, UAE. All Rights Reserved.

First published in 2016.

BENTHAM SCIENCE Bentham e Books

DEDICATION

I dedicate this book with love and gratitude to my lifelong companion Karin, our children Kim, Ted and Johke and our grand children Dihan, Mila, André, Zani and Sebastian who enrich our lives far beyond their possible understanding.

I also dedicate this book to all my mentors, especially to Alon Winnie, Dannie Moore, Dag Selander and Gale Thompson who taught me that if I understood where a nerve lives, and what membranes and fascia barriers it lives in, and how to find it, I could do any known or unknown nerve block safely and successfully. All left for me was to be a Doctor, and care for patients. That teaching inspired the creation of this textbook.

André P. Boezaart

CONTENTS

FOREWORD

I have often used the quote, attributed to my dear friend, the late Alon P. Winnie, one of the "Founding Fathers" of the American Society of Regional Anesthesia, that *"regional anesthesia is nothing more than applied anatomy."* This quote and approach to regional anesthesia has been the foundation of much of my career as a military anesthesiologist. I was therefore flattered and enthusiastic when my friend and colleague, André P. Boezaart, MD, PhD, asked me to provide a forward to this masterful work, *"The Anatomical Foundations of Regional Anesthesia and Acute Pain Medicine."*

André and I have both turned to the potential of regional anesthesia in time of war to provide safe, compassionate, and logistically sound anesthesia and analgesia to soldiers wounded in combat. André served in the South African Defense Force in 1975 during the Angola War as the only anesthesiologist for the Forward Surgical Unit. Clutching a worn copy of Daniel Moore's 1967 4th edition textbook, "Regional Block," he quickly applied the lessons therein to many war casualties in long operating room sessions. In an effort to improve efficiency and avoid repeated axillary blocks for soldiers with upper extremity wounds that required further surgery or dressing changes, André performed axillary artery cut-downs and then passed central line catheters cephalad next to the artery to where the plexus crosses the first rib to provide continuous access to the brachial plexus for re-block and continuous analgesia of the arm. These catheters would remain in place for weeks and were used for frequent dressing changes and debridements common to war wounds. André's experience likely represents the first utilization of a continuous peripheral nerve block during war. Many years later, in 2003, employing far better equipment and the same love of anatomy, I would place the first continuous peripheral nerve block in a United States soldier evacuated from Iraq after sustaining near fatal injuries that included a traumatic amputation of his left leg below the knee. As in André's experience, these continuous regional techniques provided excellent operating room anesthetic conditions, remarkable perioperative analgesia, and greatly enhanced the wounded soldiers comfort during long evacuation flights without the nausea and respiratory depression associated with the exclusive (and at the time far too common) use of morphine for pain management. I am pleased to say that regional anesthesia and continuous nerve blocks are now routine practice in American military and civilian medicine. There are few situations in medical practice that are more unforgiving and difficult than the management of polytrauma casualties in austere battlefield conditions. The "discovery" of the utility of regional anesthesia by two (much younger at the time) anesthesiologists on two very different battlefields, separated by decades, is a testimony to the power this technique affords the anesthesiologist willing to invest the time necessary to acquire the essential anatomical knowledge required to apply these techniques safely, successfully, and consistently.

It is against this background that André has produced an anatomical text that focuses on the macro-, micro-, sono-, and functional anatomy that is vital for success in the field of regional anesthesia and acute pain medicine. So much of our teaching was, and regrettably still is, focused on how to find the nerves (ultrasound, nerve stimulation, paresthesia), and by far not enough on where these nerves are and what tissues and membranes surround them. This book gives equal weight to all three of these matters. The anatomical focus and approach to regional anesthesia provided in this text is refreshingly unique and much needed. Certainly, ultrasound technology in regional anesthesia has been revolutionary in terms of our ability to place needles and deposit local anesthetics in appropriate spaces around target nerves. Unfortunately, some have leaned too heavily on this technology as a crutch to overcome a poor grasp of basic anatomy. I predict that, like André's worn copy of Daniel Moore's *"Regional Block"* saved the lives and reduced suffering of many hundreds of wounded soldiers during the 1975 Angolan War, *"The Anatomical Foundations of Regional Anesthesia and Acute Pain Medicine"* will become a cherished companion of countless anesthesiologists who desire the virtues of regional anesthesia and understand that they must apply these foundations safely and with the confidence that is borne from a detailed knowledge of human anatomy.

It is my great honor to be the first to congratulate André Boezaart on this masterful effort that is the product of, and was inspired by, a truly remarkable career in anesthesiology. André does all of us, new and old acute pain specialists and regionalists alike, a great service with this refreshing look at the modern practice of regional anesthesia and acute pain medicine based on the timeless application of gross human anatomy, also now studied through modern microscopic lenses, by ultrasound beams and defining the nerve functions with electrical stimulation – macro-, micro-, sono- and functional anatomy.

Chester 'Trip' Buckenmaier
Defense and Veterans Center for Integrative Pain Management (DVCIPM.org)
Professor Anesthesiology
Department of Military Emergency Medicine
Uniformed Services University, USU '92
USA

PREFACE

Many thousands of high quality anatomy textbooks have been written over the centuries, and this textbook does not attempt to replace any of these or to improve on any of them. As a matter of fact, many of those texts were used as source material for this book. Those books remain essential parts of our fundamental study of Medicine. They contain beautiful photographs and drawings of carefully prepared dissections of anatomical specimens. However, to make the anatomy pictures beautiful and understandable the fascia and tissue barriers that surround tissue and organs (nerves in this case) had to be removed to illustrate the structures clearly; these textbooks were written to explain the gross macroanatomy to surgeons and other physicians.

But anatomy for regional anesthesia and acute pain medicine is different. Local anesthetic agents do not readily cross over anatomical barriers, and if they did they would be highly toxic. They therefore have to be deposited in the correct spaces surrounding nerves to allow diffusion to nerve axons without harming them. To describe these spaces, the authors of this textbook make liberal use of modern microscopic and electron microscopic studies of nerves as well as new ultrasound technology to explain, not only where the nerves are, but also what structures, membranes and barriers surround them and what the functions of the nerves are. Local anesthetic agents can only be effective if they reach the axons of nerves and they can only reach the axons if they were injected into the correct tissue compartment close enough so that it can readily diffuse to the axons, while the nerve axons are still protected from its potential toxic effects.

This textbook is also not a regional anesthesia or acute pain medicine textbook. It does not attempt to instruct on the techniques or style of performing nerve blocks and the authors tried to refrain from expressing opinions, but rather reflect on the anatomical facts, as we now know them. Its quest is to teach where the nerves are (macroanatomy), what tissue membranes and barriers surround them (microanatomy), what their functions are (functional anatomy), and how to find them (sonoanatomy). If these are known and understood, any nerve block, known or unknown to us, should be easy to accomplish effectively and safely.

Some of our new understanding of the microanatomy has become apparent in only the past few years, especially the circumneural (paraneural) sheath/space, and most of the "newer" knowledge basically served to validate and emphasize our previous knowledge from the days of Keys and Retzius some 150 years ago. For the old and new understanding the authors would like to pay tribute to the contributions and influences that the groundbreaking work of Gale Thompson, Dag Selander, Daniel Moore, Henning Anderson, Manoj Karmakar, and Miguel Reina and their colleagues, among many others, had on the creation of this textbook. We finally realized that what we for many years have simply called the "sweet spot of the nerve," the place where regional anesthesiologists of yesteryear coined the phrase "*no paresthesia, no block*" for, is nothing else but the subcircumneural (subparaneural) space. It also explains why some secondary blocks work well while others fail.

With the recent introduction of ultrasound technology to our practice, we realized its tremendous value. Unfortunately, ultrasound works best when we need it least, for example, when looking at superficial nerves, and *visa versa*. Furthermore, until high-definition ultrasound is universally and readily available, the membranes and connective tissue barriers surrounding nerves will continue not to be clearly "visible" by regular ultrasound. Ultrasound scanning is dynamic, and the way to fully appreciate the image looked at is to follow a structure, a nerve for example, to see where it comes from and where it is going to, or to see pulsations of arteries, compression of veins, or shimmering of lung tissue, *etc*. For this reason, the authors present the sonoanatomy not only as still images, but also as video productions to express a particular structure's dynamic view.

Finally, the book deals with the functional anatomy of every nerve that lends itself to high yield regional block. For that we describe the motor response these nerves have to electrical stimulation, and also through video productions demonstrating the motor responses by percutaneous nerve stimulation using a human model with the surface anatomy painted on her.

The design of this textbook is such that by viewing the figures and reading their legends, together with the viewing the video productions, practitioners should gain a high level of a working knowledge of the anatomical foundations required to practice safe and effective regional anesthesia and acute pain medicine. Should the student wish to learn more, there is ample supportive text and references to study the fundamental concepts further.

André P. Boezaart
Departments of Anesthesiology and Orthopaedic Surgery and Rehabilitation
Division of Acute and Perioperative Pain Medicine
University of Florida College of Medicine
Gainesville, Florida
USA

CONTRIBUTORS

André P. Boezaart	Departments of Anesthesiology and Orthopaedic Surgery and Rehabilitation, Division of Acute and Perioperative Pain Medicine, University of Florida College of Medicine, Gainesville, Florida, USA
Paul E. Bigeleisen	Department of Anesthesiology, University of Maryland, Baltimore, Maryland, USA
Donald S. Bohannon	Department of Anesthesiology, Division of Acute and Perioperative Pain Medicine, University of Florida College of Medicine, Gainesville, Florida, USA
David A. Edwards	Vanderbilt University Medical Center, Department of Anesthesiology, Nashville Tennessee, USA
Barys V. Ihnatsenka	Department of Anesthesiology, Division of Acute and Perioperative Pain Medicine, University of Florida College of Medicine, Gainesville, Florida, USA
Linda Le-Wendling	Department of Anesthesiology, Division of Acute and Perioperative Pain Medicine, University of Florida College of Medicine, Gainesville, Florida, USA
Anastacia P. Munro	Department of Anesthesiology, Division of Acute and Perioperative Pain Medicine, University of Florida College of Medicine, Gainesville, Florida, USA
Johan P. Reyneke	Department of Maxillofacial and Oral Surgery, University of the Western Cape, South Africa; Centre for Orthognathic Surgery, Cape Town Mediclinic, Cape Town, South Africa; Department of Maxillofacial and Oral Surgery, University of the Western Cape, Cape Town, South Africa; Division of Oral and Maxillofacial Surgery, Universidad Autonoma de Nuevo Leon, Monterrey, Mexico; Department of Oral and Maxillofacial Surgery, University of Oklahoma College of Dentistry, Oklahoma City, Oklahoma, USA and Department of Oral and Maxillofacial Surgery, University of Florida College of Dentistry, Gainesville, Florida, USA
Yury Zasimovich	Department of Anesthesiology, Division of Acute and Perioperative Pain Medicine, University of Florida College of Medicine, Gainesville, Florida, USA

CHAPTER 1

Applied Macroanatomy of the Upper Extremity Nerves Above the Clavicle

André P. Boezaart[1,*] and Paul Bigeleisen[2]

[1]Departments of Anesthesiology and Orthopaedic Surgery and Rehabilitation, Division of Acute and Perioperative Pain Medicine, University of Florida College of Medicine, Gainesville, Florida, USA and [2]Department of Anesthesiology, University of Maryland, Baltimore, Maryland, USA

Abstract: In this chapter, the authors present the most common arrangement of the brachial plexus; its five roots of origin, three trunks, anterior and posterior divisions, three cords, and, finally, its terminal branches. The sensory dermatomal and osteotomal innervation of the spinal roots are discussed, as well as the neurotomal distribution of each peripheral terminal branch. Anatomical dissections of the lateral view of the neck and its posterior triangle are presented, as well as trans-sectional anatomical views at the level of the 6th cervical vertebra. Photographs of anatomical dissections of the five scalene muscles are discussed, especially the crossover of the fibers of the anterior and middle scalene muscles, which forms the paravertebral trough, and the seven most commonly found positional anomalies of the muscles with the roots of the cervical ventral rami. Finally, multiple anatomic sagittal sections of the neck, starting from the spine and ending at the mid-clavicular line, show the supraclavicular brachial plexus. These multiple sections are presented in the form of three figures of strategic positions, and also as a movie where these multiple sections have been added together to play sequentially. The authors discuss the innervation of the five joints around the shoulder girdle in some detail in this chapter.

Keywords: Anterior scalene muscle, Brachial plexus, Cervical paravertebral space, Dermatomes, Dorsal middle scalene muscle, Dorsal scapular nerve, Inferior trunk, Long thoracic nerve, Middle trunk Cords, Nerve to levator scapulae, Neurotomes, Osteotomes, Phrenic nerve, Posterior scalene muscle, Scalene minimi muscle, Shoulder joint innervation, Spinal accessory nerve, Spinal roots, Superior trunk, Suprascapular nerve, Ventral middle scalene muscle.

INTRODUCTION

The posterior triangle of the neck refers to the area between the clavicular head of the sternocleidomastoid muscle anterior and the anterior margin of the trapezius

***Corresponding author André P. Boezaart:** Departments of Anesthesiology and Orthopaedic Surgery, Division of Acute and Peri-operative Pain Medicine, University of Florida College of Medicine, 1600 SW Archer Road, Gainesville, Florida 32610, USA; Tel: 352-846-0913 (Work); Fax: 352-392-7029;
E-mail: aboezaart@anest.ufl.edu

muscle posterior; the middle third of the clavicle forms the base of the triangle. For the purposes of this chapter, the triangle extends medially to the paravertebral space, and therefore does not have a "floor."

As a good understanding of anatomy is essential for performing any regional anesthesia technique or invasive procedure for acute pain medical condition, it follows that one must understand the most fundamental principle of successful acute or perioperative pain control by regional anesthesia, namely, Hilton's Law of Anatomy [1]. The principles behind Hilton's Law were first espoused in a series of medical lectures given by John Hilton between 1860 and 1862 [1]. John Hilton (1808–1878) was a British surgeon born in Essex (UK) in 1805. He was appointed demonstrator of anatomy in 1828 at Guy's Hospital and assistant surgeon in 1845; he was appointed surgeon four years later. Ten years later, he became Professor of Anatomy and Surgery at the Royal College of Surgeons. From 1859 to 1862, he presented a series of lectures in the form of a course on "Rest and Pain" [1]. The "Law of Anatomy", which has now reached classical status, was revisited and challenged in 2013 using modern technology [2] and was found to be as sound as it was in 1860.

Hilton's Law of Anatomy states: "The same trunks of nerves whose branches supply the groups of muscles moving a joint furnish also a distribution of nerves to the skin over the insertions of the same muscles; and—what at this moment more especially merits our attention—the interior of the joint receives its nerves from the same source" [2].

Upon reflection, we realize that to move any of the joints of the upper limb, all of the muscles around that specific joint are involved. Furthermore, the skin overlying that area receives sensory innervation from branches of the brachial plexus. Because of these two facts, we know that to effectively block painful stimuli generated from any of the joints of the upper limb, we have to block the entire brachial plexus.

One common misunderstanding that needs our attention, at least in our anatomical understanding, is that if, for example, 60% of the nerves that supply sensory innervation to a joint are blocked, the pain generated from that joint would be 60% less. Through the lessons we have learned over the years, especially in obstetric anesthesia where we have seen (and our unfortunate patients have experienced) the unpleasant consequences of unblocked segments or hemi-block with epidurals, and many other clinical situations, we now realize that blocking 60% of the nerves that innervate a joint does not reduce pain by 60%. In fact, it focuses 100% of the pain into the remaining 40% of the joint, therefore, in actual fact, worsening the pain and suffering of the patient. Although well intended, it is probably not true that we are doing anything positive for the patient by blocking "some" of the nerves and therefore removing "some" of the pain. Disbelief in this misunderstanding, however, is based on clinical experience; it has yet to be challenged by formal research.

Simply put, to provide optimal pain relief caused by major surgery or trauma to a joint in the upper extremity, the entire brachial plexus must be blocked. Granted, this is not always possible, especially where the plexus is spread out, as in the lumbosacral plexus. It is most difficult to achieve during a continuous nerve block, where the catheter is placed on one specific part of the plexus; for example, the posterior cord of the brachial plexus during a continuous infraclavicular block for pain associated with major wrist or elbow surgery. When the primary block (high-volume and high-concentration initial block) wears off, the secondary block often fails because the other cords are not close enough or are not in the same circumneural (paraneural) space [3] (see Chapter 2, Fig. **1**) to allow the local anesthetic agent (now of too low a volume and concentration) to diffuse to all of the nerve axons of the other two, more distant, cords. Thus, complete coverage of the pain is not achieved (see Chapter 2).

It is also not always necessary to block all the nerves that innervate a specific joint. Most if not all of the nerves that innervate a joint reach that joint *via* its joint capsule and during synovectomy, for example, the joint capsule may be destroyed by the surgery, which in effect denervates the joint, making it necessary to block only the nerves that supply sensory innervation to the tissue outside the joint capsule.

MACROANATOMY

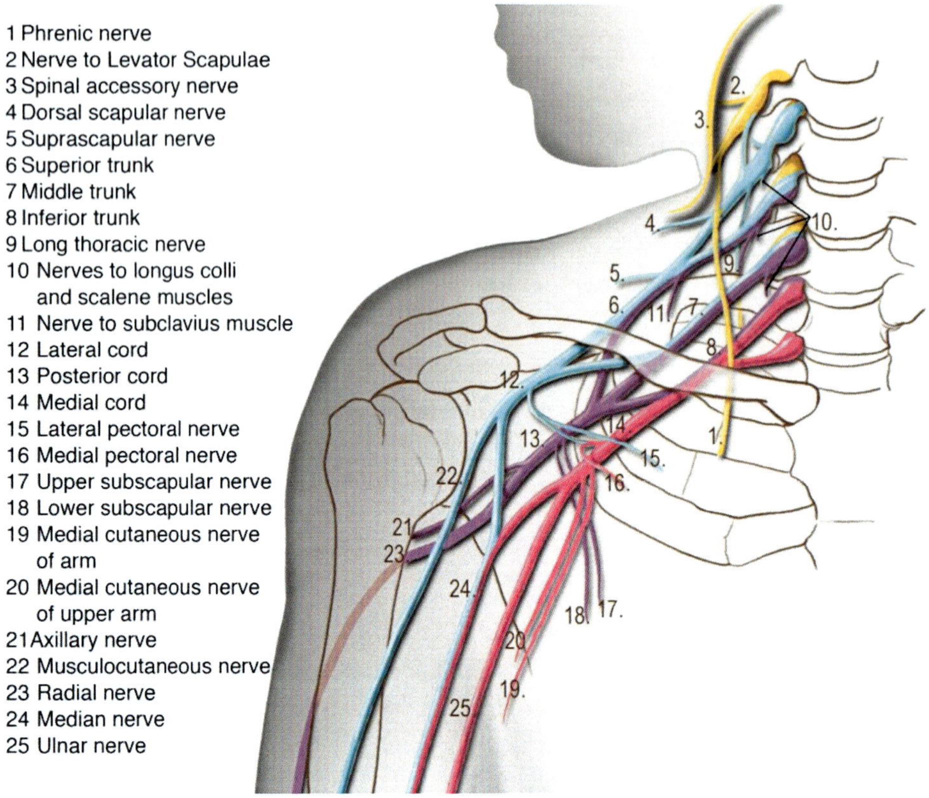

Figure 1: Schematic representation of the brachial plexus.
*The **phrenic nerve** (1) originates mainly from 4th cervical spinal root (C4) and receives a small branch from the 5th cervical spinal root (C5) of the brachial plexus and runs caudad on the belly of the anterior scalene muscle. It supplies motor innervation to the diaphragm. The **nerve to the levator scapulae muscle** (2), the **dorsal scapular nerve** (4), and the **suprascapular nerve** (5), also originate from the C4 and C5 roots. **The long thoracic nerve** (9) also stems from the C4, C5, and C6 roots. The **accessory nerve** (3) is a cranial nerve.*
*The **superior trunk** (6) forms as the C5 and C6 spinal roots join, while the **middle trunk** is a continuation from the C7 spinal root. The **inferior trunk** form as the 8th cervical (C8) and first thoracic spinal (T1) roots join. As the C5 and C6 roots come together to form the upper (superior) trunk, which gives off a small **branch to the subclavius muscle** (11). In the cervical region, the spinal roots exit the neuroforamens of the vertebra above it. Thus, C5, for example, exits the neuroforamen between the 4th and 5th cervical vertebra – above the corresponding vertebra. The first thoracic spinal root is the transition and exits below the 7th cervical vertebra and above the corresponding T1 vertebra. From there downward, all of the spinal roots of the thoracic and lumbar areas exit below the corresponding vertebra.*
*From the three trunks that usually extend to the supraclavicular area, three **divisions** split away to form the three cords of the brachial plexus: the **lateral cord** (12), the **medial cord** (13), and the **posterior cord** (14) (see Chapter 4).*

Each spinal root of the brachial plexus has its own sensory dermatomal area that it represents (Fig. **2**), as well as its own osteotomal area (Fig. **3**).

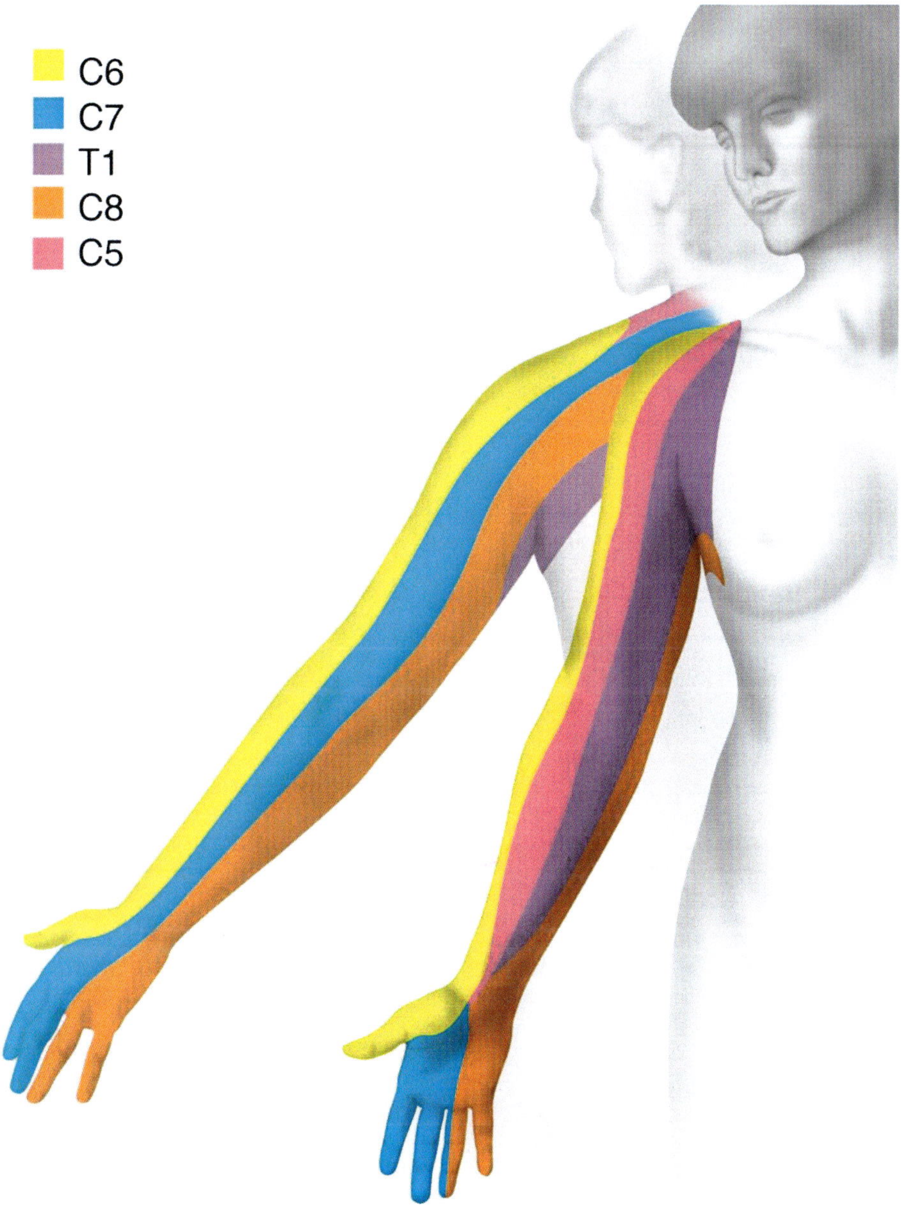

Figure 2: Schematic demarcation of the dermatomes of the upper limb.
These demarcations are not distinct segments as depicted here because there is significant overlap between adjacent dermatomes. C5, C6, C7, C8, and T1 = cervical (C5-8) and thoracic (T1) spinal roots.

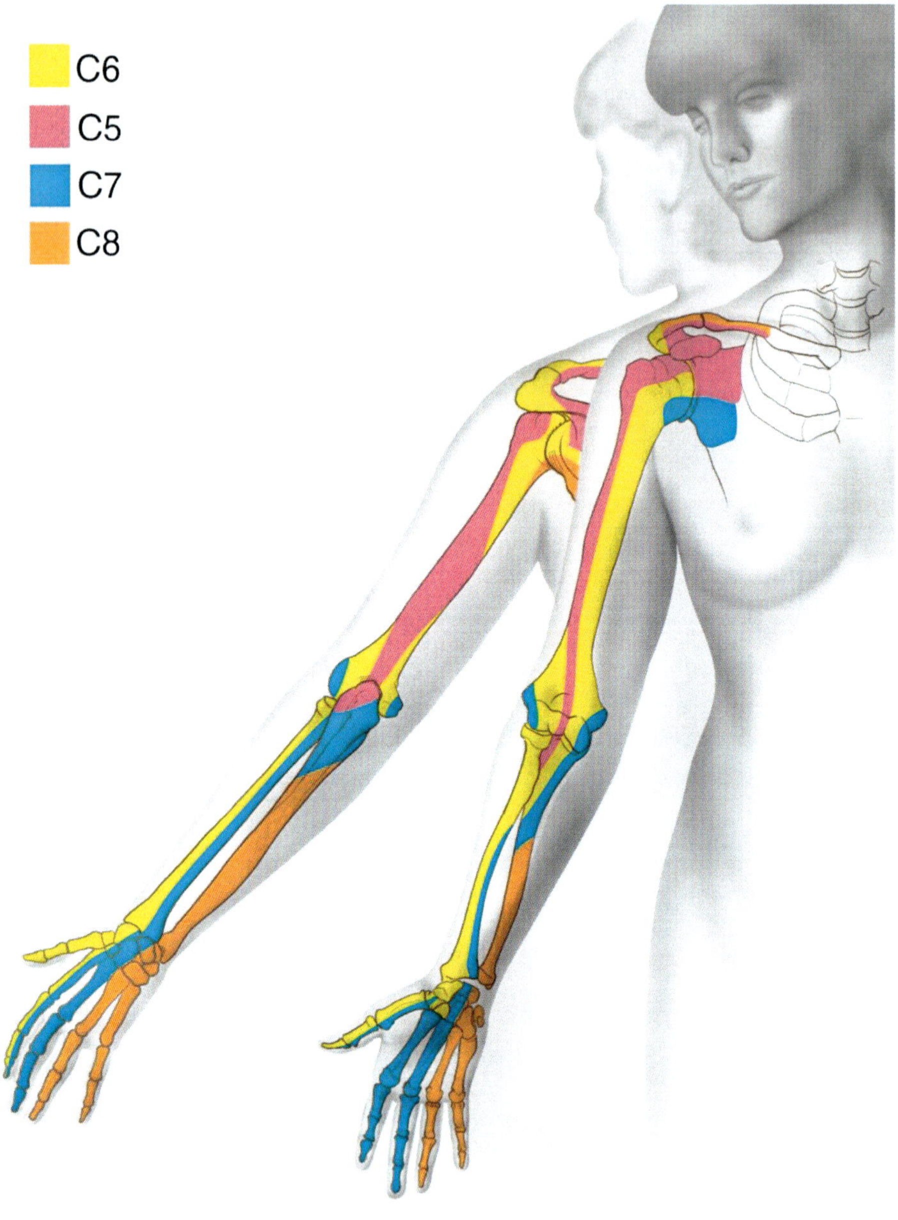

Figure 3: Schematic demarcation of the osteotomes of the upper limb.
These demarcations are not distinct segments as depicted here because there is significant overlap between adjacent osteotomes. C5, C6, C7, C8, and T1 = cervical (C5-8) spinal roots.

Although the spinal roots represent corresponding sensory dermatomes and osteotomes, the individual peripheral nerves innervate different areas of the upper limb represented by neurotomes (Fig. **4**).

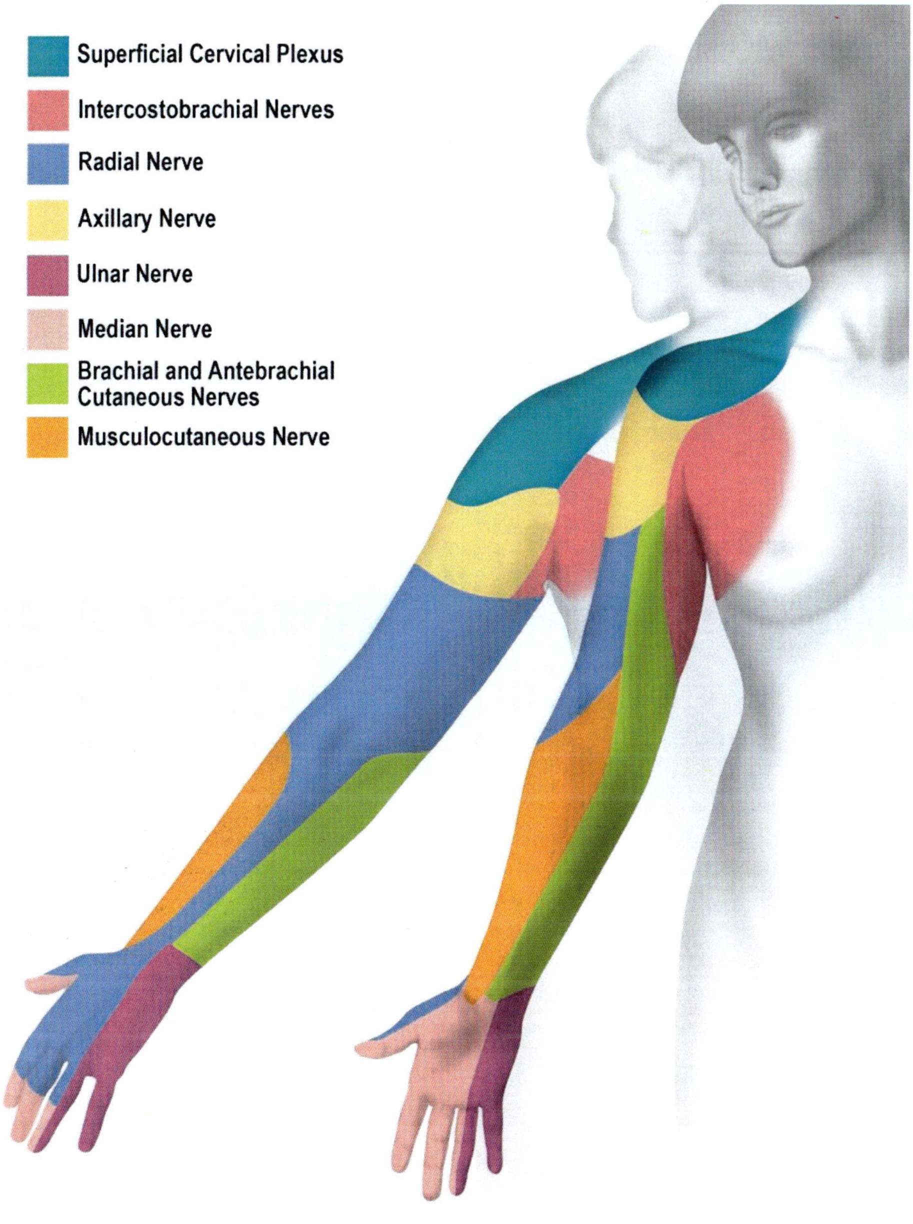

Figure 4: Schematic demarcation of the neurotomes of the upper limb.
These demarcations are not distinct areas as depicted here because there is significant overlap between adjacent neurotomes.

Please study the macroanatomy depicted in Figs. **5**, **6** and **7** below to understand the relative positions of the nerves and muscles of the posterior triangle of the neck (Figs. **5**, **6** and **7**).

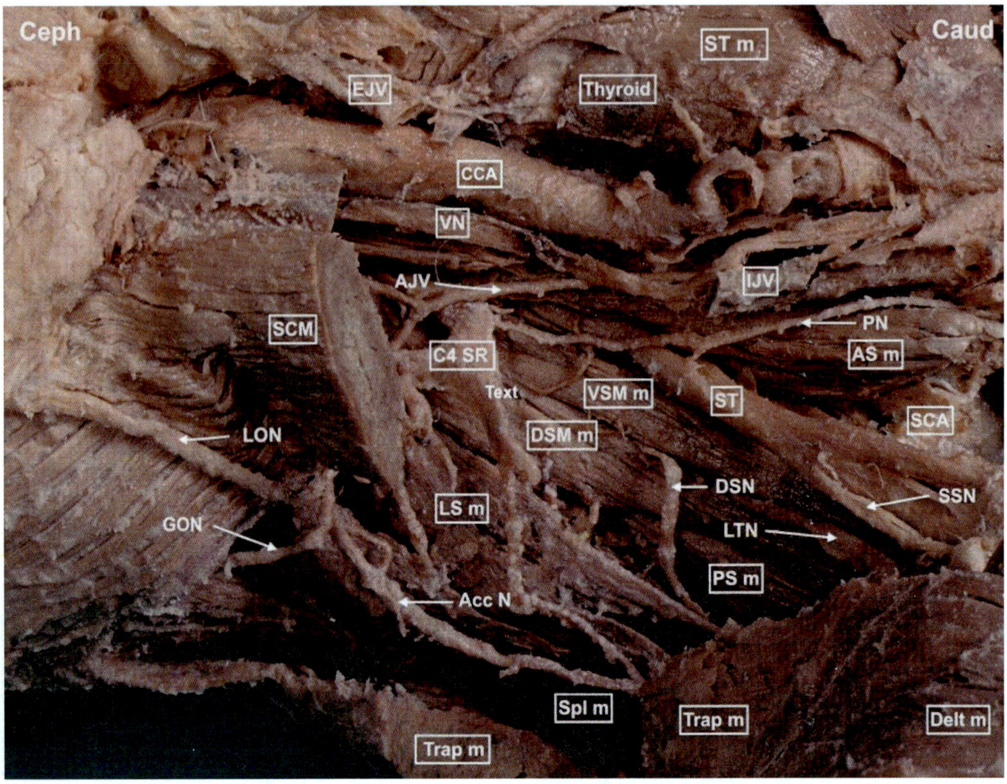

Figure 5: Anatomical dissection of the posterior triangle of the neck: lateral view.
Ceph = cephalad; Caud = caudad; SCM = sternocleidomastoid muscle (cut); Trap m = trapezius muscle (cut); Delt m = deltoid muscle; Spl m = splenius muscle; AS m = anterior scalene muscle; VSM m = ventral part of middle scalene muscle; DSM m Dorsal part of middle scalene muscle; DS m = dorsal scalene muscles m = sternothyroid muscle; LS M = levator scapulae muscle; Thyroid = thyroid gland; EJV = external jugular vein (cut); IJV = internal jugular vein (cut); AJV = anterior jugular vein; CCA = common carotid artery; SCA = subclavian artery; VN = vagus nerve (X); PN = phrenic nerve; C4 SR = 4th cervical spinal root; ST = superior trunk of the brachial plexus; DSN = dorsal scapular nerve; LTN = long thoracic nerve; SSN = suprascapular nerve; Acc = accessory nerve (XI); LON = lesser occipital nerve; GON = greater occipital nerve.

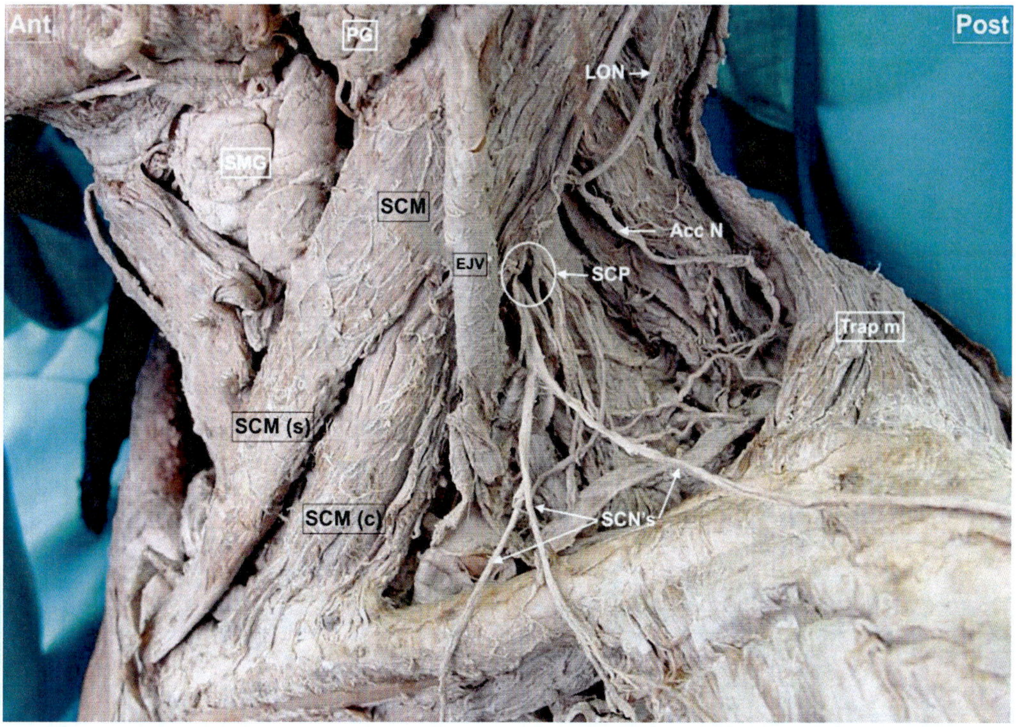

Figure 6: Anatomical dissection of the posterior triangle of the neck depicting outer structures: anterolateral view.

Ant = anterior; Post = posterior; SCM = sternocleidomastoid muscle; SCM (s) = sternal head of sternocleidomastoid muscle; SCM (c) = clavicular head of sternocleidomastoid muscle; Trap m = trapezius muscle; SMG = submandibular gland; PG = parotid gland; EJV = external jugular vein; SCP = superficial cervical plexus; SCN's = supraclavicular veins; Acc N = accessory nerve; LON = lesser occipital nerve.

We now dissect the superficial structures away (Fig. 7).

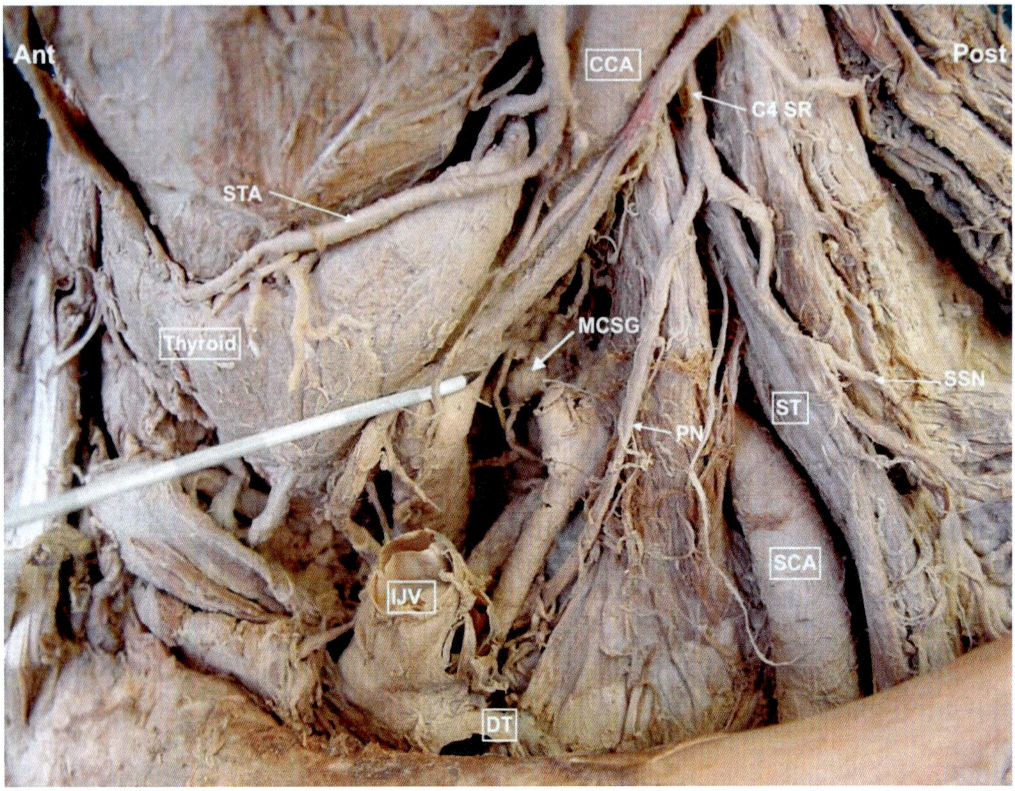

Figure 7: Anatomical dissection of the posterior triangle of the neck depicting deeper structures: anterolateral view with sternocleidomastoid muscle removed. Ant = anterior; Post = posterior; Thyroid = thyroid gland; MCSG = middle cervical sympathetic ganglion; IJV = internal jugular vein; DT = ductus thoracicus; CCA = common carotid artery; SCA = subclavian artery; STA = superior thoracic artery; ST = superior trunk of the brachial plexus; PN = phrenic nerve; SSN = suprascapular nerve; C4 SR = 4th cervical spinal root.

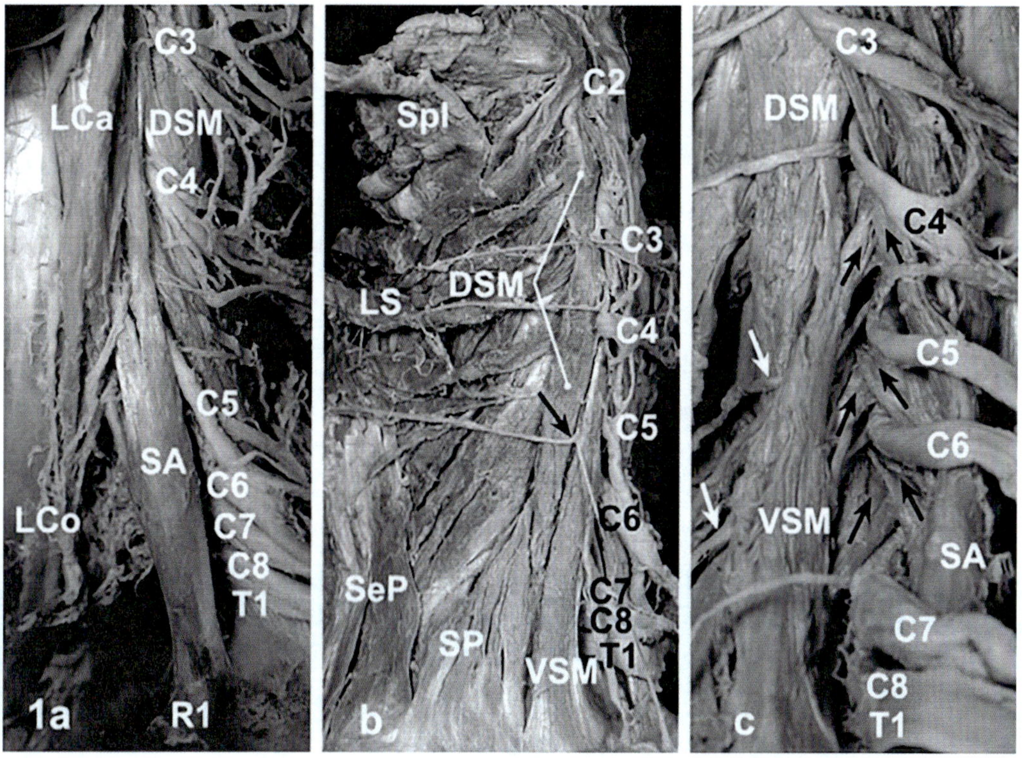

Figure 8: Dissection of 2nd to 8th ventral rami of the cervical nerve roots (C2–C8).
DSM = dorsal part of scalenus medius; LCa = longus capitis; LCo = longus colli; LS = levator scapulae; R1 = the first rib; SA = scalenus anterior; SeP = serratus posterior superior; SP = scalenus posterior; Spl = splenius capitis; T1 = the first thoracic ventral ramus; VSM = ventral part of scalenus medius.
(a) Ventral aspect of the left SA.
(b) Dorsal aspect of the right VSM, DSM and SP. Arrow indicates the common root of the dorsal scapular and long thoracic nerves.
(c) Lateral aspect of the origins of the right VSM, DSM and SA. SA and VSM attach to the anterior and posterior tubercles, and their fibers cross each other (black arrows). Upper and lower white arrows indicate the dorsal scapular and long thoracic nerves, respectively.
(Reprinted from Sakamoto [4] with permission).

It is important to note, as recently illustrated by Sakamoto [4], that muscle fibers of the anterior and middle scalene muscles cross over between the spinal roots to form an enclosed paravertebral trough medial to the cross-over (Fig. **8**). This may explain the vertical spread of local anesthetic agent along the vertebral column sometimes seen during cervical paravertebral block (Fig. **9**) [5]. Sakamoto also clarified the anatomical variations in the relationships of the five scalene muscles to the brachial plexus (Fig. **10**).

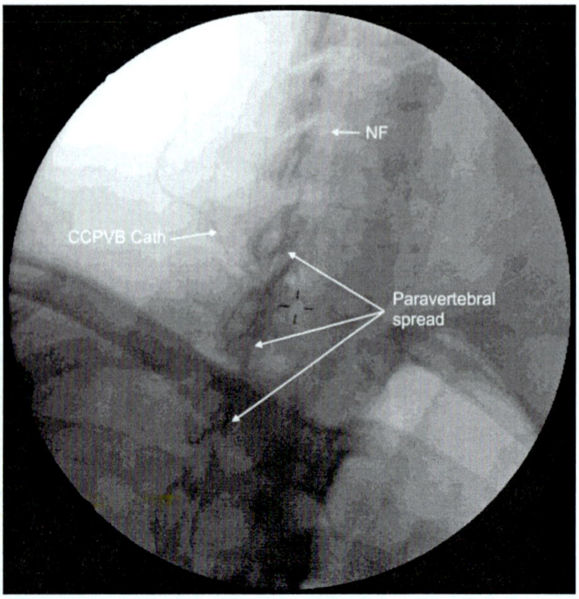

Figure 9: Oblique X-ray of cervical spine with contrast showing longitudinal paravertebral spread in the paravertebral "trough".
CCPVB Cath = catheter for continuous cervical paravertebral block placed at the level of the 7th cervical vertebra through the dorsal scalene muscle; NF = neuroforamen; arrows point to longitudinal paravertebral spread of contrast medium.

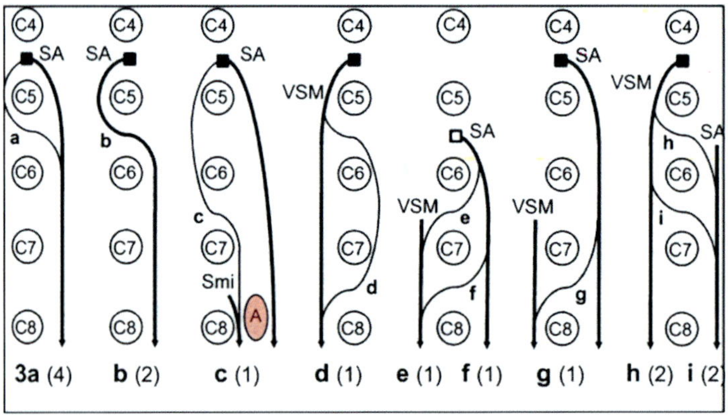

Figure 10: The schematic representations of the positional anomalies of the muscles with the roots of the cervical ventral rami.
The right hand is the ventral side, and the left one the dorsal.
A = subclavian artery; C4–C8 = the fourth to eighth cervical ventral rami; SA = scalenus anterior; Smi = scalenus minimus; VSM = ventral part of scalenus medius. Filled square = the fourth cervical vertebra; open square = the fifth cervical vertebra. The numbers in parentheses indicate the numerical quantity of the halves.
(Reprinted from Sakamoto [4] with permission)

Trans-Sectional Views of the Neck at the Level of the 6th Cervical Vertebra

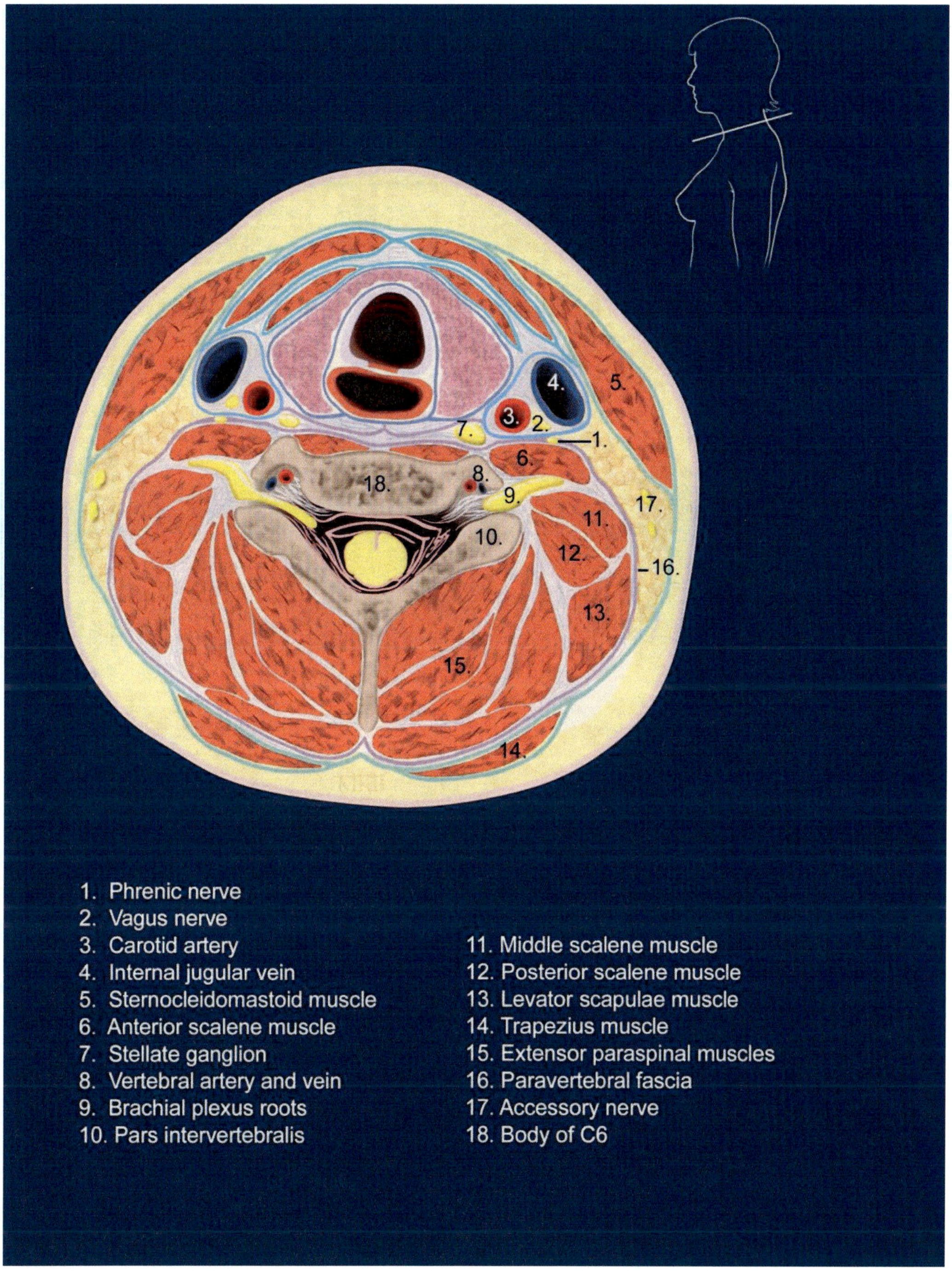

Figure 11: Trans-section of the neck through the 6th cervical vertebra area.

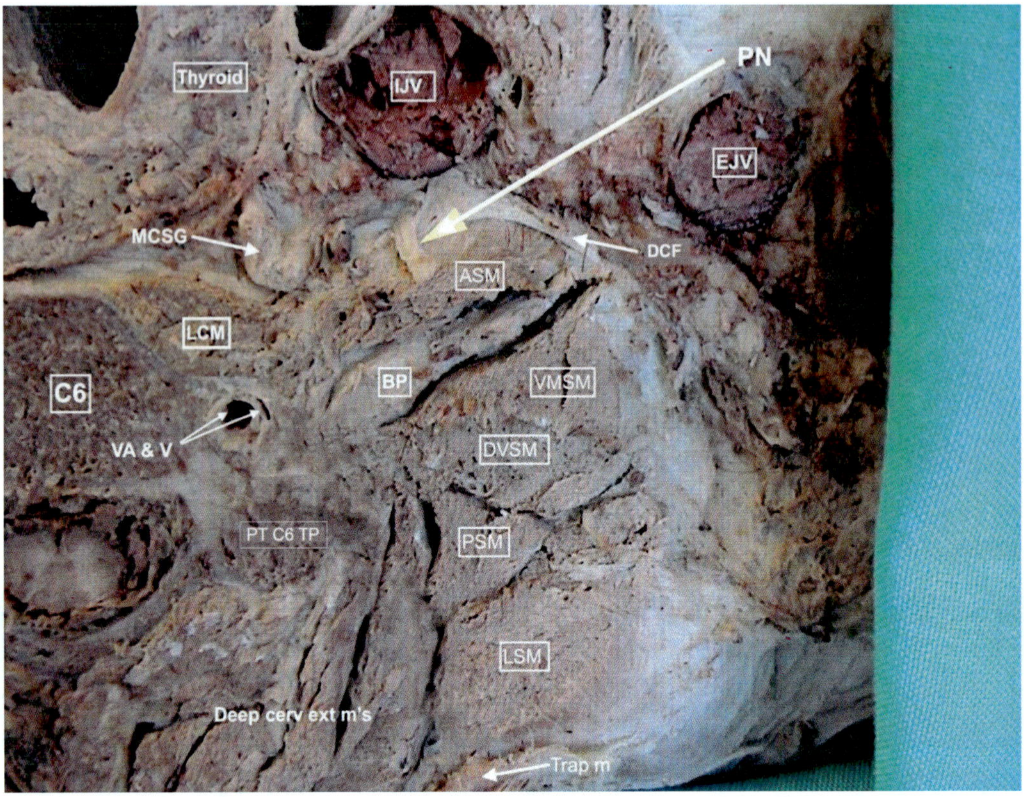

Figure 12: Anatomical axial section through the neck at the level of the 6th cervical vertebra. *C6 = body of 6th cervical vertebrae; PT C6 TP = posterior tubercle of C6 transverse process; Thyroid = thyroid gland; MCSG = middle cervical sympathetic ganglion; Deep cerv ext m's = deep cervical extensor muscles; IJV = internal jugular vein; EJV = external jugular vein; VA & V = vertebral artery and vein; ASM = anterior scalene muscle; VMSM = ventral middle scalene muscle; DVSM = dorsal middle scalene muscle; PSM = posterior scalene muscle; LSM = levator scapulae muscle; Trap m = trapezius muscle; LCM = longus colli muscle; BP = brachial plexus; PN = phrenic nerve; DCF = investing layer of deep cervical fascia.*

Sagittal Views of the Brachial Plexus

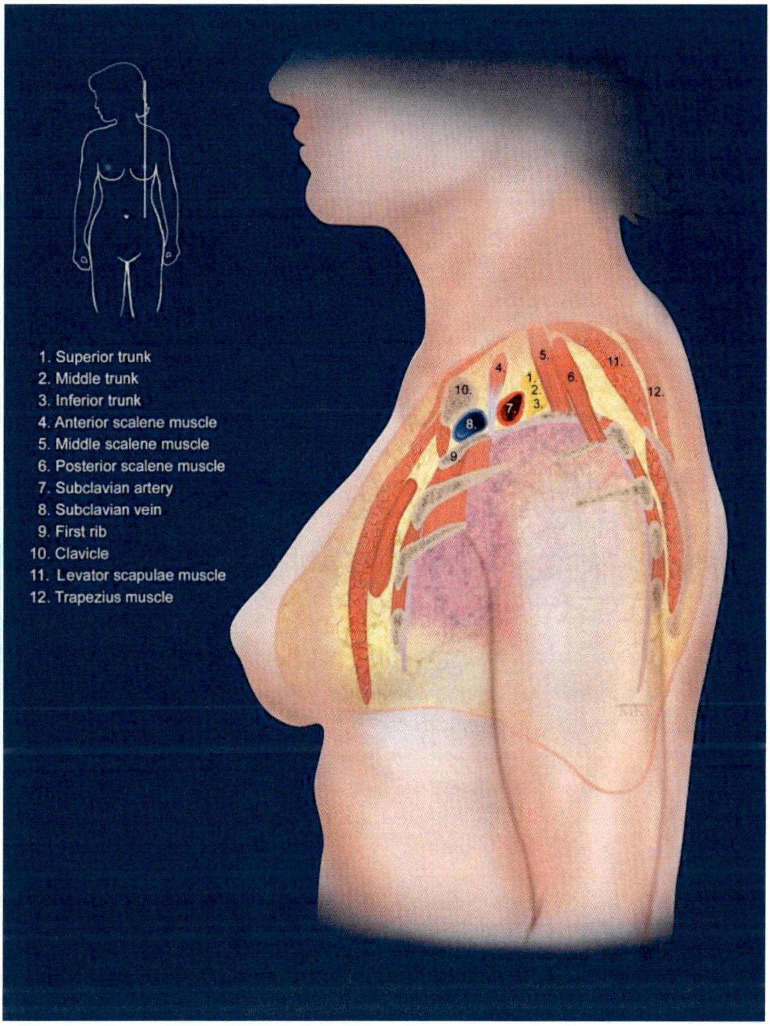

Figure 13: Sagittal view of the area where the brachial plexus crosses the first rib in the mid-clavicular plane.

*The anterior (4) and middle (5) scalene muscle implant onto the first rib (9) and the subclavian artery (7) and brachial plexus (1, 2, and 3) run between them. The posterior scalene muscle (6) implants on the second rib. The subclavian vein passes anterior to the anterior scalene muscle where it implants onto the first rib. The artery, vein, and inferior trunk course over the pleura of the dome of the lung before they reaches the first rib. In the subclavian area, therefore, the three trunks of the brachial plexus (1, 2, and 3) can be seen posterior and lateral to the artery (7) (Fig **10**) and all four of these structures are between the anterior (4) and middle (5) scalene muscles. Fig. **10** also depicts the vein (8) anterior and medial to the anterior scalene muscle and the posterior scalene muscle (6) where it implants onto the second rib. This is where the suprascapular block is typically performed.*

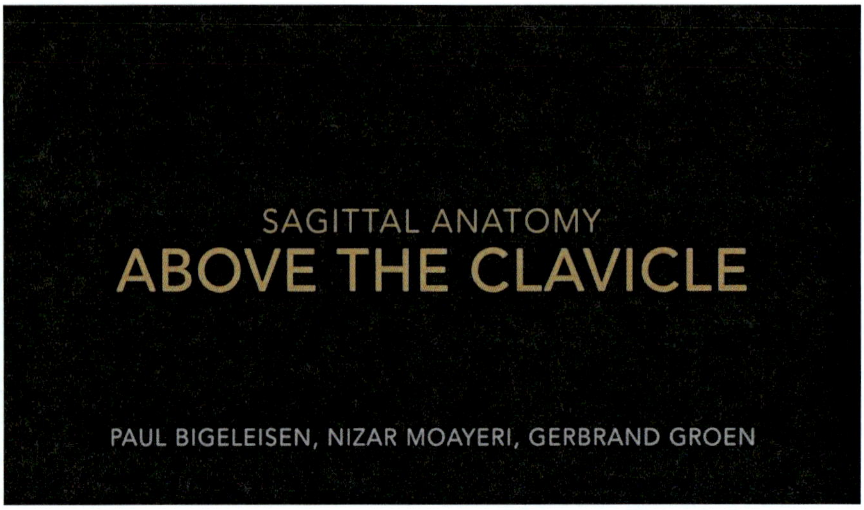

To view this movie click on this link:
https://raeducation.com/ebook

Movie 1: Sagittal sectional anatomy of the brachial plexus above the clavicle.

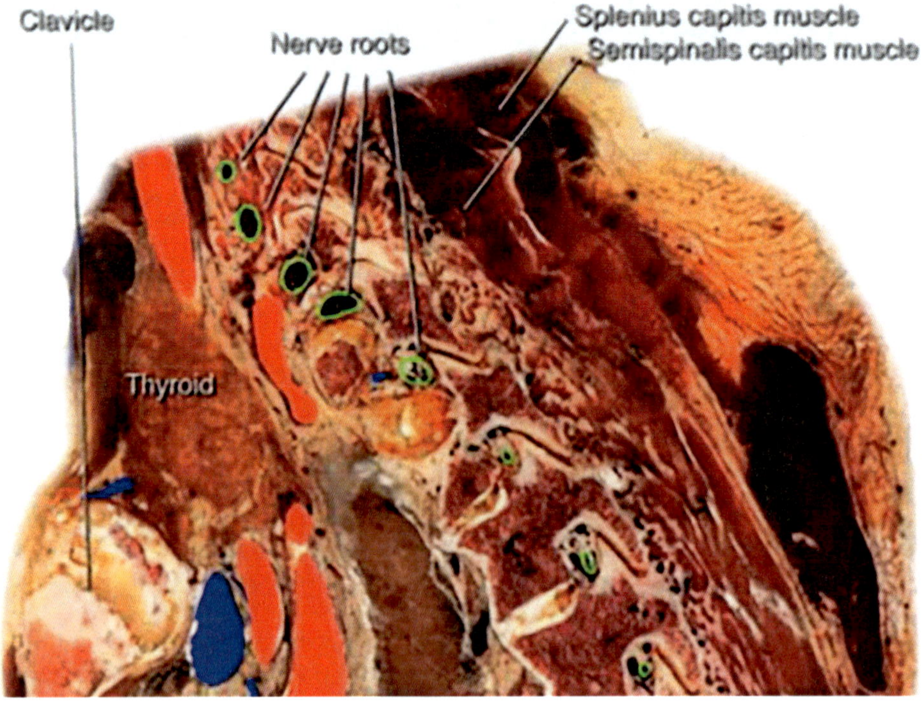

Figure 14: Anatomic sagittal section through the paramedian section showing the five roots of the brachial plexus (green).

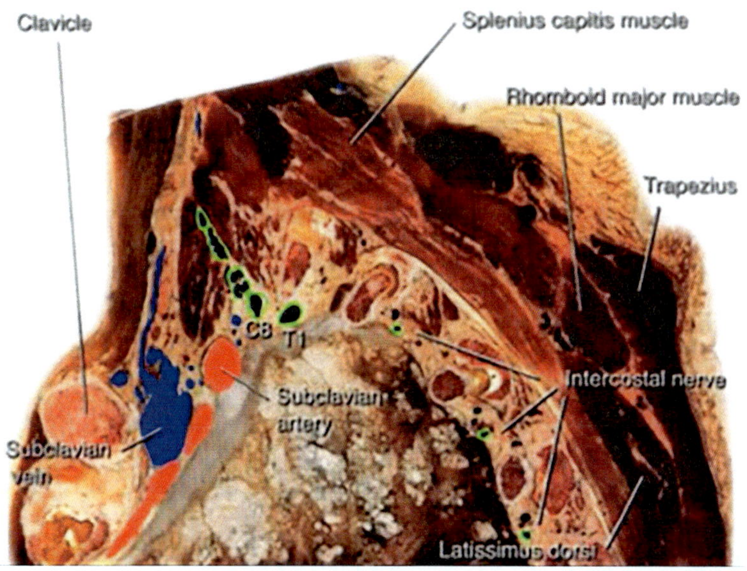

Figure 15: Anatomical sagittal section lateral to the transverse processes of the cervical vertebrae showing the 5th and 6th cervical spinal root joining to form the upper or superior trunk, the middle trunk, the 8th cervical spinal root, and the 1st thoracic spinal root not yet together to form the inferior trunk (green).
The intercostal nerves are also shown. Also, note the position of the subclavian artery and vein.

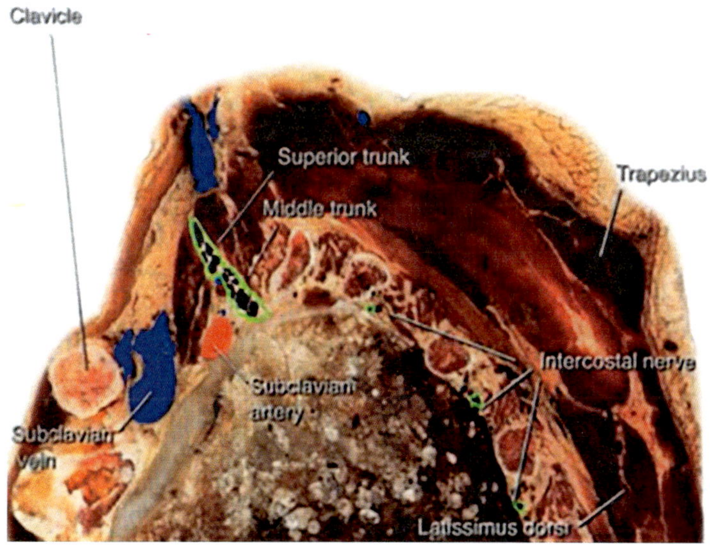

Figure 16: Anatomical sagittal section in the semi-mid-clavicular region depicting the formation of all three trunks of the brachial plexus. (Inferior trunk is not marked).

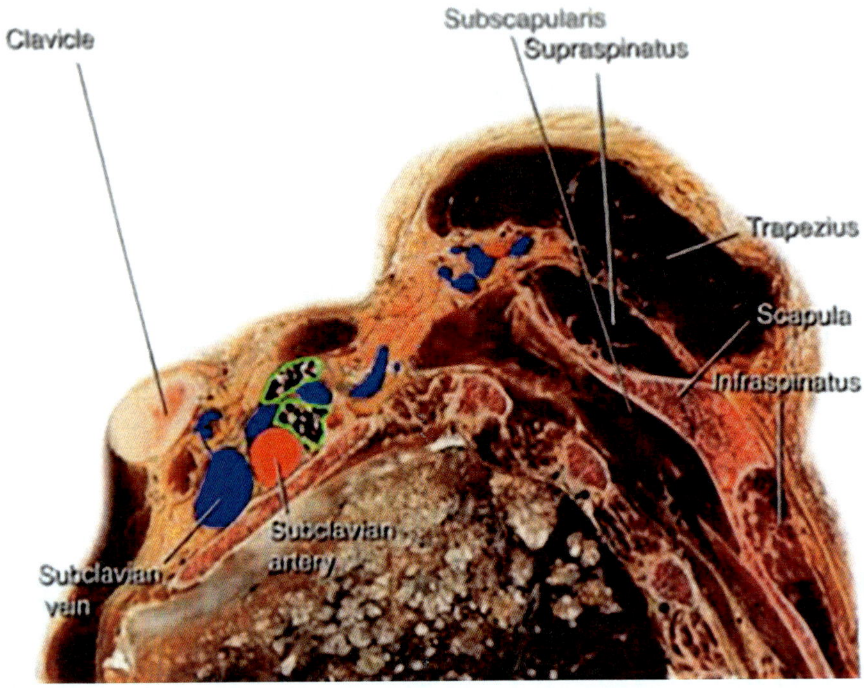

Figure 17: Anatomical sagittal section through the true mid-clavicular area depicting all three trunks (green) on the first rib and posterior and lateral to the subclavian artery.

INNERVATION OF THE SHOULDER JOINT

The shoulder girdle is highly mobile and firmly attached to the rest of the skeleton only at the sternoclavicular joint. It is able to swing 360 degrees and most of its movements shift the clavicle and brachial plexus in opposite directions; however, the position of the brachial plexus relative to the pivotal point of the shoulder girdle remains constant.

The shoulder "joint" comprises five joints: the glenohumeral, the acromioclavicular, the subacromial, the sternoclavicular, and the scapulocostal joints. Because of this, the innervation of the shoulder joint is complex, but Aszmann and his colleagues, to a large extent, unraveled it in 1996 [6].

The Glenohumeral Joint

1. ***The anterior capsule of the glenohumeral joint (GHJ)*** receives its sensory innervation from the subscapular (C5/C6), axillary (C5/C6), and lateral pectoral (C5/C6) nerves.

a. Articular branches of the subscapular nerve. There are usually three subscapular nerves that arise from the posterior cord of the brachial plexus and they give off articular branches to the anterior capsule of the GHJ.

b. Articular branches of the axillary nerve. The axillary nerve is the last nerve of the posterior cord of the brachial plexus before it becomes the radial nerve. Early in its course on the subscapular muscle, it gives off its first articular branch to the anteroinferior GHJ capsule. Further down, the axillary nerve splits into its two main branches. The medial branch supplies the sensory innervation for the scapular aspect of the anteroinferior joint capsule and parts of the axillary recess, whereas the lateral branch innervates the humeral part of the anterior capsule. The muscular branch to the teres minor muscle gives off a small articular branch to the lateral axillary recess.

c. Articular branch of the lateral pectoral nerve. The lateral pectoral nerve is the most superficial branch of the brachial plexus in the supraclavicular fossa and has a communicating branch to the medial pectoral nerve (ansa pectoralis, see Fig. **1**). Just before perforating the clavipectoral fascia, it gives off a small articular branch that runs over the acromion process where it gives off a small twig to the coracoclavicular ligament. The articular branch of the lateral pectoral nerve also innervates the anterior acromioclavicular joint. The lateral pectoral nerve further innervates the subacromial bursa and gives off an articular branch to the anterior GHJ capsule in some cases.

2. ***The posterior GHJ capsule***

a. The suprascapular nerve arises from the superior trunk of the brachial plexus and crosses the posterior triangle of the neck to the scapular notch. It gives off a relatively large superior articular branch that runs with it through the suprascapular notch underneath the transverse scapular ligament. This branch turns laterally around the base of the coracoid process where it gives off a small branch to the periostium of the coracoid process and the coracoclavicular ligament. One of its two terminal branches innervates the coracohumeral ligament and the adjacent GHJ capsule. The other terminal branch innervates the subacromial bursa and the posterior aspect of the acromioclavicular joint capsule *via* a number of smaller twigs. A large branch of the muscular branch to the supraspinatus muscle goes to the posterior GHJ capsule.

The Acromioclavicular Joint

The anterior part of the acromioclavicular joint receives its innervation from the articular branch of the lateral pectoral nerve, whereas the articular branch of the suprascapular nerve innervates its posterior part. Both of these nerves run over the coracoid process, which should theoretically make this an easily reachable position to block painful stimuli that originated from the rotator cuff, subacromial joint, or acromioclavicular joint. Note that the communicating branch from the medial pectoral nerve (ansa pectoralis) may be the reason why high interscalene blocks, especially continuous interscalene blocks, that focus on the C5 and C6 roots or upper trunk do not always provide complete analgesia for pain associated with surgery in these areas. The medial cord originates from the C8 and T1 spinal roots and inferior trunk.

The Subacromial Joint

The anterior subacromial joint and subacromial bursa receive their innervation from the articular branch of the lateral pectoral nerve, and the articular branch of the suprascapular nerve innervates mainly the posterior part of this joint and the bursa.

The Sternoclavicular Joint

The sternoclavicular joint receives its innervation from branches of the anterior supraclavicular nerve that originate from the superficial cervical plexus (C3, see Chapter 23, Fig. **12a**). It also receives its innervation from the nerve to the subclavius muscle, which is a branch of the C6 cervical spinal root or superior trunk of the brachial plexus [7].

The Scapulocostal Joint

Branches of the subscapular nerves, the long thoracic nerve and lateral cutaneous branches of the intercostal nerves, innervate the scapulocostal joint.

ACKNOWLEDGEMENTS

The authors gratefully acknowledge the following people:

- The Head of the Department of Anesthesiology of the College of Medicine of the University of Florida, Dr. Tim Morey and his department for their moral support and continuous encouragement.
- The faculty and fellows of the Division of acute and perioperative pain medicine for affording the author the time to produce this work by covering his clinical duties.
- Corey Astrom of the Department of Anesthesiology of the College of Medicine of the University of Florida for her professional and high quality text editing.
- Mary K. Bryson for her illustrations of Figs. **1**, **4**, **11** and **13**.
- Professors Gerbrand Groen and Paul Bigeleisen and Dr. Nizar Moayeri from the University Medical College in Utrecht, The Netherlands for their making of Movie **1** and providing Figs. **14-17**.
- Raeducation.com LLC for their financial support.

CONFLICT OF INTEREST

The authors confirm that this chapter contents have no conflict of Interest

DISCLOSURE

The legends of Figs. (**8** and **10**) have been copied for clarification of the figures that have been reprinted with permission from Sakamoto [4].

ABBREVIATIONS

Acc	=	accessory nerve (XI)
Acc N	=	accessory nerve
AJV	=	anterior jugular vein

Ant	=	anterior
Ao	=	aorta
AS m	=	anterior scalene muscle
ASM	=	anterior scalene muscle
BP	=	brachial plexus
C4 SR	=	4th cervical spinal root
Caud	=	caudad
CCA	=	common carotid artery
CCPVB Cath	=	catheter for continuous cervical paravertebral block placed
Ceph	=	cephalad
DCF	=	investing layer of deep cervical fascia
Deep cerv ext m's	=	deep cervical extensor muscles
Delt m	=	deltoid muscle
DS m	=	dorsal scalene muscles m
DSM	=	dorsal part of scalenus medius
DSM m	=	dorsal part of middle scalene muscle
DSN	=	dorsal scapular nerve
DT	=	ductus thoracicus
DVSM	=	dorsal middle scalene muscle
EJV	=	external jugular vein
GHJ	=	glenohumeral joint

GON	=	greater occipital nerve
IJV	=	internal jugular vein
LCa	=	longus capitis
LCM	=	longus colli muscle
LCo	=	longus colli
LON	=	lesser occipital nerve
LS	=	levator scapulae
LSM	=	levator scapulae muscle
LTN	=	long thoracic nerve
MCSG	=	middle cervical sympathetic ganglion
NF	=	neuroforamen
PG	=	parotid gland
PN	=	phrenic nerve
Post	=	posterior
PSM	=	posterior scalene muscle
PT C6 TP	=	posterior tubercle of C6 transverse process
R1	=	the first rib
SA	=	scalenus anterior
SCA	=	subclavian artery
SCM (c)	=	clavicular head of sternocleidomastoid muscle
SCM (s)	=	sternal head of sternocleidomastoid muscle

SCM	=	sternocleidomastoid muscle
SCN's	=	supraclavicular veins
SCP	=	superficial cervical plexus
SeP	=	serratus posterior superior
SHM	=	sternothyroid muscle
SMG	=	submandibular gland
SP	=	scalenus posterior
Spl	=	splenius capitis
Spl m	=	splenius muscle
SSN	=	suprascapular nerve
SSN	=	suprascapular nerve
ST	=	superior trunk of the brachial plexus
STA	=	superior thoracic artery
T1	=	the first thoracic ventral ramus
Thyroid	=	thyroid gland;
Trap m	=	trapezius muscle
VA & V	=	vertebral artery and vein
VMSM	=	ventral middle scalene muscle
VN	=	vagus nerve (X)
VSM	=	ventral part of scalenus medius
VSM m	=	ventral part of middle scalene muscle

REFERENCES

[1] Hilton, J. On Rest and Pain: A Course of Lectures on the Influence of Mechanical and Physiological Rest in the Treatment of Accidents and Surgical Diseases, and the Diagnostic Value of Pain, delivered at the Royal College of Surgeons of England in the years 1860, 1861, 1862 and 1863.

[2] Hébert-Blouin M-N, Tubbs RS, Carmichael SW, Spinner RJ. Hilton's Law revisited. Clin Anat 2014; 27: 548-55.

[3] Reina MA, Sala-Blanch X. Cross-sectional microscopic anatomy of the brachial plexus and paraneural sheaths. In: Reina MA, Ed. Atlas of functional anatomy for regional anesthesia and pain medicine. New York: Springer Science and Business Media, 2015: 185.

[4] Sakamoto Y. Spatial relationship between the morphologies and innervations of the scalene and anterior and vertebral muscles. An Anat 2012; 194: 381-88.

[5] Boezaart AP, Ihnatsenka BV. Cervical paravertebral block for elbow and wrist surgery: The jury verdict may be neither easy nor popular. Reg Anesth Pain Med 2014; 39: 361-62.

[6] Aszmann OC, Dellon AL, Birely BT, McFarland EG. Innervation of the human shoulder joint and its implications for surgery. Clin Orthop Relat Res 1996; 330: 202-7.

[7] Standring S, Ed. Gray's anatomy: The anatomical basis of clinical practice Thirty-ninth edition. New York: Elsevier Churchill Livingstone 2005; p. 827.

Chapter 2:
The Microanatomy of the Brachial Plexus and Peripheral Nerves

CHAPTER 2

The Microanatomy of the Brachial Plexus and Peripheral Nerves

André P. Boezaart*

Professor of Anesthesiology and Orthopaedic Surgery, Departments of Anesthesiology and Orthopaedic Surgery and Rehabilitation, Division of Acute and Perioperative Pain Medicine, University of Florida, College of Medicine, Gainesville, Florida, USA

Abstract: The aims of this chapter are to explain and present the older and new concepts and understanding around the microanatomy of nerve roots, trunks, and peripheral nerves. More recent work over the past 3 or 4 years looked at nerves with high-definition ultrasound and electron microscopy and illustrated that the paraneural or circumneural sheath is what neurosurgeons for years have been calling the "gliding apparatus" of the nerve. The space just deep to this layer is the subcircumneural (subparaneural) space, which should most probably be the target space for successful and safe single-injection block and catheter placement for continuous nerve block. The different microanatomical features of spinal roots, plexus trunks, and peripheral nerves are discussed and compared, as well as the microanatomical explanation of the different sonographical appearance of these three types of nerves.

Keywords: Anterior motor spinal root, Anterior scalene muscle, Arachnoid mater, Arachnoid villi, Arachnoid villus, Circumneural sheath, Circumneurium, Cross-over of muscle fibers, Dorsal middle scalene muscle, Dorsal scapular nerve, Dura mater, Epimysium, Epineurium, Long thoracic nerve, Paraneural cyst, Paraneural sheath, Phrenic nerve, Pia mater, Posterior scalene muscle, Posterior sensory spinal root, Prevertebral layer of deep cervical fascia, Scalene minimi muscle, Subcircumneural space, Subepimyseal space, Subparaneural space, Ventral middle scalene muscle.

INTRODUCTION

For effective regional anesthesia and nerve blocks in acute pain medicine, it is not only vital to understand the cross-anatomical positioning of plexuses and nerves (macroanatomy) and how to find the nerves (sonoanatomy and functional

***Corresponding author André P Boezaart:** Professor of Anesthesiology and Orthopaedic Surgery, Departments of Anesthesiology and Orthopaedic Surgery, Division of Acute and Peri operative Pain Medicine, University of Florida College of Medicine, 1600 SW Archer Road, Gainesville, Florida 32610, USA; Tel: 352-846-0913 (Work); Fax: 352-392-7029; E-mail: aboezaart@anest.ufl.edu

anatomy), but also what membranes and tissue layers surround them and how the nerves are connected to each other and to the central nervous system.

This becomes especially crucial in acute pain medicine, where not only the primary block, during which a high volume of a high concentration of local anesthetic agent is usually injected, but also the secondary block must succeed. The secondary block comes into play when the effect of the primary block wears off; the continuous (secondary) block must take effect thereafter. Local anesthetic agents have their effect by blocking the electrical activity of the nerve axons (by blocking the sodium channels) and can only reach the axons after being directly injected onto the axons in the same fascial compartment, which has certain inherent dangers, or by diffusing through the various tissue layers to the axons against a concentration gradient. This gradient is not constant or static, but changes regularly as the blood stream continuously and at a variable rate, depending on the regional blood flow, removes the drug on both sides of the tissue membrane.

Drug diffusion over membrane and fascia barriers follows Fick's Law [1] (simplified as $dQ/dt = P \times \Delta C$, where dQ/dt is the rate of diffusion (flux), P is the permeability constant of the drug and membrane conductance, and ΔC is the concentration gradient over the membrane. This is simplified, but the membrane conductance (P) will obviously change as the thickness and permeability of the membrane changes and the permeability constant of the drug changes (see also http://en.wikipedia.org/wiki/Fick's_laws_of_diffusion).

There is an optimal place where a local anesthetic drug must be placed for optimal primary block as used in regional anesthesia, or where a catheter for continuous nerve block has to be placed for continuous nerve block for ongoing pain. Over the years, this has been referred to as the "sweet spot of the nerve," a term with different meanings at different times. In the era when nerve blocks were mainly done for local and regional anesthesia for surgery, the quest was to have a safe and dense motor and sensory block with a fast onset and relatively long duration of action for use as the sole anesthetic, replacing general anesthesia. At that time, the practitioners of yesteryear used paresthesia to identify the "sweet spot" and the phrase "no paresthesia, no anesthesia" was coined [2].

In later years, when nerve stimulators become popular in identifying the "sweet spot" of the nerve, different currents were proposed to explain why certain nerve blocks were more successful than others with their quicker onset and longer duration than others using the same dose of local anesthetic agent. It was generally thought that a nerve stimulator output between 0.2 and 0.5 mA put the needle tip on the correct side of the relevant membranes around the nerves, but not deep enough so that the needle was inside the nerve fascicles where the raw unprotected axons are. This notion was never met with undisputable scientific verification, but was popularized by expert opinion. Experience over many years taught us that this was indeed most probably the case.

Enter the era of continuous nerve block, first in an effort to improve regional blood flow, and later for the management of ongoing acute perioperative pain [3]. Initially, it was thought that if a catheter were placed near enough to a nerve [4], the continuous secondary block would be successful. This was met with failure and disappointment; it was later realized that the catheter also had to be placed in the "sweet spot" of the nerve [3]. Practitioners applied a nerve stimulator to the catheter and found that if the motor response to nerve stimulation continued unchanged or improved during advancement of the catheter, the primary and secondary blocks would be optimal [3]. If, however, the motor response did not continue during placement, the primary block may still be successful, but the secondary block would invariably fail.

When ultrasound was introduced, it essentially supplanted the use of any other technique for the placement of nerve blocks in regional anesthesia. However, it did not live up to its promises for continuous nerve blocks because the identification of the "sweet spot" of the nerve and visualization of the tip of catheter placed into that spot were not clear. Very recently, Anderson and coworkers [5], with anatomical dissection, and Karmakar and colleagues [6] with high-definition ultrasound identified what they called the paraneurium of the nerve and its sub-paraneural space. This was nothing else than what neurosurgeons for years have called the "gliding apparatus" of a nerve [7] and it was etymologically more correctly named the circumneurium and the sub-circumneural space [8] (see Fig. **1**, Fig. **1** of chapter 7, Fig. **1** of chapter 11, and Fig. **1** of chapter 14). Many, including the current author, now believe that the sub-circumneural space is in fact the "sweet spot" of the nerve. What practitioners do not yet agree upon is on how to identify this space when high-definition ultrasound is not readily available. There seems to be agreement for when it is available, which is currently very seldom the case. Most, including the current author, now use ultrasound to identify the nerve and then nerve stimulation to place a catheter for a continuous nerve block. This is the so-called "dual-guidance technique" [9], which will no doubt be replaced in the near or not so near future as more ultrasound-"visible" catheters become available and high-definition ultrasound technology becomes more widely available.

MICROANATOMY

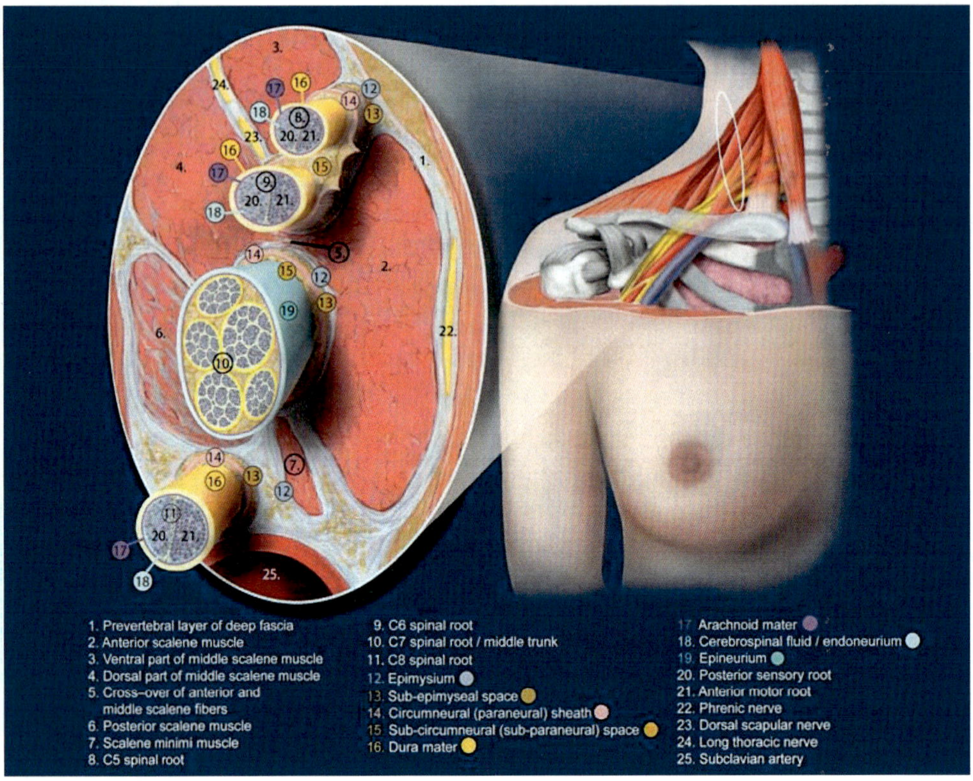

Figure 1: Sagittal microanatomy of the brachial plexus and scalene muscles.
Note in this figure:
This parasagittal view is of a longitudinal "cut" as illustrated on the figure on the right.

1. *The phrenic nerve (22) is in the prevertebral layer of the deep fascia and lies anterior on the belly of the anterior scalene muscle (2). This is the epimysium (12) between the muscles and the nerve roots and is connected to the sub-epimyseal space (13), which forms the "doughnut" around the roots if "hydro-dissected" with fluid.*
2. *The middle scalene muscle has a ventral part (3) and dorsal part (4), and the dorsal scapular nerve (23), which innervates the rhomboid muscles, and long thoracic nerve (24, which innervates the serratus anterior muscle lie between them.*
3. *The posterior scalene muscle slips of origin (6) are aponeurosis here, thus more of a tendon.*
4. *The fibers of the anterior and middle scalene muscles cross over between the spinal roots (5). See Chapter 1.*
5. *The scalene minimi muscle (7) often separates the middle trunk (10) from the C8 root (11).*
6. *At the level of this "cut" the T1 spinal root has not yet joined the C8 spinal root to form the inferior trunk.*
7. *The nerve roots are covered by dura (16) and arachnoid (17) mater and the endoneurium contain cerebrospinal fluid.*
8. *The spinal roots have a posterior (dorsal) sensory root (20) and an anterior (ventral) motor root (21).*

9. *The middle trunk (10) has epineurium (10) around it. The dura here form septae, which later close to form nerve fascicles.*
10. *All spinal roots and trunks have a circumneural (paraneural) sheath (14) that surrounds them and a sub-circumneural space between the dura (16) and the sheath (14). For continuous nerve block catheter placement within this space would be ideal.*
11. *Outside the circumneural sheath is a sub-epimyseal space (13), which is surrounded by the epimysium (12).*
12. *The subclavian artery (25) is in close relationship to the lower spinal roots and trunks.*

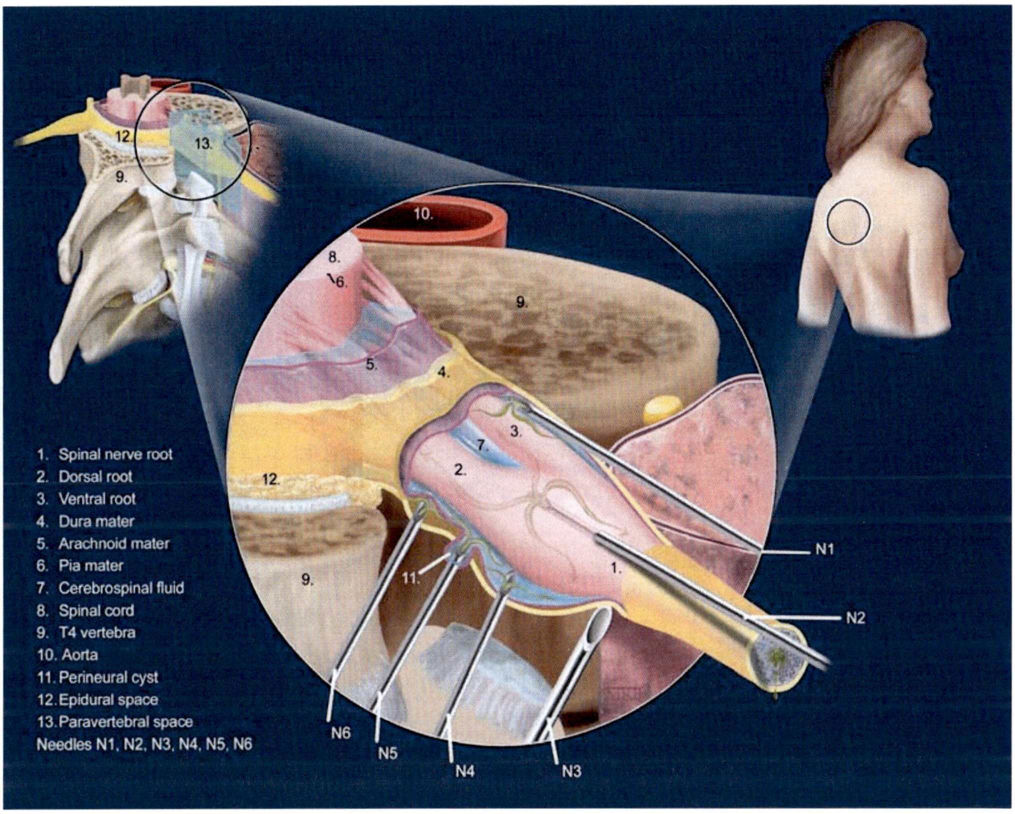

Figure 2: Schematic representation of the thoracic paravertebral space and the meninges surrounding the spinal root.

Six possible needle placements are illustrated:

Needle 1 (N1): Subarachnoid placement of a relatively thin needle during transforaminal injection (usually steroids).

Needle 2 (N2): Intraparenchymal placement of relatively thin needle during nerve root block (e.g., interscalene block at cervical level) or intercostal nerve block.

Needle 3 (N3): Extradural Tuohy needle during paravertebral block.

Needle 4 (N4): Subarachnoid placement of relatively thin needle during paravertebral block.

Needle 5 (N5): Needle placement into a perineural cyst during paravertebral block.

Needle 6 (N6): Subdural (extra-arachnoid) needle placement during paravertebral block.

Catastrophic outcomes following paravertebral blocks at the cervical [10-13], thoracic [14], and lumbar levels [15-17] have been reported, some of which were reversible cases of extensive epidural/subdural blocks with total spinal anesthesia [15, 17]. Unfortunately, other cases resulted in paraplegia, quadriplegia, and even death [16]. The explanation for these catastrophes focused on intra-cord injection, which complicated the blocks performed on patients under general anesthesia [18]. Interscalene block has also been blamed for disastrous outcomes [19-23]. The report of four cases of spinal injury after an interscalene block described by Benumof [18], who served as expert witness in the legal challenges associated with these cases, attracted much attention. It generated a fierce debate on the safety of performing blocks on patients under general anesthesia [9]. The conclusions reached by Benumof, that blocks should not be performed under general anesthesia, were, regrettably, largely incorrect. These tragic outcomes, like many others, were most likely caused by intra-root injection, and had no relation to the fact that the patients were under general anesthesia when the blocks were placed. Benumof's conclusions were largely based on not taking into account the microanatomy of the connective tissue framework of the nervous system. All of these cases of catastrophic outcomes had two things in common: they all followed root level nerve blocks with thin, relatively sharp needles [11-24].

Microanatomy of the Peripheral Nervous System

Our understanding of the microanatomy of the peripheral nervous system is over 140 years old. In 1876, Key and Retzius [25] (Richardson's stain) and Horster and Whitman in 1931 (Trypan Blue) [26] studied the spread of intraneurally injected solutions. In 1948, French repeated this work with radiopaque contrast medium in dogs [27]. Moore [28] used methylene blue-stained exocaine in 1954, and in 1978, Selander [29] used radioactive local anesthetic with fluorescent dye to study the microanatomy of the sciatic nerve in rabbits (Figs. **3** and **4**). In the interval, electron microscopy [30, 31] was used to basically verified what was known [31]. A very recent publication on the ultrastructure of nerves confirmed that our fundamental understanding was in fact correct [31].

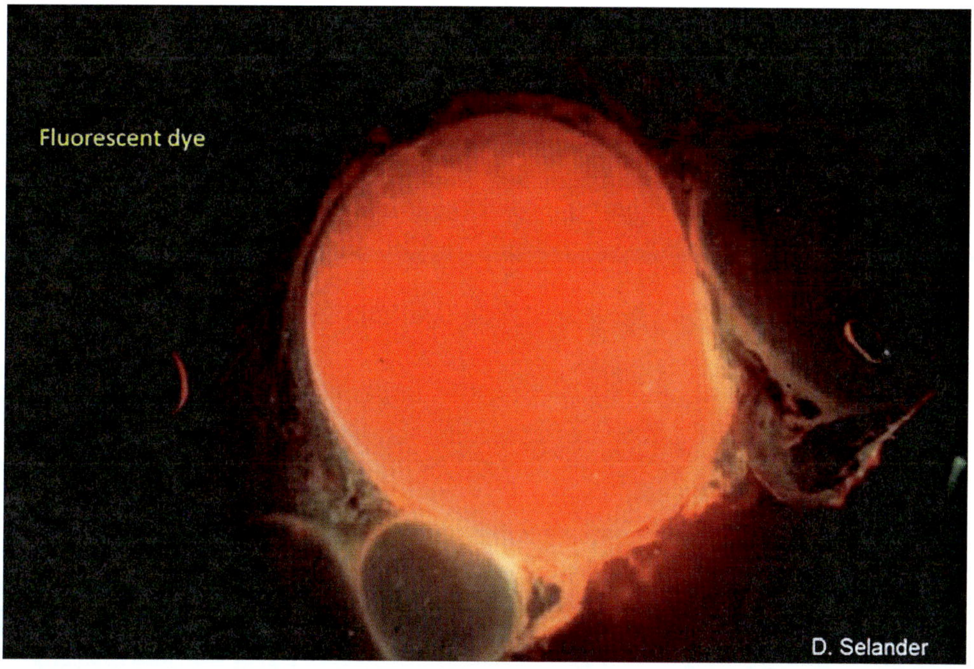

Figure 3: Intrafascicular spread of fluorescent dye.
(Figure supplied by Dr. Selander in personal communication with author)

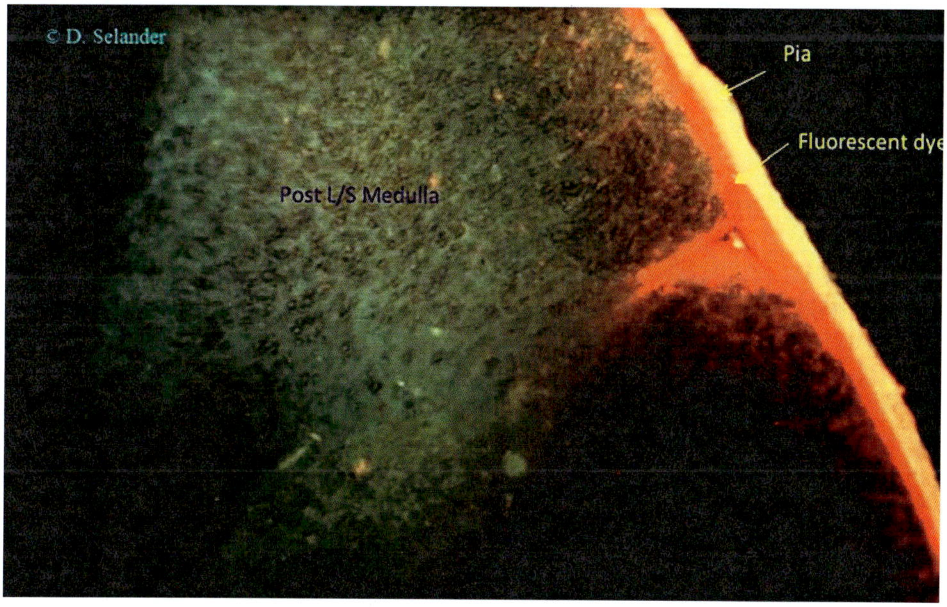

Figure 4: Central spread of fluorescent dye: subpial distribution on spinal cord *via* posterior root.
Post L/S Medulla = posterior lumbar spinal medulla
(Figure supplied by Dr. Selander in personal communication with author)

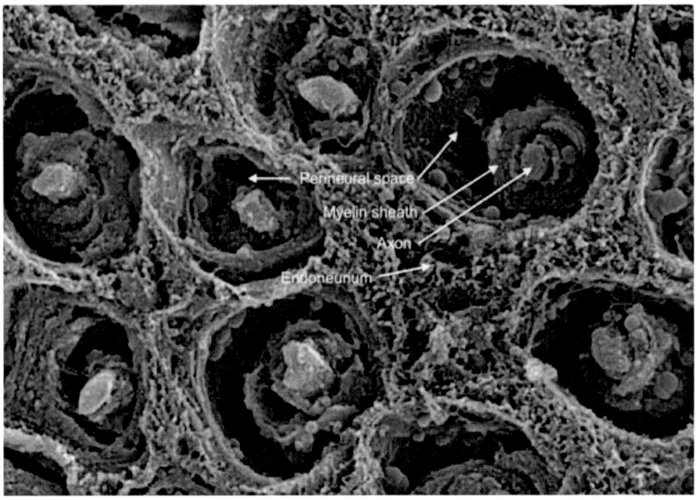

Figure 5: Perineural spaces. Scanning electron microscopy, magnification × 2000.
(Annotations by author)
(Reprinted from Reina, et al. [31] *with permission)*

The Circulation of Cerebrospinal Fluid

George B. Hassin brought the "modern" concept of cerebrospinal fluid (CSF) circulation to our attention in 1948 [34]. He criticized the teachings of CSF circulation as follows:

> *"The orthodox teaching is, on the whole, still the dominating one: The CSF originates from the choroid plexus (its tuft cells or blood vessels); is discharged into the cerebral ventricles; leaves them through the foramina of Luschka and Magendie; gathers in the cisterns of the base of the brain whence it flows to the villi or pacchionian bodies, and from these structures into the dural sinuses to be discharged from there into the peripheral venous circulation."*

This "theory" was convincingly disproved in 1948 [34], as the driving force behind the movement of CSF was pressure, and if the heart contracts during systole, the brain and spinal cord expand and the pressure in the CSF rise. But it rises equally throughout, leaving us to wonder: why would CSF flow from one area of high pressure to another area with the same pressure? The "modern" understanding of CSF circulation can be summarized as follows:

- CSF represents the tissue fluids (extracellular fluid) of the brain and spinal cord.

- It includes the contents of the Virchow-Robin spaces. The fluid in these spaces originates as the tissue fluid and is discharged into the cerebral ventricles and the subarachnoid spaces.

- The absorption of CSF is not through the villi or pacchionian bodies, but through the perineural villi of the cranial nerves and spinal roots (see Fig. **10** of chapter 21).

- The function of the choroids plexuses is not to secrete fluid but to excrete or eliminate from it noxious substances and to make it absorbable by the perineural villi [34, 35].

- There is no central force that sets CSF in circulation. A pressure differential does not exist under normal conditions but is a passive process set in motion by a lumbar or other puncture, which probably formulated the scientific basis of our earlier understanding.

- The force that manipulates the forward propulsion of the spinal fluid out through the spinal roots is the collapsing and expanding movements of the brain and spinal cord during the cardiac cycle.

- The hematoencephalic barrier is the Virchow-Robin spaces.

- The tissue fluid deep to the epineuria of peripheral nerves, but outside the perineuria covering the nerve fascicles, is lymph and drains *via* lymph vessels to the regional lymph nodes, whereas the tissue fluid inside the fascicles deep to the perineuria is the tissue fluid or extracellular fluid of the nerve axons, namely CSF.

Longitudinal flow within the fascicle is inhibited minimally, whereas lateral extension is restricted by the relatively non-compliant perineurium [27]. Injection into peripheral nerve fascicles, which is difficult to achieve in the first place, (depending on the volume and pressure of the injectate) has direct access to the CSF and the interstitium (medulla) of the spinal cord [28, 29] *via* the perineurial spaces (Fig. **5**). The channels by which this progression occurs have been called perineurial spaces and have been demonstrated by the studies of Dag Selander, *et al.* [29] and Moore, *et al.* [28]. More recent work by Reina has verified the earlier work of Selander [31-33] (Figs. **3** through **5**).

Injection into a spinal root, on the other hand, is relatively easy, because the nerve roots are relatively large compared to the needle, and the pressure inside the roots is low - basically equivalent to that of the subarachnoid space of the spinal cord (Fig. **2**). The injectate, therefore, similarly has direct access to the CSF and spinal cord interstitium - the clinical consequences of which depend on the volume, rate, and pressure of the injection and the path taken *via* the perineurial spaces of the axons (Fig. **5**). If a relatively high volume of local anesthetic agent, say approximately 10 mL, were injected into the subarachnoid space, the result would be a total spinal block with immediate respiratory arrest [12-15]. If, however, the same volume and drug were injected inside the parenchyma of the spinal nerve, the spread would occur distally and centrally, as outlined by needle number 2 in Fig. (**2**) *via* the perineural spaces, thus delaying respiratory arrest [11, 16, 18, 22, 23] because the drug must, according to Moore [28], first diffuse over the pia mater in sufficient quantities to enter the CSF; from there, it can reach the respiratory centers in the brain. Any injectate will generally follow the path of least resistance and has even been found as far distant as the cerebellum of one of the animals studied by Selander, where it was injected into a fascicle of the popliteal section of the animal's sciatic nerve [29].

Ultrastructure of Peripheral Nerves

Although the development of peripheral nerves occurs embryologically later than that of roots and trunks, for ease of understanding, the peripheral nerves will be considered first here. Peripheral nerves are composed of numerous fasciculi; each is surrounded by a dense perineurium and held together by a looser epineurium [25, 26, 31-33]. The circumneurium (paraneurium) has been purposefully left out of Fig. (**6**) because it is discussed in more detail in Chapters 7, 11, and 14 with the ultrastructures of specific peripheral nerves.

The ***endoneurium*** (Fig. **6**, No. 9) is a fine cylindrical lamina that encloses groups of axons with their respective Schwann cells. The axons consist of different axon fiber types, depending of the type of nerve in question (see Table **1**). Both myelinated and unmyelinated axons are surrounded by the collagen fibers of the endoneurium, but the endoneurium is permeable and thus does not interfere with molecule passage through it. The single-layered endothelial cells of the capillaries in the endoneurium contribute to the blood-nerve barrier [31]. The term endoneurium is sometimes incorrectly used to denote the intrafascicular compartment of the nerve. Its use should be restricted to refer to intrafascicular connective tissue, excluding the perineurial partitions that may subdivide fascicles [25]. Approximately 40% to 50% of the intrafascicular space is occupied by non-neural elements and anywhere from 20%to 30% of this is endoneurial fluid (CSF) and connective matrix - the endoneurium [25, 31].

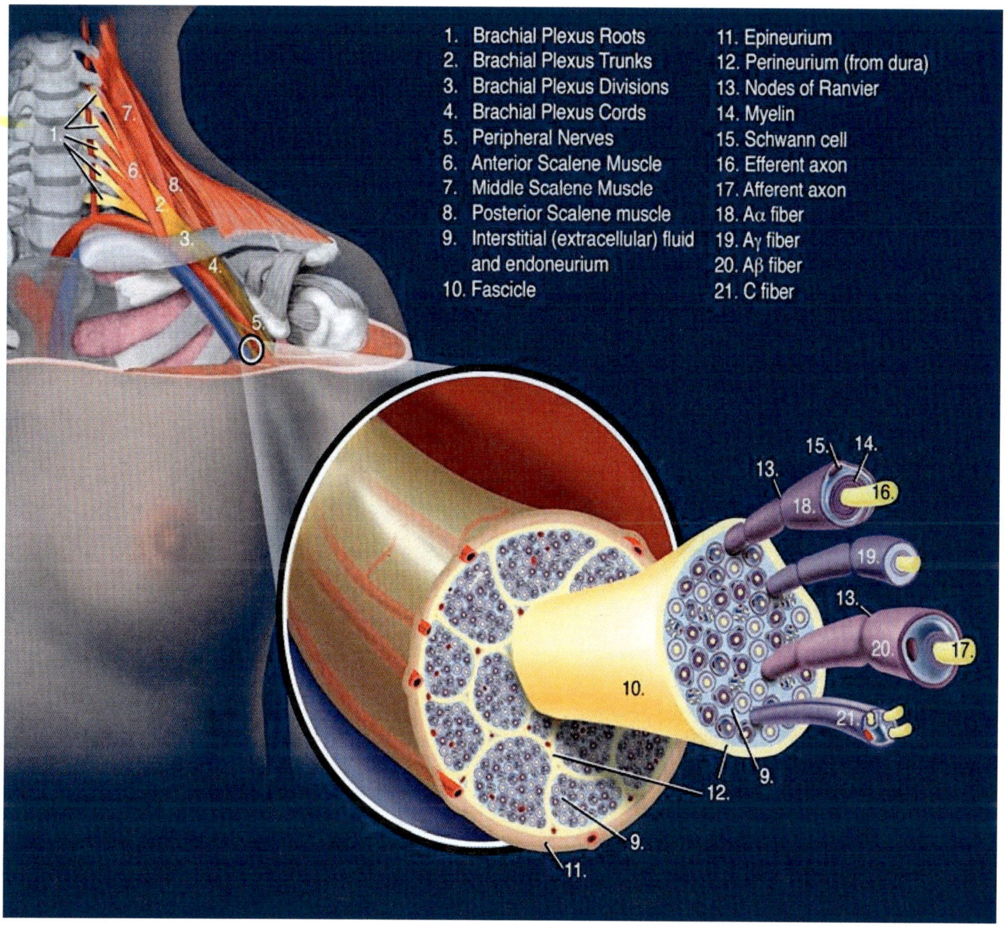

Figure 6: Ultrastructure of a peripheral nerve. [Circumneural (paraneural) sheath not depicted] (see Fig. **1** of chapter 2, Fig. **1** of chapter 7, Fig. **1** of chapter 11, and Fig. **1** of chapter 14).

The ***perineurium*** (Fig. **6**, No. 12) comprises multiple single-cell layers that enclose individual nerve fascicles [31]. They become progressively thinner as the number of fascicles increase. As Key and Retzius [25] describe, the essential structure of the perineurium is a lamellated arrangement of flattened cells separated by layers of collagenous connective tissue that provides an ensheathment for both the somatic and peripheral autonomic nerves and their ganglia. The cellular lamellae are composed of concentric sleeves of flattened polygonal cells that are equipped to function as a metabolically active diffusion barrier, although they do not have the morphologic features of a true epithelium.

Table 1. Classification, diameter, conduction velocity, and function of nerve axons in a peripheral nerve.

Type	Erlanger-Gasser classification	Diameter	Myelin	Conduction velocity	Motor fibers/sensory receptors
α	Aα	13-20 μm	Yes	80-120 m/s	Extrafusal muscle fibers
γ	Aγ	5-8 μm	Yes	4-24 m/s	Intrafusal muscle fibers
Ia	Aα	13-20 μm	Yes	80-120 m/s	Proprioception
Ib	Aα	13-20 μm	Yes	80-120 m/s	Golgi tendon organ
II	Aβ	6-12 μm	Yes	33-75 m/s	Secondary receptors of muscle spindle; All cutaneous mechanoreceptors
III	Aσ	1-5 μm	Thin	3-30 m/s	Free nerve endings of touch and pressure; Nociception of neospinothalamic tract; Cold thermoreceptors
IV	C	0.2-1.5 μm	No	0.5-2.0 m/s	Nociceptors of paleospinothalamic tract; Warmth receptors
Pregangl	B	1-5 μm	Yes	3-15 m/s	(Preganglionic fibers)
Postgangl	C	0.2-1.5 μm	No	0.2-1.5 m/s	(Postganglionic fibers)

(*From:* http://en.wikipedia.org/wiki/Nerve_conduction_velocity)

The ***epineurium*** (Fig. **6**, No. 11) consists of a condensation of areolar connective tissue that surrounds the perineurial ensheathment of the fascicles of uni- and multifascicular nerves [27, 31]. The attachment of the epineurium to surrounding connective tissue is loose, allowing the nerve to be relatively mobile except where tethered by entering blood vessels or branches [27]. Greater amounts of connective tissue are normally present where nerves cross over joints. In general, the more fascicles there are, the greater the quantity of epineurium.

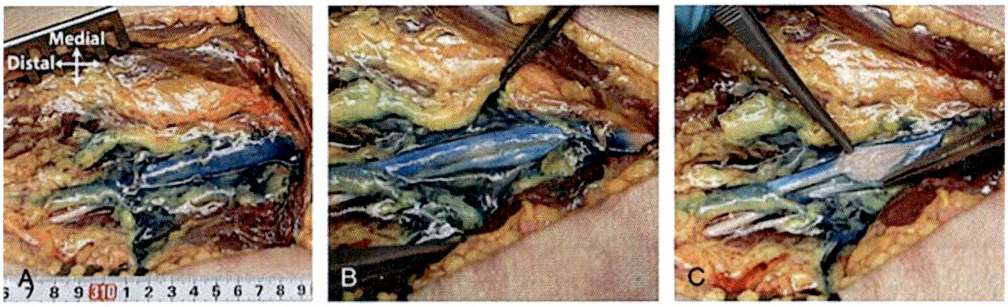

Figure 7: Gross dissection after an ultrasound-guided injection of diluted methylene blue.
A. The transparent shiny circumneural (paraneural) sheath is expanded by the injectate around the sciatic nerve and along the tibial nerve. The blue stripe proximal to the bifurcation is the injection site.
B. The paraneural sheath is cut open and split aside by two pairs of tweezers. The sciatic nerve is exposed, and the epineurium is colored by the injectate.
C. The sciatic nerve is opened through a cut in the epineurium to verify that the injection was not intraneural. (Reprinted from Anderson, et al., [5] with permission)

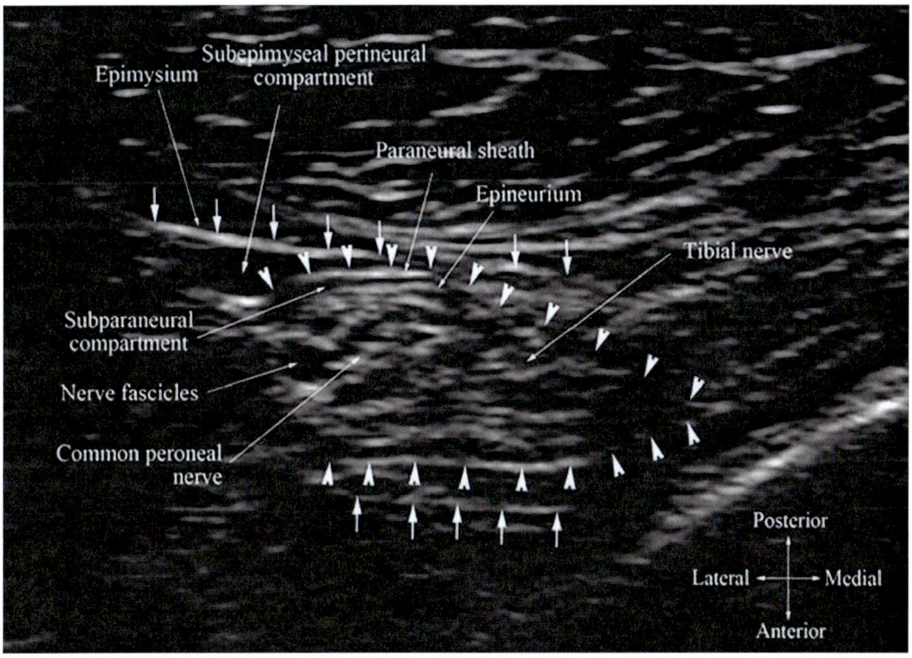

Figure 8: High-definition (and zoomed) transverse sonogram of the sciatic nerve at the level of its bifurcation into the tibial and common peroneal nerve at the popliteal fossa.
The paraneural sheath (white arrowheads) is interposed between the epimysium (short white arrows) of the surrounding muscles and the outer surface of the sciatic nerve (epineurium), which also appears hyperechoic. The subepimyseal (perineural) and subparaneural compartments are seen as hypoechoic areas between the epimysium and the paraneural sheath, and between the paraneural sheath and the epineurium, respectively. (Reprinted from Karmakar, et al., [6] with permission)

Variable quantities of adipose tissue are also present in the epineurium, particularly in the larger nerves. After studying the distribution of fat in human nerves and finding predominance in the sciatic nerve, researchers feel that this tissue probably has a protective function in cushioning the fascicles against injury by compression. The susceptibility to compression injury is likely to be less in large multifascicular nerves with considerable quantities of epineurium and fat than in smaller and unifascicular nerves.

The ***vasa nervorum*** (Fig. **9**) enter the epineurium, where they communicate with a longitudinal anastomotic network of arterioles and venules [27]. The epineurium also contains lymphatic vessels, which are not present within the fascicles. These lymphatic channels accompany the arteries of the peripheral nerves and pass into the regional lymph nodes [34].

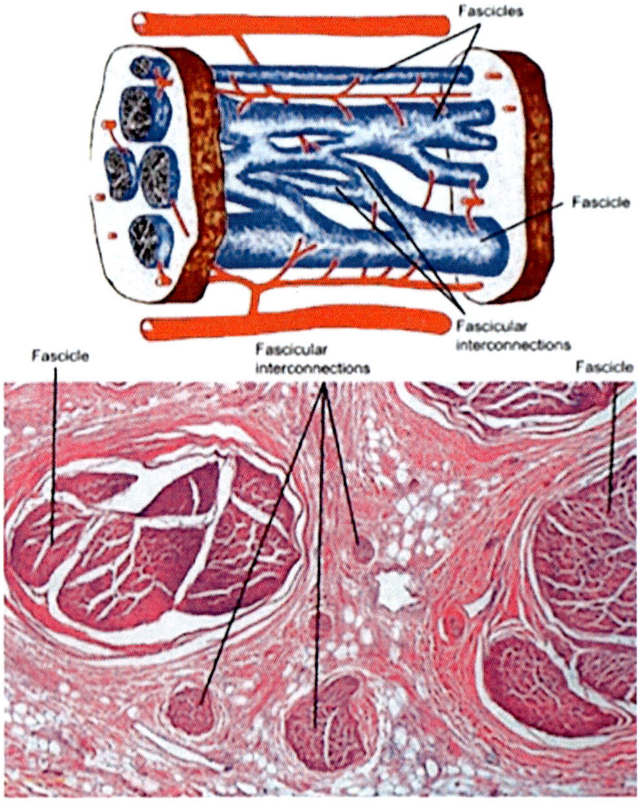

Figure 9: Intraneural plexus.
a. Diagram showing fascicular interconnections; b. Fascicular interconnections
Nerve fascicles are interconnected inside of individual nerves by a complex intraneural plexus. (Reprinted from Reina [33] with permission)

Anderson and colleagues [5] recently demonstrated the ***circumneural (paraneural) sheath*** [8] in dissections, while Karmakar and his colleagues [6] described the appearance of the circumneural sheath with high-definition ultrasound. In neurosurgical texts, it has been known as the "gliding apparatus" of the nerve [7]. We now know that injection of a local anesthetic agent or catheter placement in the subcircumneural space (subparaneural space) is ideal for single-injection and continuous nerve block, respectively [8]. Reina and colleagues stained sections through the brachial plexus and peripheral nerves with Masson's trichrome staining to convincingly demonstrate the microscopic ultrastructure of the circumneural (paraneural) sheaths (Fig. **10**) [32].

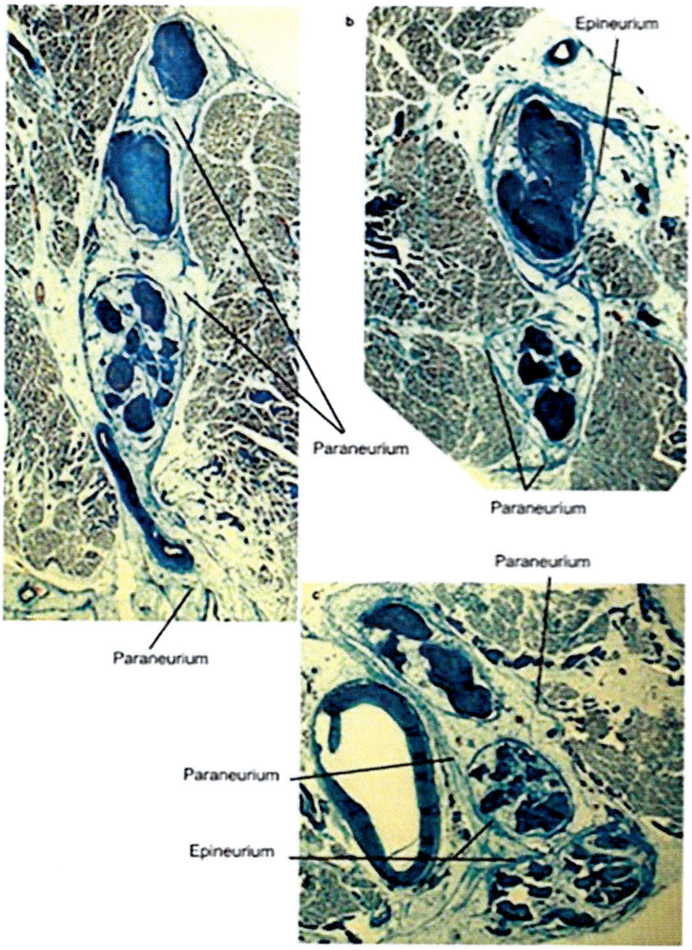

Figure 10a: Internal structure of a nerve root in the interscalene region.
Masson's trichrome stained to show paraneurium
(Reprinted from Reina and Sala-Blanch [32] with permission)

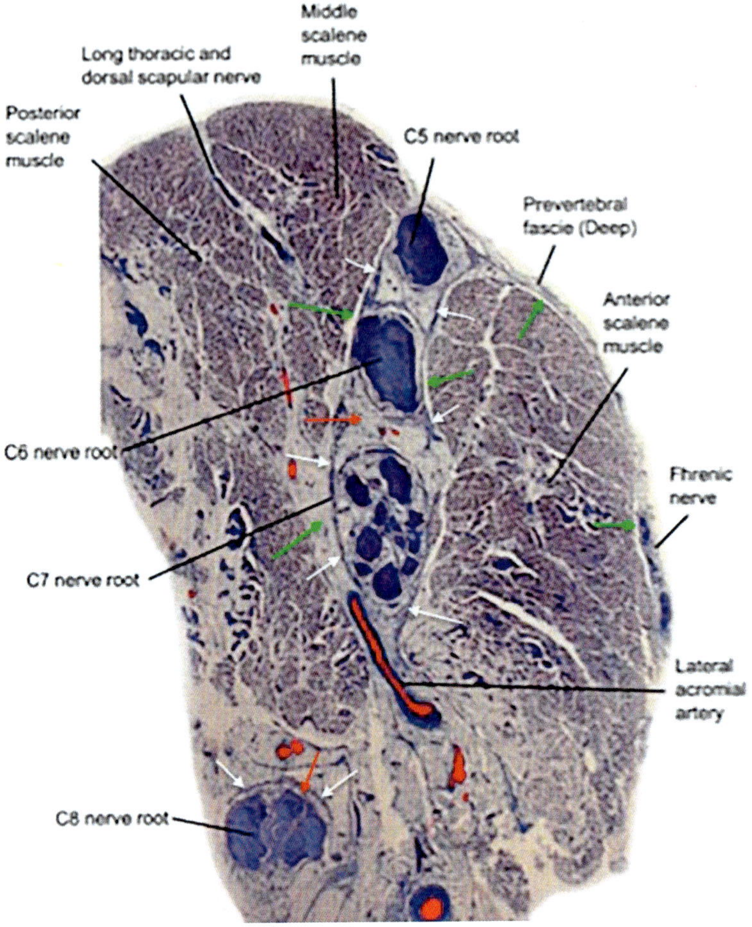

Figure 10b: Cross sectional microanatomy of the brachial plexus at the interscalene region.
Masson's trichrome stained.
Note paraneurium (circumneurium) - white arrows, subepimyseal space - green arrows, and subcircumneural (subparaneural) space - red arrows (Arrows placed by author).
(The long thoracic and dorsal scapular nerves lie between the ventral and dorsal parts of the middle scalene muscles)
(Posterior scalene muscle in this figure should read Dorsal medial scalene muscle).
Reprinted from Reina and Sala-Blanch [32] with permission
The Experimental Work of Selander, et al. [29] on Intraneural Injections into Rabbit Sacral Nerves Demonstrated the Following:

Epineurial injection: An irregular bleb formed around the injection site upon intraneural injection deep to the epineurium but outside the perineurium. The tracer spread for a short distance within an easily expanding epineurium, which often ruptured. When 50 to 100 μL was injected at 100 μL/min, the injection pressure rose within a few seconds to 30 to 60 mmHg and thereafter quickly decreased to a steady 10 to 30 mmHg. As soon as the injection stopped, the pressure returned to zero.

Intrafascicular injection: When Selander injected blue tracer into a fascicle of rabbit sciatic nerves, the tracer spread rapidly, both proximally and distally, within the fascicle. In another study, while being injected deep to the perineurium of the sciatic nerve, a blue tracer was seen to spread rapidly, proximally and distally, inside the fascicle. The longitudinal spread varied, but in all cases, it reached the sacral plexus. Distally, the tracer colored the tibial nerve, sometimes even reaching the foreleg. In the studies of French and colleagues [27], the tracer (radiopaque contrast medium) reached the lumbar plexus *via* the injected fascicle; it is possible that it may even track distally *via* an entirely different nerve originating from the plexus. They also showed that high-pressure intrathecally injected contrast medium spread down the fascicles of peripheral nerves.

Selander and coworkers [29] demonstrated that if the injection was made into a small fascicle, the injectate did not extend beyond the sacral plexus, but if the injection was made into a large fascicle, the injectate easily passed the sacral plexus and reached the spinal cord. During slow injection, the spread in the medulla was superficially under the pia mater. In some of the experimental animals, the spread was into the CSF, and the dura and arachnoid were also colored. In one animal, the blue stain extended to the cerebellum. The animal died shortly after the injection.

In cross-sections of the spinal medulla, the fluorescent tracer used by Selander and Sjöstrand was mainly seen in the thin subpial space. Accumulation of the tracer was noted in the dorsal root-medulla junction area, extending into the substantia gelatinosa of the anterior horns, and into the anterior median fissure (Figs. **3** and **4**).

Selander and Sjöstrand recorded pressures between 435 and 675 mmHg when injecting 50 to 100 µL at a rate of 100 µL/min. After cessation of the injection, the pressure remained above the estimated capillary perfusion pressure (50 mmHg) for at least 10 minutes [29].

Ultrastructure of the Brachial Plexus Trunks

The trunks of the plexuses should be seen as transitional areas from roots to peripheral nerves. The perineuria surrounding the fascicles start to split away and axons are separated by perineurial sheath interdigitations or septae (Fig. **11**). There seems to be interindividual variation on the level at which the septae form, but functionally and practically from a regional anesthesia viewpoint, the trunks should be regarded as transitional areas between clearly defined fasciculi with rigid perineurial of the peripheral nerves to the root area where perineuria are not present and all the perineuria have joined to form the dura.

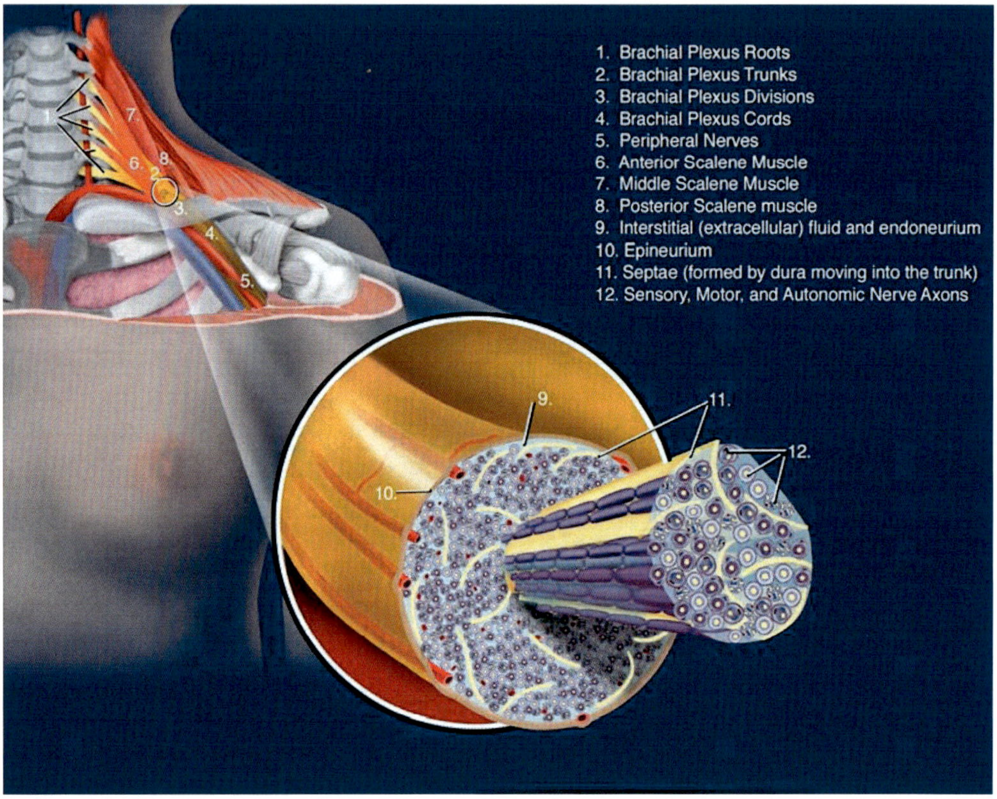

Figure 11: Ultrastructure of a brachial plexus trunk.

Ultrastructure of the Spinal Roots

After splitting away from the fascicles, the perineurium, at the level of the nerve roots, thickens and fuses with the dura. The perineuria of the peripheral nerves, therefore, are continuations of the dura mater. As a consequence, the axons inside the roots are no longer protected by the perineurium, and the extracellular fluid or tissue fluid, is the CSF.

The mesothelial cells of the arachnoid membrane become hyperplastic at the point of exit of the nerves and form a cuff around the roots just after they penetrate the dura mater. Beyond this cuff, no tissue can be seen that is recognized as arachnoid.

The connective tissue framework of the peripheral nervous system, therefore, arises entirely from a continuation of the perineurium, starting at the dura mater. As the nerve progresses peripherally, it is more and more subdivided by perineural interdigitations until each fascicle of nerve axons eventually has its own perineurial sheath.

At the root level, as the spinal roots leave the spinal cord *via* the intervertebral foramen, the roots are covered by all three meningeal layers: the pia mater, which continues distally as the perineural epithelium of the peripheral nerves [34] (see Fig. **7** of chapter 19), the arachnoid mater, which seems to continue with the pia layer (as the pia-arachnoid membrane distally as the perineural epithelium of the peripheral nerve [35]), and the dura mater, which continues distally as the septae in the trunk areas and the perineurium in the peripheral nerves [35]. Injections deep to the arachnoid at the spinal roots are subarachnoid injections with similar consequences as spinal subarachnoid injections (Fig. **2**).

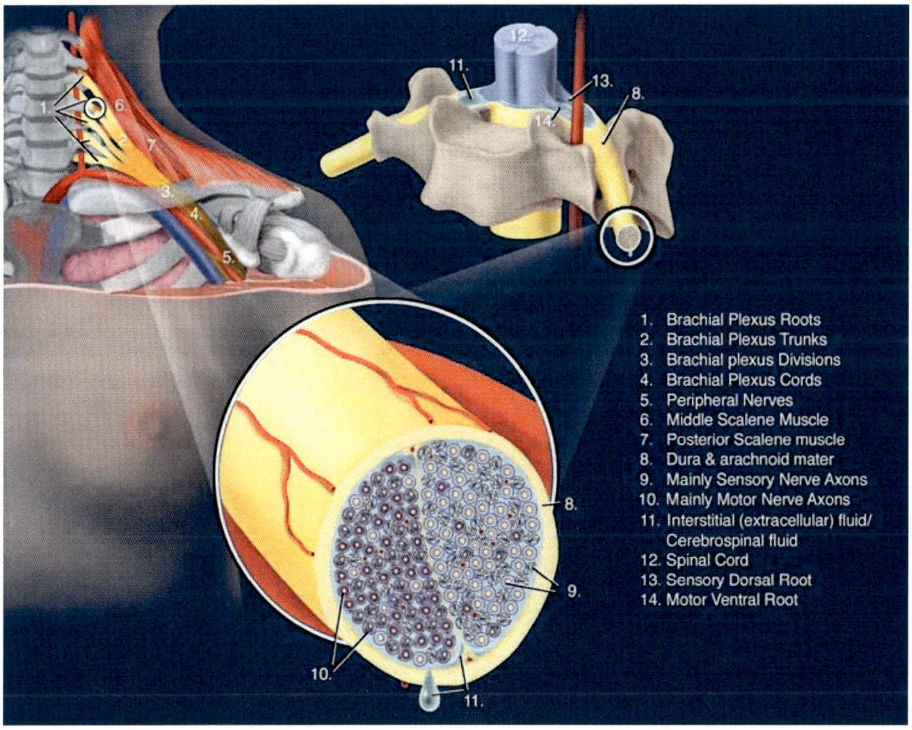

Figure 12: Ultrastructure of a spinal root nerve.

Practical Clinical Implications of Nerve Ultrastructure

With the recent introduction of ultrasound, it has become clear that nerves can be either hyper- or hypoechoic. Furthermore, nerve circumneural sheaths can be visualized with high-definition ultrasound [6, 36] (Fig. **8**), whereas regular clinically used ultrasound technology fails to show this sheath in most instances. When studying this ultrasonographic appearance of nerves, it can be seen that the spinal roots are hypoechoic (Fig. **13**). More distally, the trunks are more hyperechoic (Fig. **14**), and most distal nerves appear hyperechoic (Fig. **15**), resembling the so-called "honeycomb" appearance. Clearly, the "honeycomb" represents the fascicles surrounded by thick dense perineuria at this level (Fig. **15**), which are absent at the more central root levels (Fig. **13**). The root and trunk level appear hypoechoic basically because they are fluid-filled - with CSF in this case.

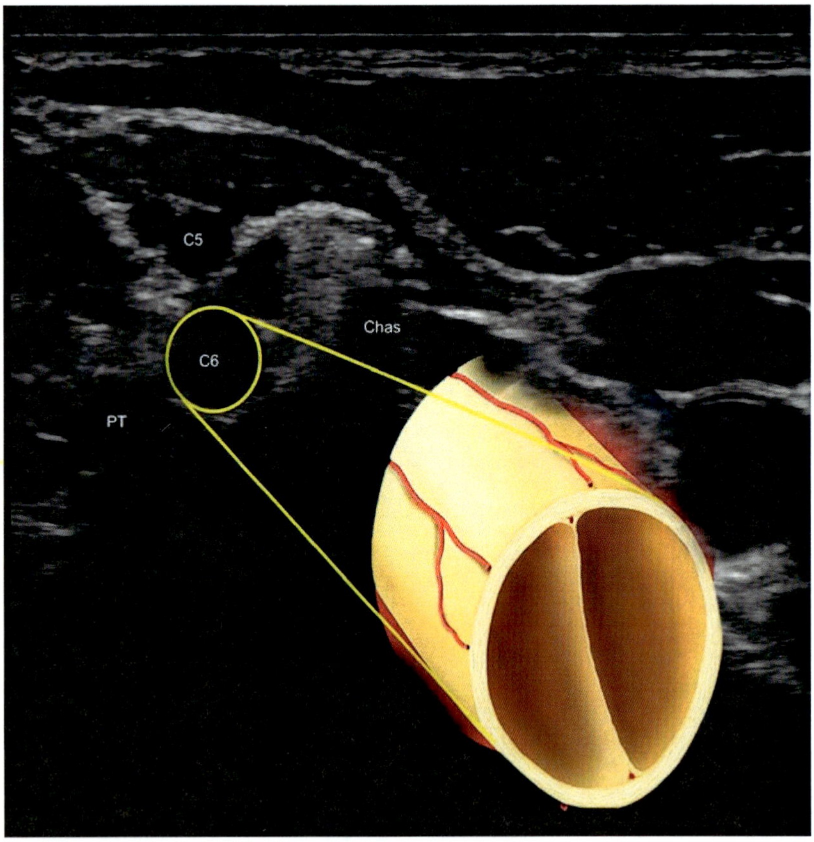

Figure 13: Hypoechoic appearance of spinal root nerve.
C5 = 5th cervical nerve root; C6 = 6th cervical nerve root; Chas = Chassaignac's tubercle of the transverse process of the 6th cervical vertebra; PT = posterior tubercle of the transverse process of the 6th cervical vertebra.

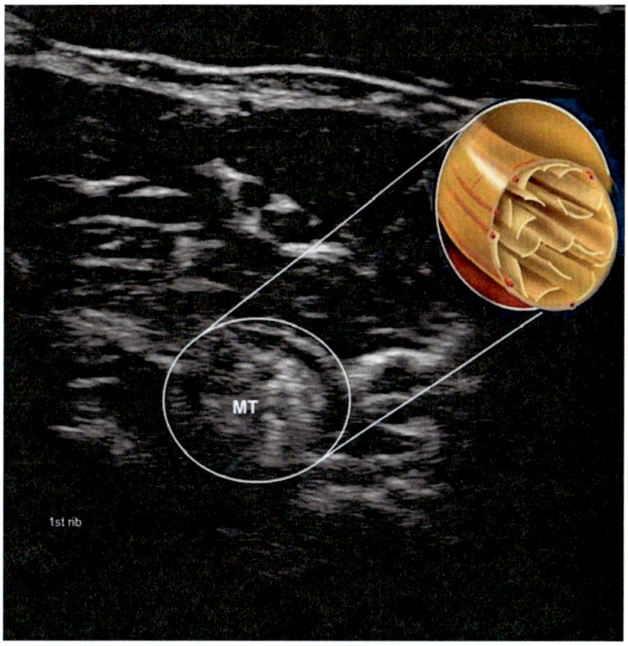

Figure 14: More hyperechoic appearance of a brachial plexus trunk nerve.
MT = middle trunk.

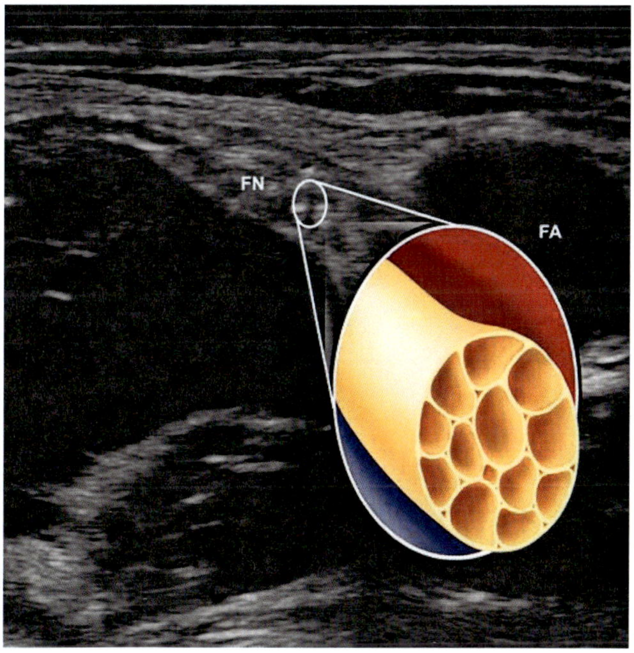

Figure 15: "Honeycomb" appearance of a peripheral nerve.
FN = femoral nerve; FA = femoral artery.

Recent ultrasound work during axillary nerve blocks has also confirmed that "intraneural injections" have no untoward consequences as long as the injection is deep to the circumneurium or epineurium, but remains *outside* the perineurium [37]. Although intrafascicular injections are difficult to achieve and are undesirable, the work of French, *et al.* [27], where the contrast medium they injected into the fascicles remained in the fascicle for up to 5 weeks, makes it understandable that we may encounter an occasional numb area (a thumb, for example) a few weeks after peripheral a nerve block.

It is clear, then, that injections at the root level (and trunk level of some individuals) should be regarded as epidural injections because the injection is made directly outside of the dura (or extradural or peridural or epidural [10]) surrounding the spinal roots. All of the time-tested safety practices for spinal epidural injections should therefore logically also apply for root level, paravertebral, or paraspinal epidural injections. These safety practices should include the avoidance of sharp or thin needles [38]; the use of large-bore Tuohy needles (for continuous *and* single-injection blocks) [39, 40]; the use of similar test doses to test for intravascular or intrathecal injection; fractionation of the main dose; and perhaps even similar guidelines for anticoagulation, although this is open to debate and can be expected to be contested [41].

ACKNOWLEDGEMENTS

The author gratefully acknowledge the following people:

- The Head of the Department of Anesthesiology of the College of Medicine of the University of Florida, Dr. Tim Morey and his department for their moral support and continuous encouragement.

- The faculty and fellows of the Division of acute and perioperative pain medicine for affording the author the time to produce this work by covering his clinical duties.

- Corey Astrom of the Department of Anesthesiology of the College of Medicine of the University of Florida for her professional and high quality text editing.

- Mary K Bryson for her illustrations of Figs. **1, 2, 6, 11** and **12**.

- Fig. (**2**) was redrawn from an original drawing of Barys V. Ihnatsenka, M.D., which is regarded as a "preprint" that he used for his lectures. It has not been peer reviewed, nor has it had any other value added to it by a publisher (such as formatting, copyright, technical enhancement *etc.*).

- Raeducation.com LLC for their financial support.

CONFLICT OF INTEREST

The author invented the "stimulating catheter" and receives royalties from TeleFlex for its sales.

DISCLOSURE

Parts of this work has been previously published in Boezaart AP. That which we call a rose by any other name would smell as sweet- and its thorns would hurt as much. Reg Anesth Pain Med 2009; 34: 3-7 [39].

"Parts of this work has been previously published in Boezaart AP, Tighe P. New trends in regional anesthesia for shoulder surgery: Avoiding devastating complications. Int J Shoulder Surg 2010; 4: 1-8 (www.internationlshoulder journal.org) [40].

Parts of this work have been previously published in Boezaart AP. Microanatomy of the peripheral nervous system revisited, and its implications for paravertebral (para-neuraxial) blocks. Proceedings of the 10th Annual pre-ASA Meeting, Orthopedic Anesthesia Pain Rehabilitation Society (www.OAPRS.org); 2013 October 11; San Francisco, California. United States of America [42].

ABBREVIATIONS

Chas	=	Chassaignac's tubercle of the transverse process of the 6th cervical vertebra
CSF	=	cerebrospinal fluid
FA	=	femoral artery
FN	=	femoral nerv
MT	=	middle trunk

Post L/S Medulla	=	posterior lumbar spinal medulla
Postgangl	=	postganglionic
Pregangl	=	preganglionic
PT	=	posterior tubercle of the transverse process of the 6th cervical vertebra

REFERENCES

[1] Mather LE, Tucker GT. Properties, absorption and disposition of local anesthetic agents. In: Cousins MJ, Horlocker TT, Car DB, Bridenbaugh PO, Eds. Neural Blockade in Clinical Anesthesia and Pain Medicine. Philadelphia: Wolter Kluwer/Lippincott Williams & Wilkins; 2009: p.53.

[2] Moore DC. Regional Block, 4th edition. Springfield Illinois, Charles C. Thomas Publisher, 1967, p.241.

[3] Boezaart AP, de Beer JF, Du Toit C, van Rooyen K: A new technique of continuous interscalene nerve block. Can J Anaesth 1999; 46: 275-81.

[4] Enneking FK, Close counts. Reg Anesth Pain Med 2007; 32: 280-81.

[5] Andrerson HL, Anderson SL, Tranun-Jensen J. Injecting inside the paraneural sheath or the sciatic nerve: Direct comparison among ultrasound imaging, macroscopic anatomy and histologic analysis. Reg Anesth Pain Med 2012; 37: 410-14.

[6] Karmakar MK, Shariat AN, Pangthipampai P, Chen J. High-definition ultrasound imaging defines the paraneural sheath and the fascial compartments surrounding the sciatic nerve at the popliteal fossa. Reg Anesth Pain Med 2013; 38: 447-51.

[7] Millesi H, Zoch G, Rath T. The gliding apparatus of peripheral nerve and its clinical significance. Ann Chir Main Memb Super. 1990; 9: 87-97.

[8] Boezaart AP. The Sweet Spot of the Nerve: Is the "Paraneural Sheath" Named Correctly, and Does It Matter? Reg Anesth Pain Med 2014; 39: 557-8.

[9] Aveline C, Le Roux A, Le Hetet H, Vautier P, Cognet F, Bonnet F. Postoperative efficacies of femoral nerve catheters sited using ultrasound combined with neurostimulation com-pared with neurostimulation alone for total knee arthroplasty. Eur J Anaesthesiol 2010; 27: 978-84.

[10] Boezaart AP, Lucas SD, Elliott CE. Paravertebral block: cervical, thoracic, lumbar and sacral. Curr Opin Anaesthesiol 2009; 22: 637-43.

[11] Voermans NC, Crul BJ, de Bondt BJ, Zwarts MJ van Engelen BG. Permanent loss of cervical spinal cord function associated with the posterior approach. Anesth Analg 2006; 102: 330-1.

[12] Aramidah M, van den Oever HLA, Walstra GJ, Dzoljic M. Spinal anesthesia as a complication of brachial plexus block using the posterior approach. Anesth Analg 2002; 94: 1338-9.

[13] Grefkens JM, Bürger K. Total spinal anesthesia after an attempted brachial plexus block using the posterior approach. Anaesthesia 2006; 61: 1105-8.

[14] Lekhak B, Bartley C, Conacher ID, Nouraei SM. Total spinal anaesthesia associated with insertion of a paravertebral catheter. Br J Anaesth 2001; 86: 280 - 2.

[15] Gentili M, Aveline C, Bonnet F. Total spinal anesthesia after posterior lumbar plexus block. Ann Fr Anesth Reanim 1998; 17: 740 - 2.

[16] Houten J. Paraplegia after lumbosacral nerve root block, report of three cases. The Spine J 2002; 2: 70 - 5.

[17] Pousman RM, Mansoor Z, Sciard D. Total spinal after continuous posterior lumbar plexus block. Anesthesiology 2003; 98: 1281-2.

[18] Benumof JL. Permanent loss of spinal cord function associated with interscalene block performed under general anesthesia. Anesthesiology 2000; 93: 1541-4.

[19] Ross S, Scarborough CD. Total spinal anesthesia following brachial plexus block. Anesthesiology 1973; 39: 458.

[20] Dutton RP, Eckhardt III WF, Sunder N. Total spinal anesthesia after interscalene blockade of the brachial plexus. Anesthesiology 2004; 80: 939-41.

[21] Tetzlaff JE, Yoon HJ, Dilger J, Brems J. Subarachnoid anesthesia as a complication of an interscalene brachial plexus block. Case report. Reg Anesth 1994; 19: 357-9.

[22] Passannante AN. Spinal anesthesia and permanent neurological deficit after interscalene block. Anesth Analg 1996; 82: 873-4.

[23] Lee JL. Catastrophic complications of interscalene nerve block. Anesthesiology 2001; 95: 1301.

[24] Borgeat A, Ekatodramis G, Gaertner E. Performing an interscalene block during general anesthesia must be the exception. Anesthesiology 2001; 95: 1302-3.

[25] Key A, Retzius G. Studies in the anatomy of the nervous system and connective tissue. Stockholm: Samson and Wallin, circa; 1876.

[26] Horster H, Whitman L. The method of intraneural injection. [Die Methode der intraneuralen Injektion]. Z Hygiene 1931; 113: 113.

[27] French JD, Strain WH, Jones GE. Mode of extension of contrast substances injected into peripheral nerves. J Neuropathol Exp Neurlogy 1948; 7: 47 - 58.

[28] Moore DC, Hain RF Ward A, Bridenbaugh LD. Importance of the perineural spaces in nerve blocking. JAMA. 1954; 156: 1050-5.

[29] Selander D, Sjöstrand J. Longitudinal spread of intraneurally injected local anesthetics. Acta Anaesth Scand 1978: 22: 622-34.

[30] Röhlich P, Knoop A. Elektronenmikroskopische Untersuchenen an den Hüllen des N. Ischiadicus der Ratte. Z Zellforsch Mikrosk Anat 1961; 53: 299-305.

[31] Reina MA, Navarro RA, Mateos EMD. Ultrastructure of myelenated and unmyelenated axons. In: Reina MA, Ed. Atlas of functional anatomy for regional anesthesia and pain medicine. New York, NY, Springer 2015; pp. 3-18.

[32] Reina MA, Sala-Blanch X. Cross-sectional microscopic anatomy of the brachial plexus and paraneural sgheaths. In: Reina MA, Ed. Atlas of functional anatomy for regional anesthesia and pain medicine. New York, NY, Springer 2015; pp.161-88.

[33] Reina MA, Dominquez MF, Tardieu I. Origin of the fascicles and intraneural plexus. In: Reina MA, Ed. Atlas of functional anatomy for regional anesthesia and pain medicine. New York, NY, Springer 2015; pp. 99-126.

[34] Hassin GB. Cerebrospinal fluid: Its origin, nature and function. J Exp Neuropath Axp Neurol 1948; 7: 172-81.

[35] Shantha TR, Evans JA. The relationship of epidural anesthesia to neural membranes and arachnoid villi. Anesthesiology 1972; 37: 443-557.

[36] Karmakar MK. High-definition and three-dimensional volumetric ultrasound imaging of the sciatic nerve. In: Reina MA, Ed. Atlas of functional anatomy for regional anesthesia and pain medicine. New York, Springer 2015; pp. 355-81

[37] Bigeleisen PE. Nerve puncture and apparent intraneural injections during ultrasound-guided axillary block does not invariably result in neurologic injury. Anesthesiology 2006; 105: 779-83

[38] Boezaart AP, Franco CD. Thin sharp needles around the dura (Letter). Reg Anesth Pain Med 2006; 31: 388-9

[39] Boezaart AP. That which we call a rose by any other name would smell as sweet- and its thorns would hurt as much. Reg Anesth Pain Med 2009; 34: 3-7.

[40] Boezaart AP, Tighe P. New trends in regional anesthesia for shoulder surgery: Avoiding devastating complications. Int J Shoulder Surg 2010; 4: 1-8.

[41] Chelly JE. Perineural infusions of local anesthetics: more to the review (Letter). Anesthesiology 2006; 106: 191.

[42] Boezaart AP. Microanatomy of the peripheral nervous system revisited, and its implications for paravertebral (para-neuraxial) blocks.Proceedings of the 10th Annual pre-ASA Meeting, Orthopedic Anesthesia Pain Rehabilitation Society (www.OAPRS.org); 2013 October 11; San Francisco, California. United States of America.

Chapter 3:
Sonoanatomy of the Posterior Triangle of the Neck

CHAPTER 3

Sonoanatomy of the Posterior Triangle of the Neck

Barys V. Ihnatsenka[1], André P. Boezaart[2,*], Yury Zasimovich[1] and Anastacia P. Munro[3]

[1]Department of Anesthesiology, Division of Acute and Perioperative Pain Medicine, University of Florida College of Medicine, Gainesville, Florida, USA; [2]Departments of Anesthesiology and Orthopaedic Surgery and Rehabilitation, Division of Acute and Perioperative Pain Medicine, University of Florida College of Medicine, Gainesville, Florida, USA and [3]Department of Anesthesiology, Division of Acute and Perioperative Pain Medicine, University of Florida College of Medicine, Gainesville, Florida, USA

Abstract: With this chapter, the authors discuss the sonoanatomy of the posterior triangle of the neck. The basic sonoanatomy is approached from two angles, the first from a static ultrasound point of view to give the reader the opportunity to study the different structures in detail. Secondly, a video production has been produced to explain the dynamic ultrasound of this area. In both instances, the ultrasound transducer probe is placed so that the initial view is that of a known structure. In the anterolateral approach, the probe is placed on the cricoid cartilage and moved posterior to bring the thyroid gland into view; slightly more posterolateral, the common carotid artery comes into view, followed by the large anterior tubercle of the transverse process of the 6th cervical vertebra. From this known position, the probe is moved cephalad and caudad to identify the other structures of the cervical vertebrae and brachial plexus. In the lateral approach, the probe is placed in the supraclavicular area where the subclavian artery and vein are clearly visible, and from there, the trunks of the brachial plexus are followed cephalad to view the transverse processes of the vertebrae and the spinal nerve roots and trunks as they exit the neuroforamens and form the trunks. The sonoanatomy of the supraclavicular fossa is discussed in detail.

Keywords: Anterior scalene muscle, Brachial plexus, Brachial plexus trunks, Cervical paravertebral block, Cervical spinal roots, Chassaignac's tubercle, Circumneural sheath, Dorsal scapular artery, Dorsal scapular nerve, Dynamic ultrasound, Interscalene block, Longus colli muscle, Middle cervical sympathetic ganglion, Middle scalene muscle, Neuroforamens, Paraneural sheath, Phrenic nerve, Posterior scalene muscle, Sonoanatomy, Static ultrasound, Stellate ganglion, Sternocleidomastoid muscle, Superficial cervical plexus, Transverse process, Ultrasound.

***Corresponding author André P Boezaart:** Departments of Anesthesiology and Orthopaedic Surgery, Division of Acute and Peri-operative Pain Medicine, University of Florida College of Medicine, 1600 SW Archer Road, Gainesville, Florida 32610, USA; Tel: 352-846-0913 (Work); Fax: 352-392-7029; E-mail: aboezaart@anest.ufl.edu

INTRODUCTION

Ultrasound is a dynamic process whereby structures can and should be followed to their origins and destinations for optimal identification [1]. It is therefore not always satisfactory to study static ultrasound images. When studying the sonoanatomy of the neck [2], the authors strongly advise readers to study the macro- and microanatomy first and then to view the accompanying video (Movie **1**) and functional anatomy video production that illustrate the dynamic and static sonoanatomy of the posterior triangle of the neck.

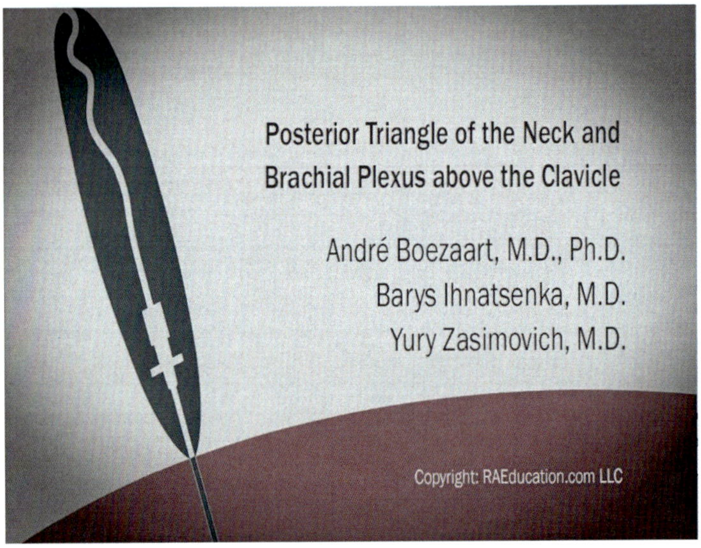

To view this movie click on this link:
https://raeducation.com/ebook

Movie 1: The dynamic sonoanatomy of the brachial plexus above the clavicle.

SONOANATOMY

Anterolateral View

To obtain the ultrasound images in this section, the authors positioned the model ("patient") in the lateral position with the head raised 30 to 45 degrees. This allows the veins in the neck to collapse. For the first seven images, the ultrasound probe was placed in an anterolateral position and scanning took place from the known position of the thyroid gland anterior, or the trachea or carotid artery, and the scanning depicted took place from cephalad to caudad starting at the 3rd cervical spinal root and moving down toward the 8th cervical root. It is important to understand the numbering of the spinal roots. Cervical spinal roots 1 through 7 exit ***above*** the corresponding vertebra, whereas the 8th cervical spinal root exits ***below*** the 7th cervical vertebra. From the 1st thoracic spinal root (T1) to the 5th lumbar spinal root (L5), they all exit **below** the corresponding vertebra.

The ultrasound probe that was used was a 6- to 13-MHz linear probe with a 38 mm footprint (HFL - 38, SonoSite Fujifilm, Bothell, WA, USA) [2].

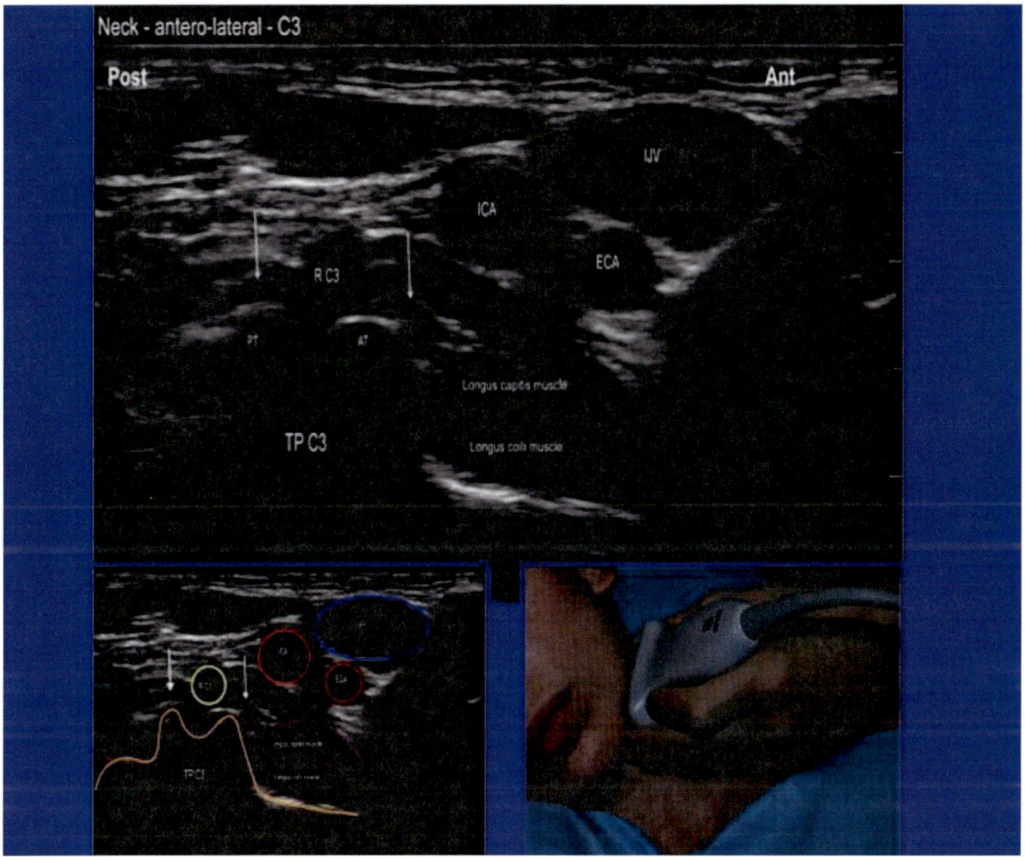

Figure 1: Sonoanatomy of the posterior triangle of the neck - C3 - anterolateral view.
Post = posterior, Ant = anterior, ICA = internal carotid artery, ECA = external carotid artery, IJV = internal jugular vein (Valsalva maneuver applied), R C3 = 3rd cervical spinal nerve root (C3) emerging from between the anterior and posterior tubercles of the transverse process of C3, TP C3 = transverse process of the 3rd cervical vertebra (C3), PT = posterior tubercle of the transverse process of the tubercle of C3, AT = anterior tubercle of the transverse process of the tubercle of C3. The arrows indicate the slips of origin of the anterior and middle scalene muscles.

Note: At this level of C3, we can see the longus capitis muscle, which runs from the occiput to the anterior tubercles of the 1st (C1) to those of the 5th (C5) cervical vertebrae, and the longus colli muscle, which lies just anterior to the transverse processes and runs from the bodies of C1 to that of the 4th cervical vertebra (C4) to the bodies of C5 to that of the 3rd thoracic vertebra (T3). Lower down, below C4 and C5, only the longus colli muscle is present [3].

This is the patient positioning in which the authors would typically prefer to perform a posterior approach interscalene nerve block (although not at this level) [4-6].

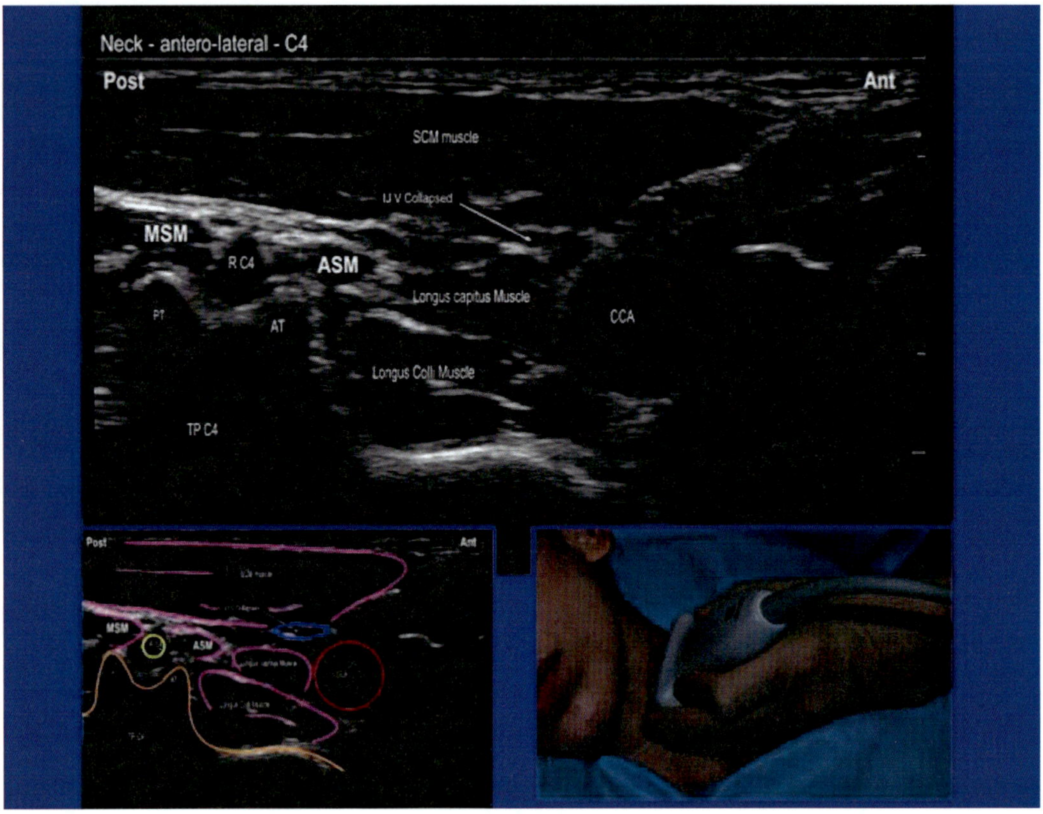

Figure 2: Sonoanatomy of the posterior triangle of the neck - C4 - anterolateral view.
Post = posterior, Ant = anterior, CCA = common carotid artery, IJV = internal jugular vein (collapsed), R C4 = 4th cervical spinal nerve root (C4), TP C4 = transverse process of the 4th cervical vertebra (C4), PT = posterior tubercle of the transverse process of C4, AT = anterior tubercle of the transverse process of C4, ASM = anterior scalene muscle (slips of origin), MSM = middle scalene muscle (slips of origin), SCM = sternocleidomastoid muscle.

*The long thoracic nerve (see Chapter 1, Fig. **1**) also originates at this level from C4, C5, and C6 and runs with the DSN where it exits between the ventral and dorsal middle scalene muscles. Injury to either/both of these nerves during a nerve block here is possible.

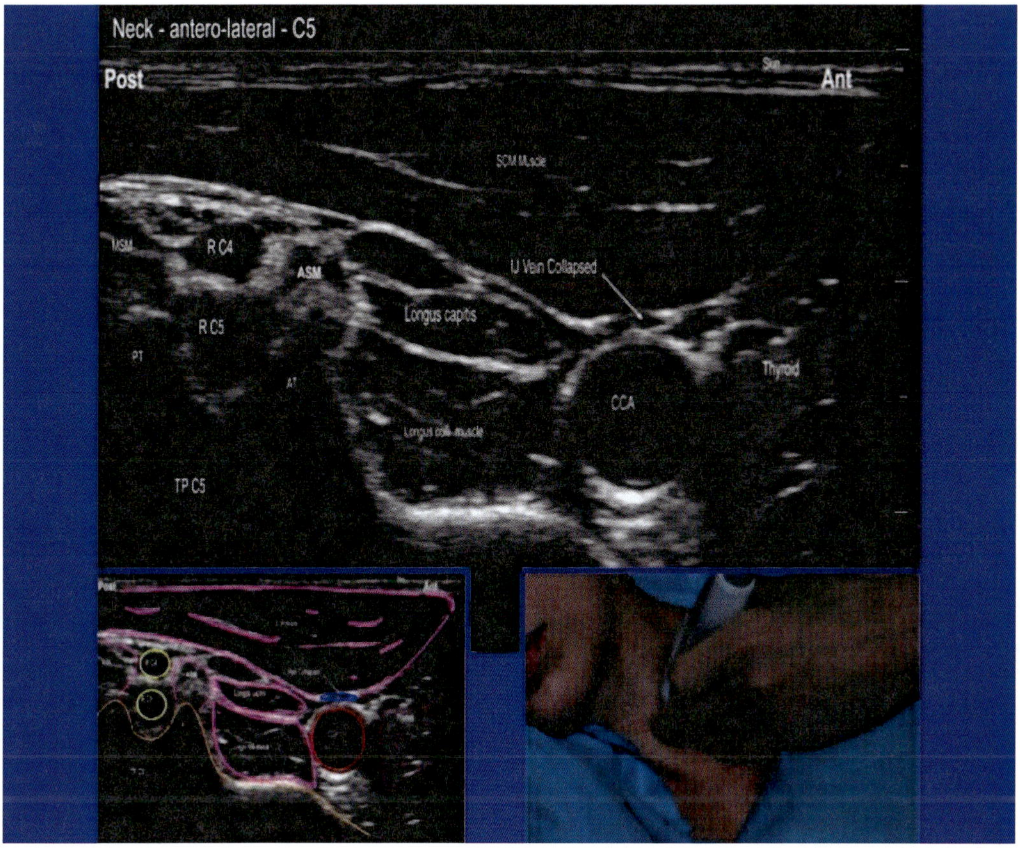

Figure 3: Sonoanatomy of the posterior triangle of the neck - C5 - anterolateral view.
Post = posterior, Ant = anterior, CCA = common carotid artery, IJV = internal jugular vein (collapsed), R C4 = 5th cervical spinal nerve root (C4), R C5 = 5th cervical spinal nerve root (C5), TP C5 = transverse process of the 5th cervical vertebra (C5), PT = posterior tubercle of the transverse process of C5, AT = anterior tubercle of the transverse process of C5, ASM = anterior scalene muscle (slim at origin), MSM = middle scalene muscle (slim at origin), SCM = sternocleidomastoid muscle, Thyroid = thyroid gland.

Note: Both longus capitis and longus colli muscles are present at this level [2].

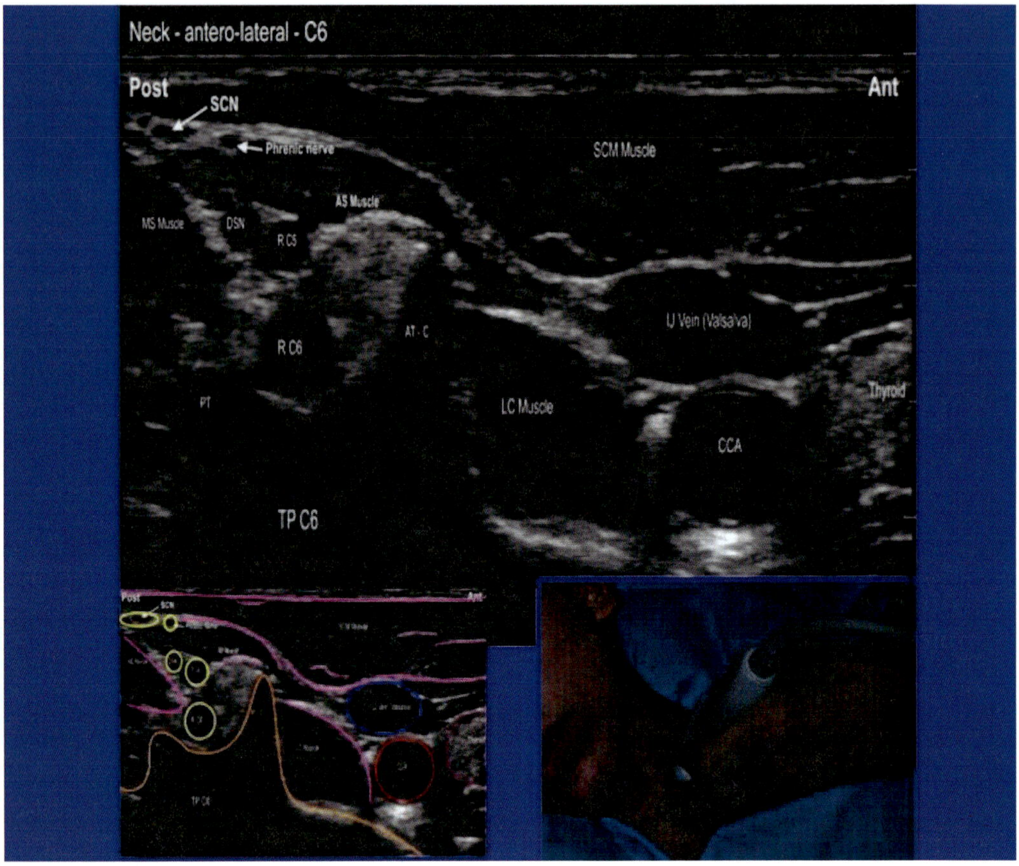

Figure 4: Sonoanatomy of the posterior triangle of the neck - C6 - anterolateral view.
Post = posterior, Ant = anterior, CCA = common carotid artery, IJV = internal jugular vein (Valsalva maneuver applied), R C5 = 5th cervical spinal nerve root (C5), R C6 = 6th cervical spinal nerve root (C6), DSN = dorsal scapular nerve originating from the C5 spinal root, TP C6 = transverse process of the 6th cervical vertebra (C6), PT = Posterior tubercle of the transverse process of C6, AT C = large anterior tubercle of the transverse process of C6 (also known as the Carotid tubercle or Chassaignac's tubercle), AS Muscle = anterior scalene muscle, MS Muscle = middle scalene muscle, LC muscle = longus colli muscle (longus capitis muscle is not present at this level), SCM muscle = sternocleidomastoid muscle, SCN = supraclavicular nerves.*

Note the phrenic nerve on the anterior belly of the anterior scalene muscle.

At this level, the SCN, which are part of the superficial cervical plexus, can be seen under the posterior edge of the SCM.

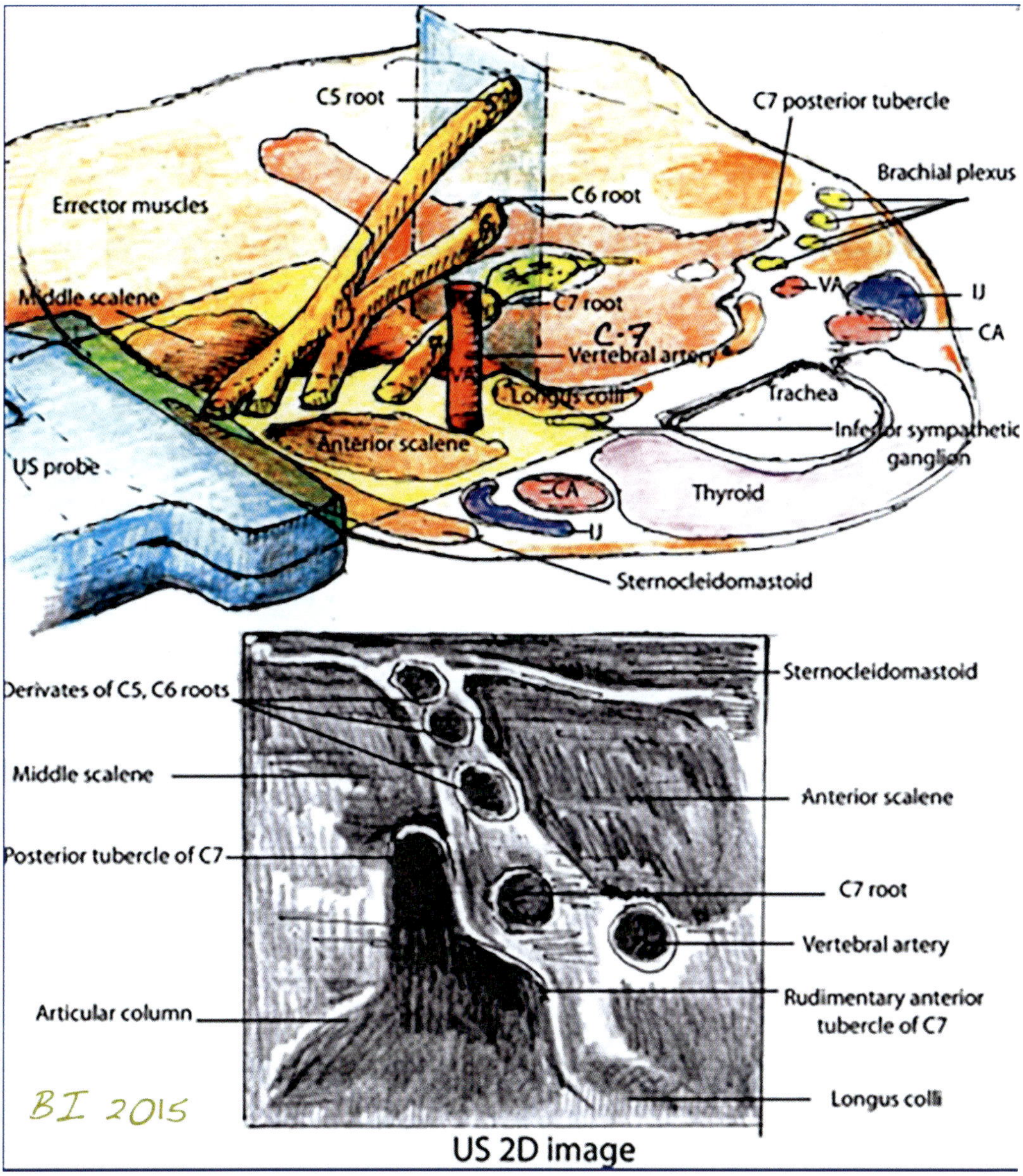

Figure 5a: Schematic three-dimensional view of the posterior triangle of the neck through the transverse process of the 7th cervical vertebra.

CA = carotid artery; VA = vertebral artery; IJ = internal jugular vein; US probe = ultrasound transducer probe;

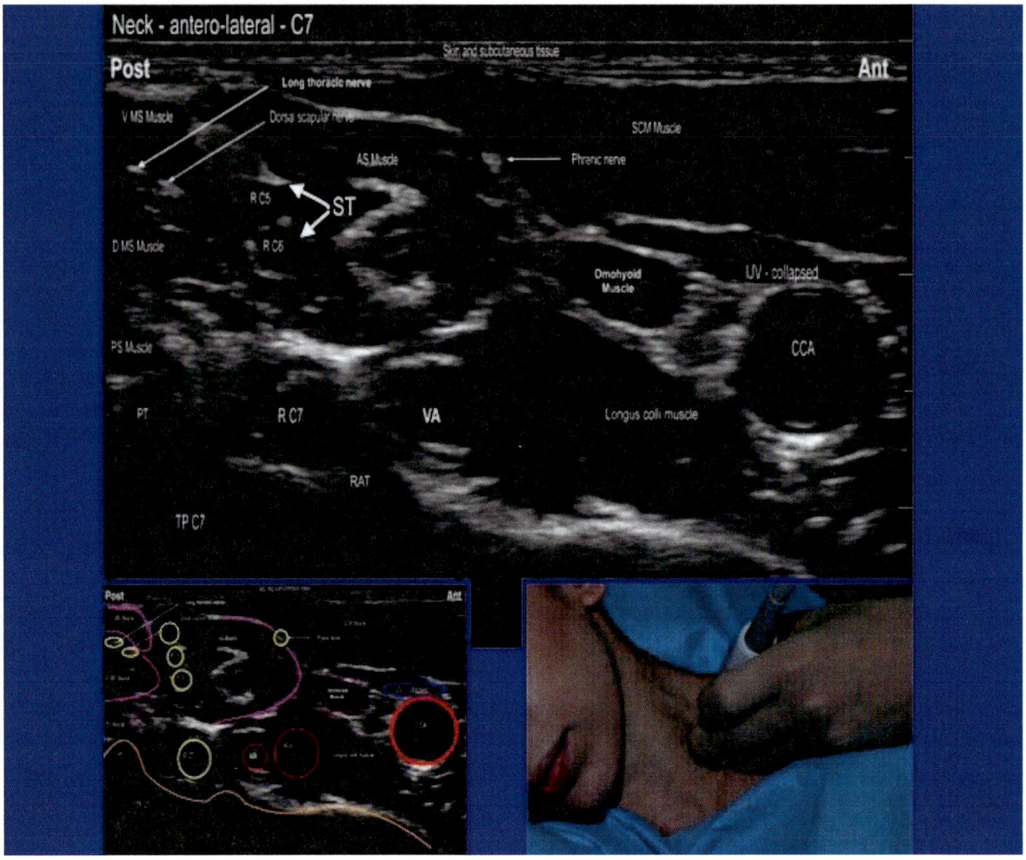

Figure 5b: Sonoanatomy of the posterior triangle of the neck - C7 - anterolateral view.
Post = posterior, Ant = anterior, CCA = common carotid artery, IJV = internal jugular vein (collapsed), R C5 = 5th cervical spinal nerve root (C5), R C6 = 6th cervical spinal nerve root (C6), R C7 = 7th cervical spinal nerve root (C7), TP C7 = transverse process of the 7th cervical vertebra (C7), PT = posterior tubercle of the transverse process of C7, RAT = rudimentary anterior tubercle (which is mostly absent), AS Muscle = anterior scalene muscle (note the phrenic nerve on its belly), VMS Muscle = ventral middle scalene muscle (note the dorsal scapular nerve between the ventral and dorsal scalene muscles. The long thoracic nerve also runs here), DMS Muscle = dorsal middle scalene muscle, PS Muscle = posterior scalene muscle, SCM muscle = sternocleidomastoid muscle, VA = vertebral.*

Note: The long thoracic nerve exits with the DSN between the VMS and DMS (see Chapter 1, Fig. **1**), and can often be identified with dynamic ultrasound. Please refer to the Movie **1** illustrating the dynamic sonoanatomy of the posterior triangle of the neck.

*C5 and C6 are generally in a common circumneural sheath here as they join to form the upper or superior trunk.

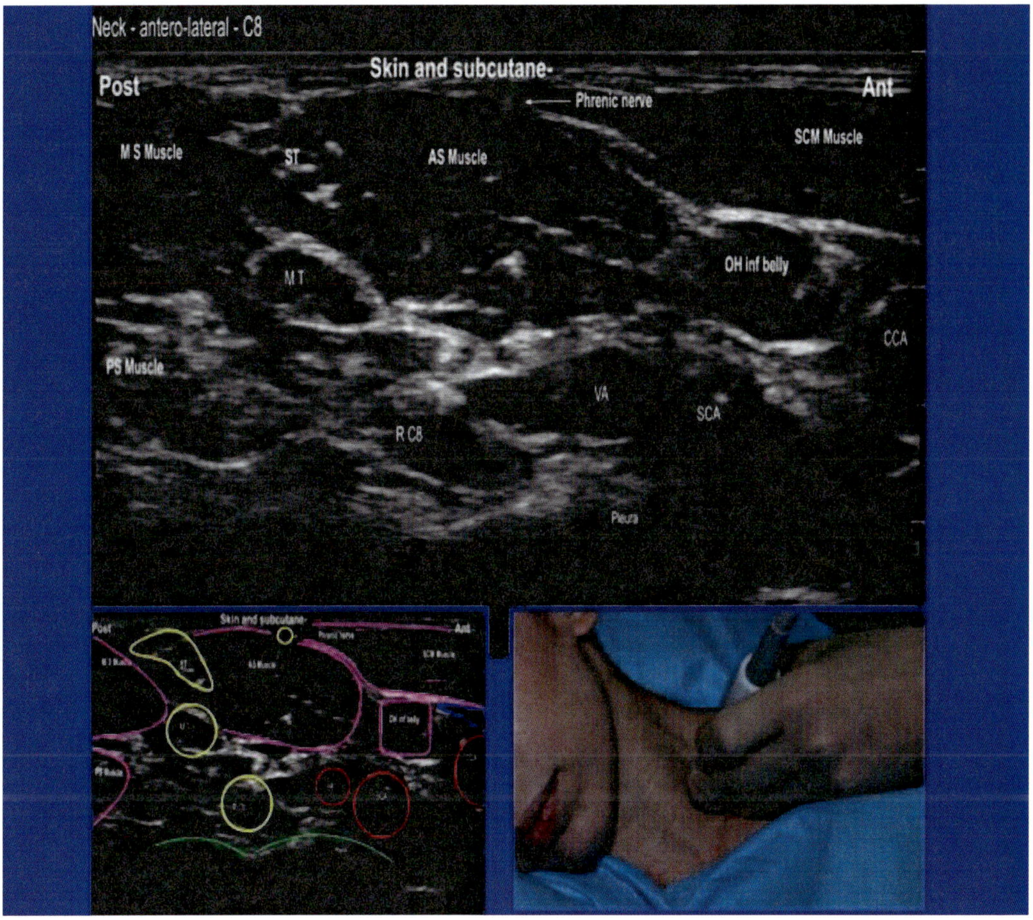

Figure 6: Sonoanatomy of the posterior triangle of the neck - C8 - anterolateral view.
Post = posterior, Ant = anterior, CCA = common carotid artery, OH Muscle = omohyoid muscle, ST = superior or upper trunk of the brachial plexus, MT = medial or middle trunk of the brachial plexus, R C8 = 8th cervical spinal nerve root (C8) (Note that the 1st thoracic spinal nerve root has not yet joined from underneath the first rib to form the inferior or lower trunk. Also note the position of the C8 nerve root on the pleura of the dome of the lung), AS Muscle = anterior scalene muscle (note the phrenic nerve on its belly), MS Muscle = middle scalene muscle, PS Muscle = posterior scalene muscle, SCM muscle = sternocleidomastoid muscle, SCA = subclavian artery, VA = vertebral artery.

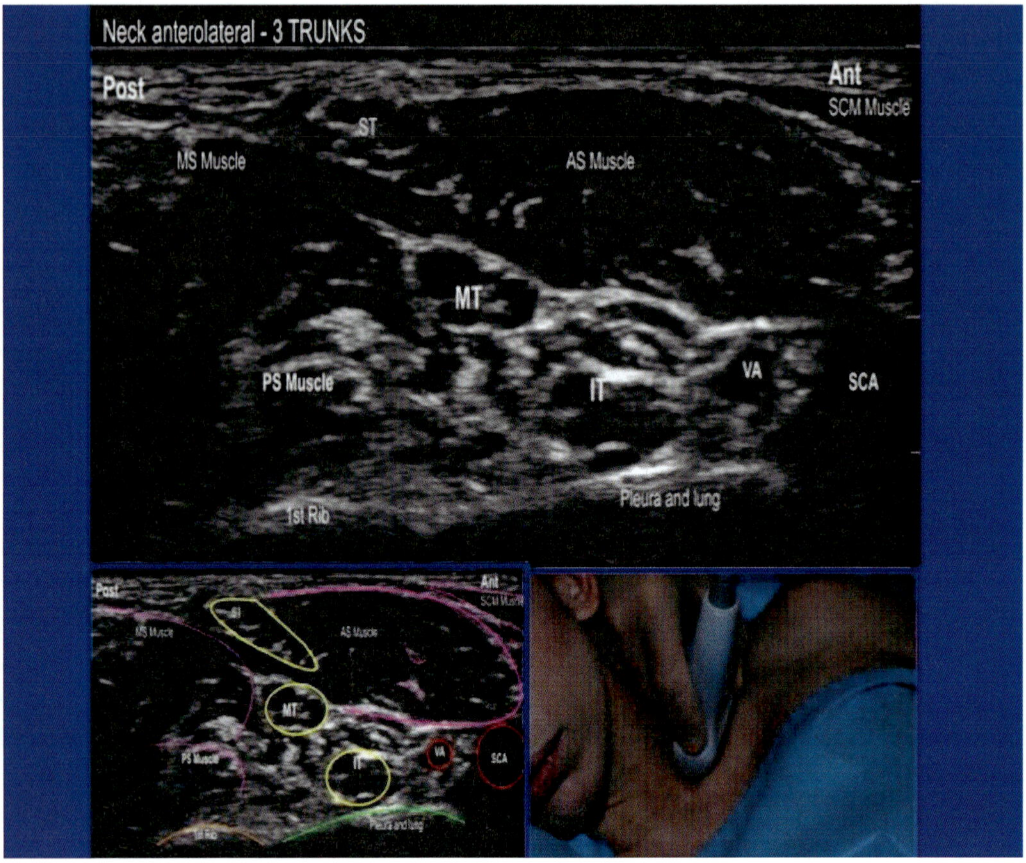

Figure 7a: Sonoanatomy of the posterior triangle of the neck - all three trunks -anterolateral view. *Post = posterior, Ant = anterior, ST = superior or upper trunk, MD = medial or middle trunk, IT = inferior or lower trunk, AS Muscle = anterior scalene muscle (note the large size of the scalene muscles at this level), MS Muscle = middle scalene muscle, PS Muscle = posterior scalene muscle (Note the tendonous appearance), SCM muscle = sternocleidomastoid muscle, SCA = subclavian artery, VA = vertebral artery.*

Note the position of the inferior trunk on the pleura of the dome of the lung. From the level of the 7th cervical vertebra, the entire brachial plexus can be visualized by slight up and down movement of the ultrasound transducer (Fig. **7b**).

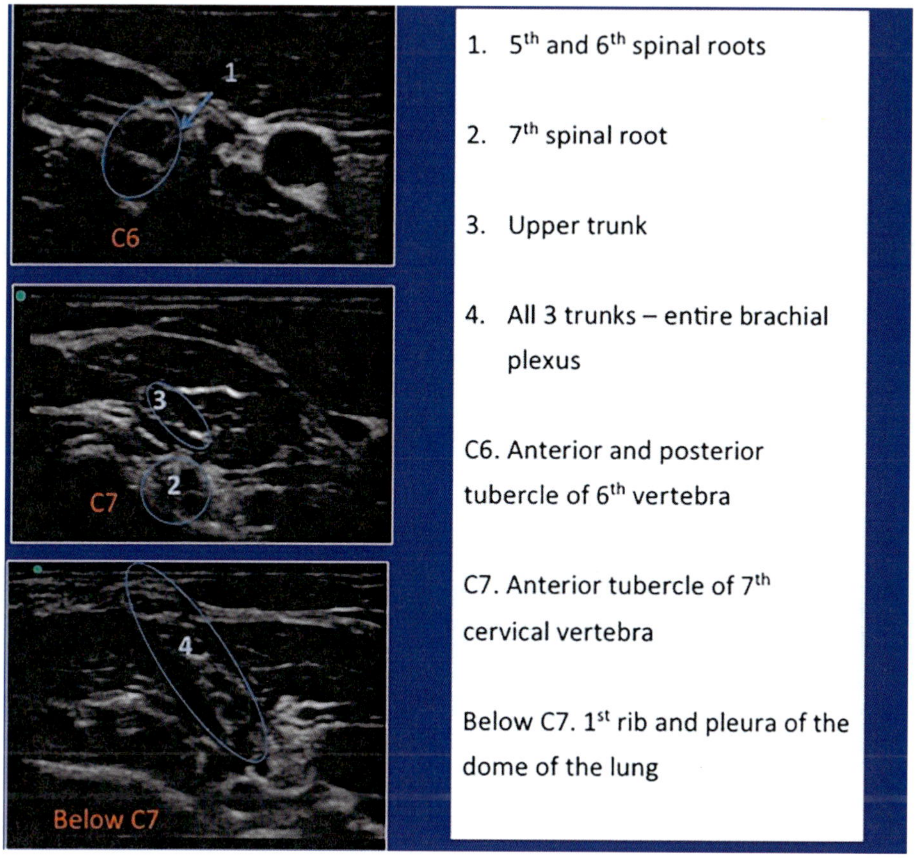

Figure 7b: Summary of the visualization of the brachial plexus from anterolateral.

Lateral View

To obtain the ultrasound images in this section, the authors positioned the model in the lateral position with the head slightly raised. For the next five images, the ultrasound probe was placed in a lateral position and scanning took place from the known position of the subclavian artery in the supraclavicular area moving the probe cephalad while keeping the transverse processes of the vertebrae in the center of the image. Unlike the previous section, where scanning was from C3 downward to C8, in this section, scanning is from C8 up toward C4, keeping the transverse processes of the vertebrae in the center of the probe. The ultrasound probe that was used was a 6- to 13-MHz linear probe with a 38-cm footprint (HFL - 38, SonoSite Fujifilm, Bothell, WA, USA) [2].

It may be of value to study the drawing of the ultrasound images of Fig. (**8a**) first before studying the more detailed supraclavicular ultrasound images of Figs. (**8b**, **9**).

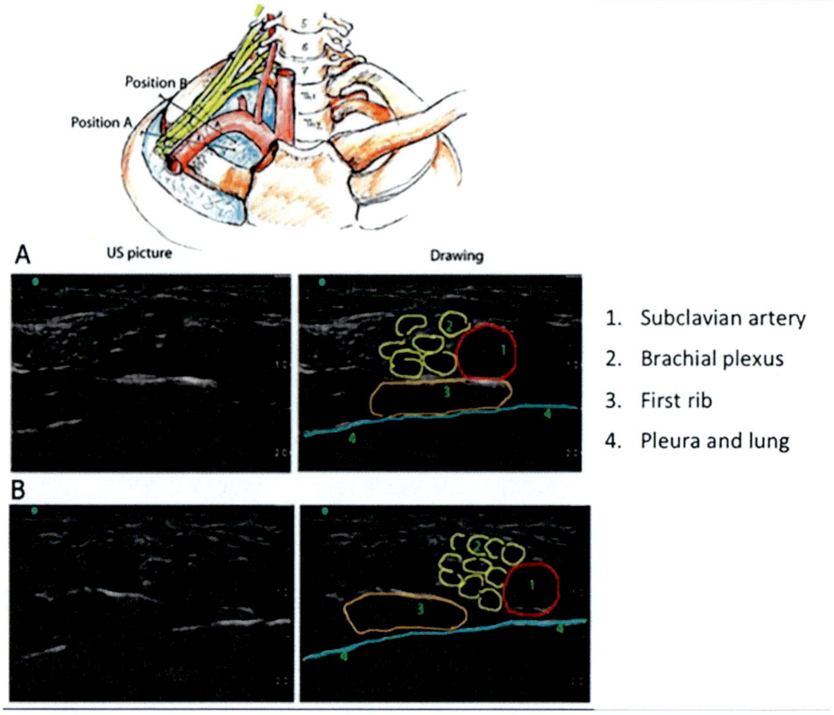

Figure 8a: Sonoanatomy of the supraclavicular area.

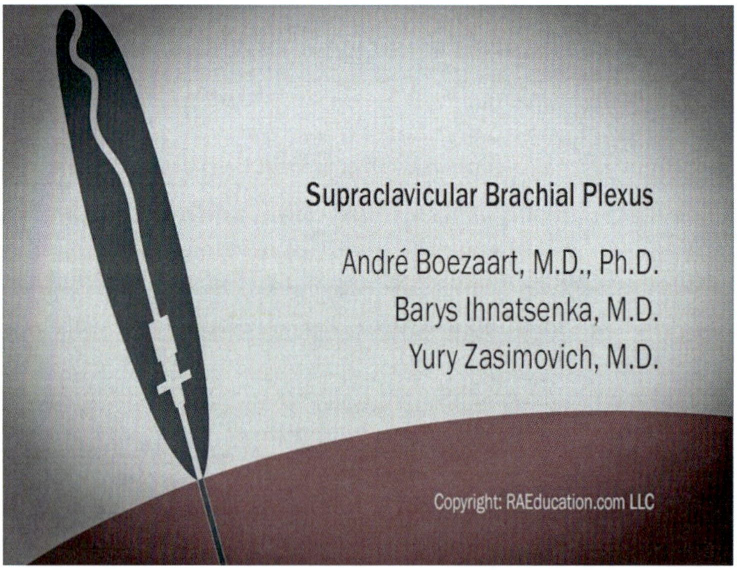

To view this movie click on this link:
https://raeducation.com/ebook

Movie 2: The dynamic sonoanatomy of the brachial plexus in the supraclavicular fossa.

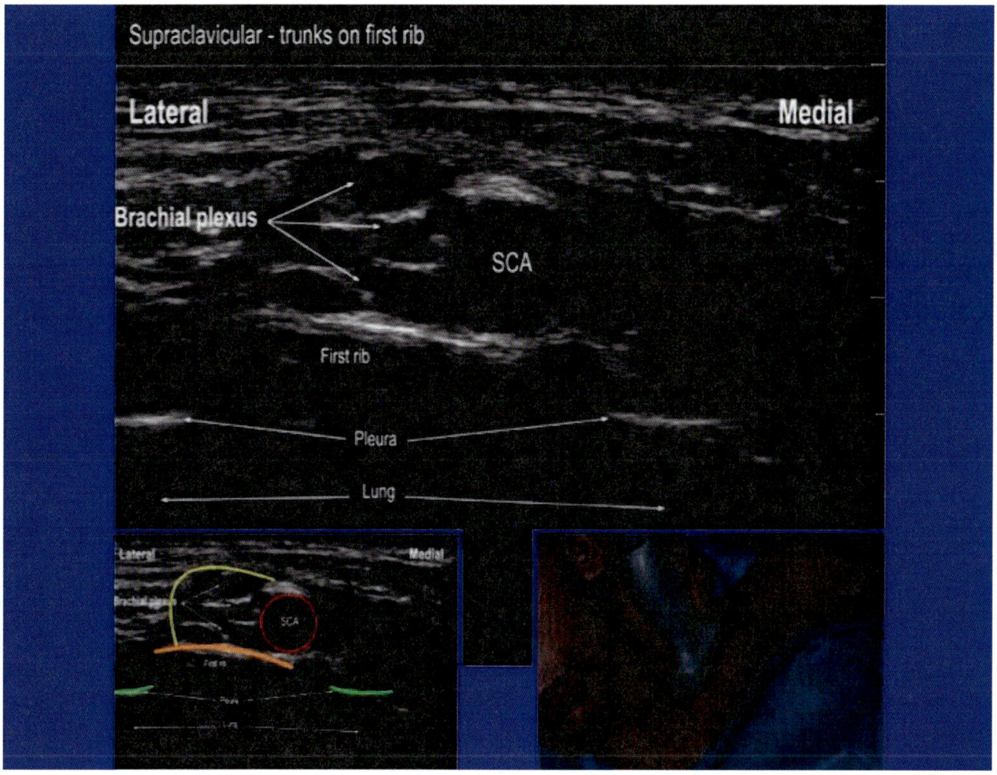

Figure 8b: Sonoanatomy of the supraclavicular brachial plexus - subclavian artery viewed on the first rib. *SCA = subclavian artery.*

With the ultrasound probe in the supraclavicular fossa just lateral to the sternal head of the sternocleidomastoid muscle, the subclavian artery can be easily visualized. Lateral to it is the brachial plexus - and commonly the three trunks of the brachial plexus, but these structures can also be divisions of the brachial plexus. Inferolateral to the brachial plexus, the long thoracic nerve can often be seen and superficial, and also lateral to the brachial plexus is the suprascapular artery vein and nerve [7]. These neurovascular bundles and nerves can often be identified separately. Please view the dynamic sonoanatomy video (Movie **2**) to see the relationship of the dorsal scapular artery, which is a branch of the subclavian artery, and the brachial plexus at this level. This artery commonly splits the brachial plexus into superficial and deep portions. It usually lies between the upper and middle trunks.

With the ultrasound beam tilted anterior (ventrally; the probe handler dorsally or posterior and the beam directed underneath the clavicle) and the shoulder joint pushed down, the subclavian artery can be visualized on the first rib. This adds some safety to the supraclavicular block, as will be explained in more detail with the next figure, where the subclavian artery is visualized on the pleura.

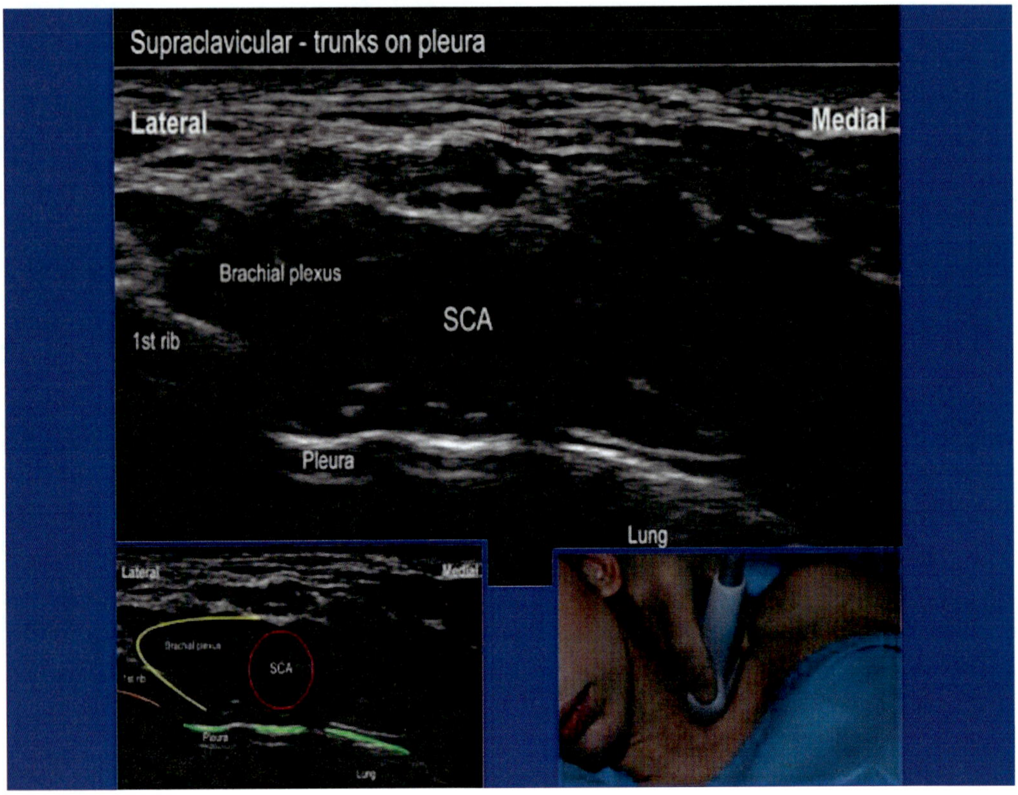

Figure 8c: Sonoanatomy of supraclavicular brachial plexus - subclavian artery viewed on the pleura.
SCA = subclavian artery.

Note the position of the ultrasound probe. The ultrasound beam is now tilted more toward the posterior or dorsally toward the neck and the cupola of the lung, or the shoulder joint is somewhat elevated. It can now be seen that the subclavian artery and the brachial plexus are visualized on the pleura of the dome of the lung, which is vulnerable to needle injury during a supraclavicular nerve block and the obvious complication of pneumothorax.

A popular ultrasound-guided technique for a supraclavicular block is to place the needle into the so-called "corner pocket" between the subclavian artery and the first rib [8]. If there is confusion between where the first rib is and where the pleura is, the dangerous complication of pneumothorax could occur, which was a common complication before ultrasound was introduced.

The authors would encourage the reader to view the associated dynamic sonoanatomy video (Movie **2**) that illustrates this point better.

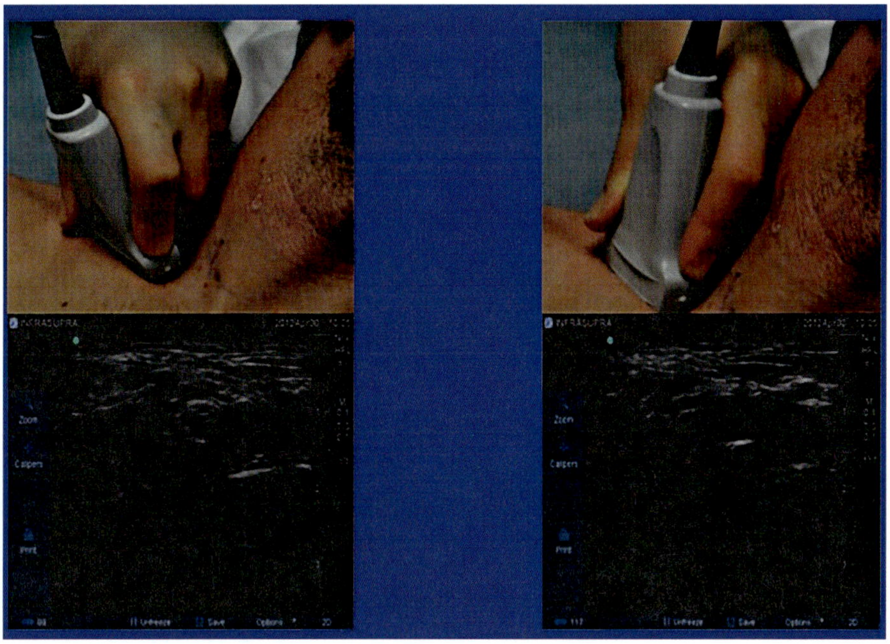

Figure 8d: Ultrasound transducer positioning for supraclavicular block.
On the left hand top photograph, the ultrasound beam is pointed dorsally or posterior and the ultrasound image below it illustrate the subclavian artery where it is situated on the pleura of the lung. In the right hand photograph the probe is tilted such that the ultrasound beam is directed ventrally or anterior, and the image below it (right) is now of the subclavian artery situated on the first rib.

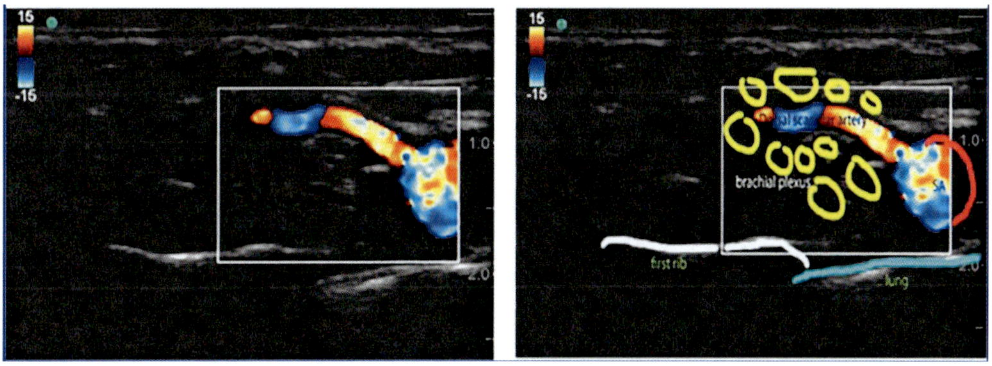

Figure 9: Dorsal scapular artery.
When the Doppler function of the ultrasound is applied we can clearly see the dorsal scapular artery where it comes off of the subclavian artery. It frequently courses between the nerves of the brachial plexus where it splits it into superficial and deeper parts - most commonly the upper and medial trunks.

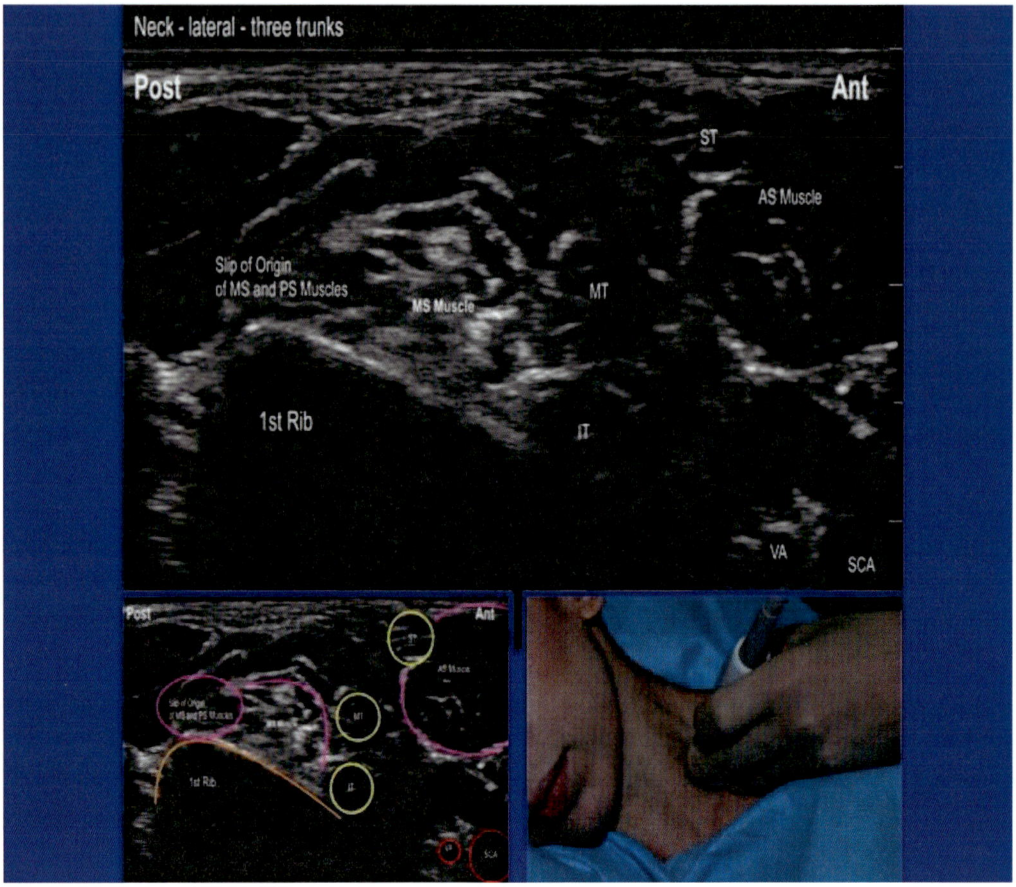

Figure 10: Sonoanatomy of the posterior triangle of the neck - three trunks - lateral view.
Post = posterior, ant = Anterior, SCA = subclavian artery, VA = vertebral artery, ST = superior trunk of the brachial plexus where C5 and C6 have fused, MT = middle trunk, which is formed from the 7th spinal nerve root, IT = inferior or lower trunk, which is formed by the fusion of the 8th cervical and 1st thoracic spinal nerve roots, AS Muscle = anterior scalene muscle, MS Muscle = middle scalene muscle, PS Muscle = posterior scalene muscle.

Sliding the probe more cephalad, the middle trunk comes into view, and if we follow this trunk further cephalad we can see where it exits just anterior to the posterior tubercle of the transverse process of the 7th cervical vertebra (Fig. **11**). See also video:

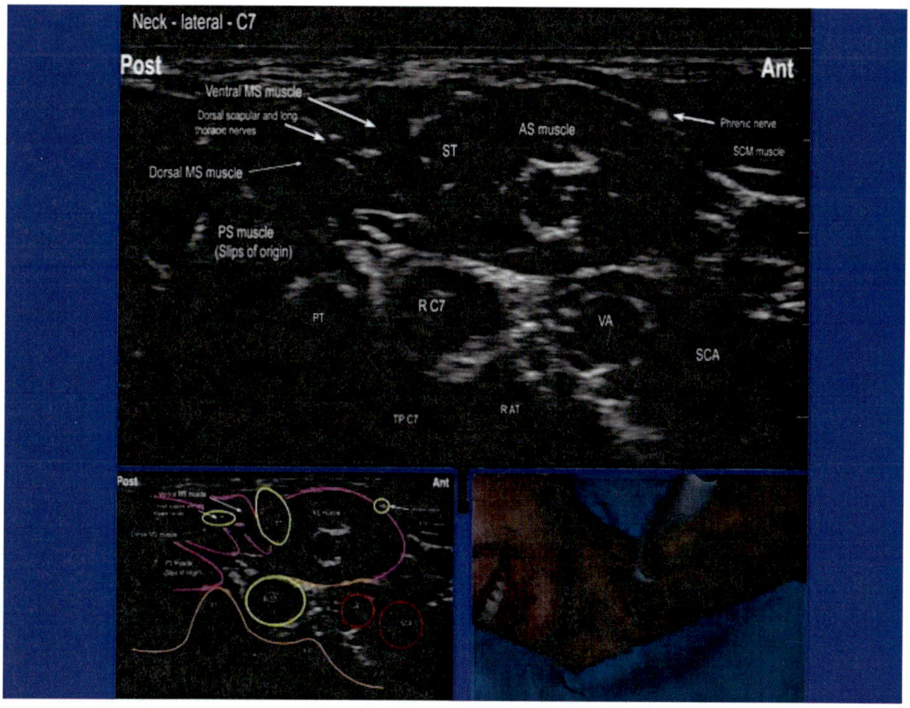

Figure 11: Sonoanatomy of the posterior triangle of the neck - C7 - lateral view.
Post = posterior, Ant = anterior, SCA = subclavian artery, VA = vertebral artery, R C7 = 7th cervical spinal nerve root (C7), ST = superior trunk of the brachial plexus where C5 and C6 have fused. Note, in this image, these two roots are about to fuse together to form the upper or superior trunk, TP C7 = transverse process of the 6th cervical vertebra, R AT = rudimentary anterior tubercle of the transverse process of C7, PT = posterior tubercle of the transverse process, AS Muscle = anterior scalene muscle, Ventral MS muscle = ventral middle scalene muscle, Dorsal MS muscle = dorsal middle scalene muscle (Note the dorsal scapular nerve between the ventral MS and dorsal MS muscles. The long thoracic nerve also exits here with the dorsal scapular nerve), PS muscle = posterior scalene muscle (slips of origin), SCM Muscle = sternocleidomastoid muscle.*

*This is typically the position in which the authors would prefer to perform a cervical paravertebral block [9-13] on patients. We would aim for the C6 root after "walking off" of the posterior tubercle of C7 and advancing through the slips of origin of the posterior scalene muscle. For shoulder surgery placing the catheter in the sub-circumneural space (also called the sub-paraneural space) of C6 (or that of the upper trunk) (please see Chapter 2) would be ideal, while and the C7 root (or middle trunk) would be ideal for elbow and wrist surgery (see Chapter 9). The posterior scalene muscle is more aponeurotic or tendonous at its slips of origin from the posterior tubercles of the transverse processes of the 5th, 6th, and 7th vertebrae [3], which provides a handy landmark for the loss of resistance to air technique combined with electrical stimulation when ultrasound is not used (air obscures ultrasound picture) or with ultrasound (triple guidance) where 5% dextrose in water is used instead of air. We can also choose to advance more lateral and between the posterior and dorsal part of the middle scalene muscles. Whatever approach is used to block the brachial plexus roots or trunks, it is important to avoid injury to the long thoracic and dorsal scapular nerves (see Chapters 1 and 2). The 6th cervical root should be clearly visible from the level of the C7 transverse process, and following it upward (cephalad) will bring the transverse process of the 6th cervical vertebra into view. It usually has a large anterior tubercle called the Carotid tubercle of Chassaignac's tubercle and the C6 spinal root exits the neuroforamen just posterior to it (Fig. **12**).

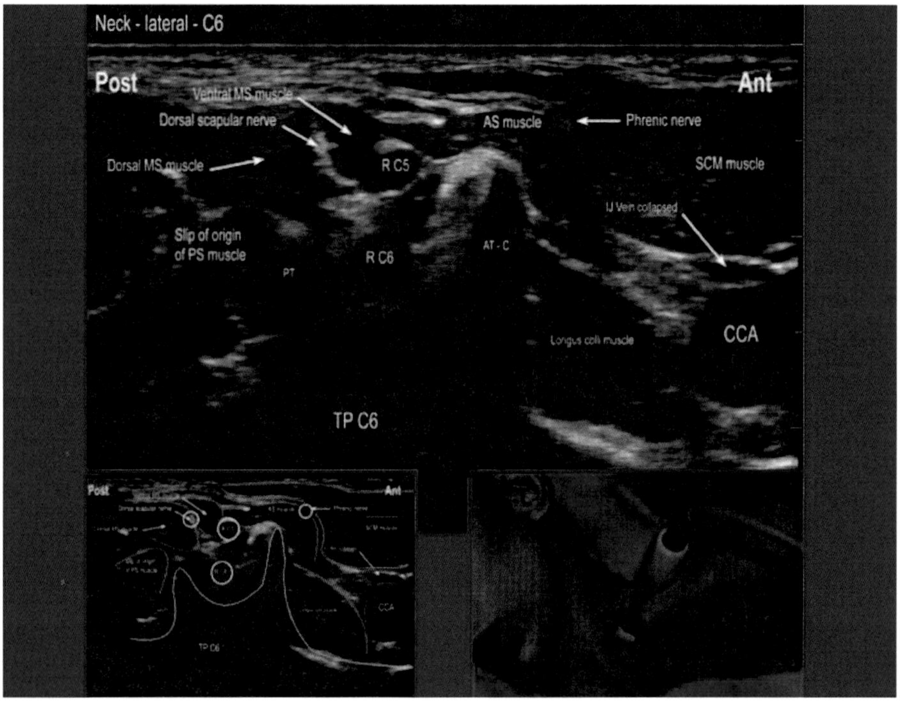

Figure 12: Sonoanatomy of the posterior triangle of the neck - C6 - lateral view.
Post = posterior, Ant = anterior, CCA = common carotid artery, IJ Vein = internal jugular vein (collapsed), R C5 = 5th cervical spinal nerve root (C5), R C6 = 6th cervical spinal nerve root (C6), TP C6 = transverse process of the 6th cervical vertebra, AT C = large anterior tubercle of the transverse process also called the carotid tubercle or Chassaignac's tubercle, PT = posterior tubercle of the transverse process, AS Muscle = slips of origin of the anterior scalene muscle, Ventral MS muscle = ventral middle scalene muscle, Dorsal MS muscle = dorsal middle scalene muscle (Note the dorsal scapular nerve between the ventral and dorsal MS muscles. The long thoracic nerve also exits here with the dorsal scapular nerve), PS muscle = slips of origin of the posterior scalene muscle [3], SCM Muscle = sternocleidomastoid muscle.

Note the absence of the longus capitis muscle at this level; only the longus colli muscle is visible at the level of C6. The middle cervical sympathetic ganglion is situated deep to the fascia of the longus colli muscle, which is situated just anterior to the large anterior tubercle of the transverse process of the 6th cervical vertebra. The cervicothoracic ganglion (or stellate ganglion), which is lower down at the level of the 7th cervical vertebra, just behind the subclavian artery, is commonly also approached from here - counting on caudal spread of local anesthetic agent in the ventral fascial plane of the longus colli muscle.

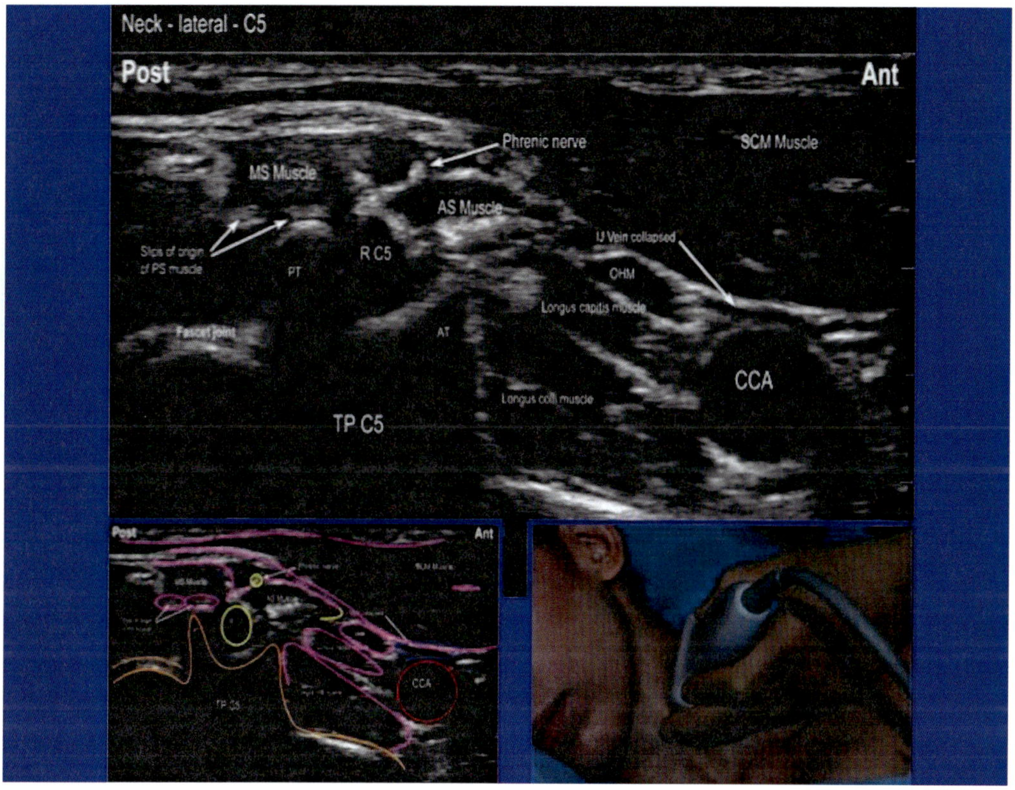

Figure 13: Sonoanatomy of the posterior triangle of the neck - C5 - lateral view.
Post = posterior, Ant = anterior, CCA = common carotid artery, IJ Vein = internal jugular vein (collapsed), R C5 = 5th cervical spinal nerve root (C5), TP C5 = transverse process of the 5th cervical vertebra, AT = anterior tubercle of the transverse process, PT = posterior tubercle of the transverse process, AS Muscle = anterior scalene muscle (Note the phrenic nerve on its belly close to the, C5 spinal nerve root at this level), MS Muscle = middle scalene muscle, PS Muscle = slips of origin of the posterior scalene muscle, SCM Muscle = sternocleidomastoid muscle.

Immediately lateral to the C6 spinal root the C5 spinal root should be clearly visible, and following this root further cephalad brings the transverse process with its similar-looking anterior and posterior tubercles into view. The 5th spinal root exits the neuroforamen between these to tubercles, and, if one follows the C5 spinal root caudad or laterally, one can usually see the dorsal scapular nerve coming off of it. This nerve can be followed posteriorly as it courses with the long thoracic nerve between the ventral and dorsal bellies of the middle scalene muscle.

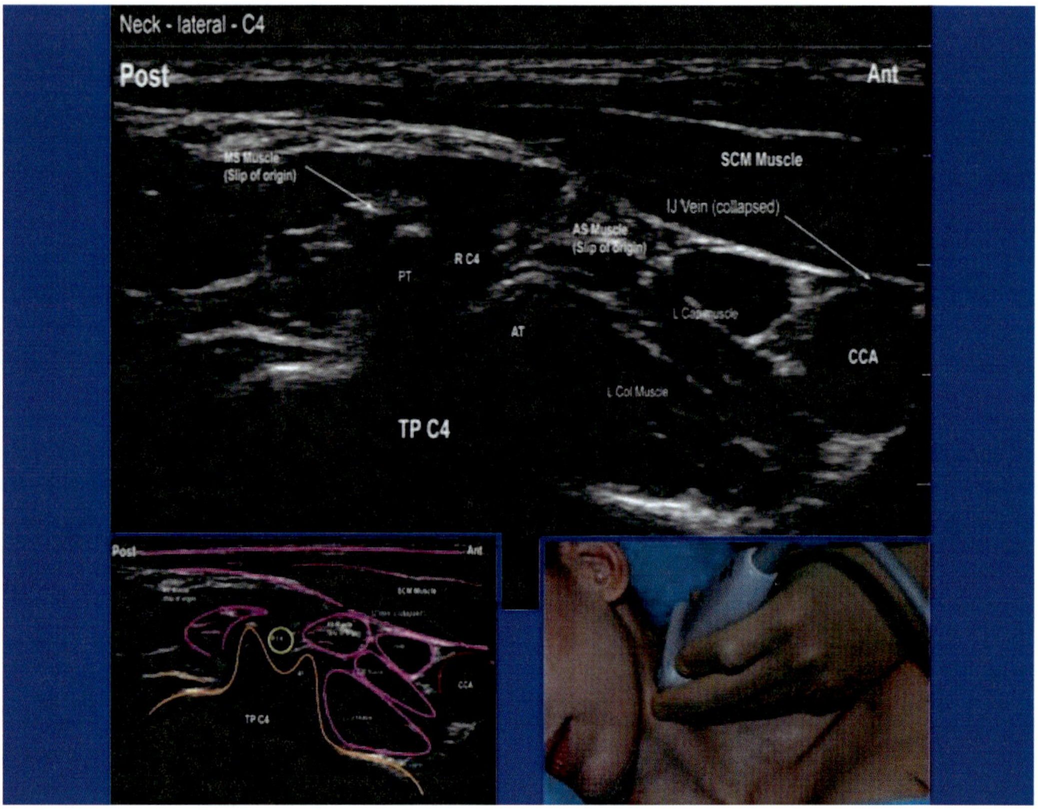

Figure 14: Sonoanatomy of the posterior triangle of the neck - C4 - lateral view.
Post = posterior, Ant = anterior, CCA = common carotid artery, IJ Vein = internal jugular vein (collapsed), R C4 = 4th cervical spinal nerve root (C4), TP C4 = transverse process of the 4th cervical vertebra, AT = anterior tubercle of the transverse process, PT = posterior tubercle of the transverse process, AS Muscle = slips of origin of the anterior scalene muscle, MS Muscle = slips of origin of the middle scalene muscle, L Cap Muscle = longus capitis muscle, L Col Muscle = longus colli muscle, SCM Muscle = sternocleidomastoid muscle.

Further cephalad are the transverse processes and equal anterior and posterior tubercles of the 4th and 3rd cervical vertebrae with their corresponding spinal roots exiting between the tubercles. Note that at the level of C3 the common carotid artery has split into its internal and external branches, and again note the presence of the longus capitis and longus colli muscles at this level. This, of course is where the deep cervical plexus block is performed [14].

The C5 spinal nerve root is often targeted during the longitudinal approach to the interscalene block [15,16], although the more classical approach as described by Winnie in 1970 [17] targets the upper trunk lower down. Because the phrenic nerve is so close to the C5 spinal root at this level, phrenic nerve palsy due to local anesthetic overflow or phrenic nerve needle injury are potential complications of both of these approaches to an interscalene block [18].

ACKNOWLEDGEMENTS

The authors gratefully acknowledge the following people:

- The Head of the Department of Anesthesiology of the College of Medicine of the University of Florida, Dr. Tim Morey, and his department for their moral support and continuous encouragement.

- The faculty and fellows of the Division of acute and perioperative pain medicine for affording the authors the time to produce this work by covering their clinical duties.

- Professors Gerbrand Groen and Paul Bigeleisen and Dr. Nizar Moayeri from the University Medical College in Utrecht, The Netherlands for their making of Movie **3** and providing Figs. **21**-**23**.

- Corey Astrom of the Department of Anesthesiology of the College of Medicine of the University of Florida for her professional and high quality text editing.

- Nancy Hagen of the Iowa Public Radio for her narration of the movies.

- Raeducation.com LLC for their financial support.

CONFLICT OF INTEREST

The authors confirm that this chapter contents have no conflict of Interest.

ABBREVIATIONS

Ant	=	anterior
AS Muscle	=	anterior scalene muscle
ASM	=	anterior scalene muscle
AT	=	anterior tubercle
AT C6	=	large anterior tubercle of the transverse process of C6
CCA	=	common carotid artery
DSN	=	dorsal scapular nerve
ECA	=	external carotid artery
ICA	=	internal carotid artery
IJV	=	internal jugular vein
LC muscle	=	longus colli muscle
MS Muscle	=	middle scalene muscle
MSM	=	middle scalene muscle
Post	=	posterior
PT	=	posterior tubercle
R C3	=	3rd cervical spinal nerve root (C3)
R C4	=	4th cervical spinal nerve root (C4)
SCM	=	sternocleidomastoid muscle
SCM muscle	=	sternocleidomastoid muscle
SCN	=	supraclavicular nerves

TP C3 = transverse process of the 3rd cervical vertebra (C3)

TP C4 = transverse process of the 4th cervical vertebra (C4)

TP C6 = transverse process of the 6th cervical vertebra (C6)

US probe = ultrasound transducer probe

REFERENCES

[1] Ihnatsenka BV, Boezaart AP. Ultrasound: Basic understanding and learning the language. Int J Shoulder Surg. 2010; 4: 55-62.
[2] Ihnatsenka BV, Boezaart AP. Applied sonoanatomy of the posterior triangle of the neck. Int J Shoulder Surg. 2010; 4; 63-74.
[3] Netter FH. Atlas of human anatomy. 2nd ed. East Hanover, NJ: Novartis; 1997: plate 25.
[4] Antonakakis JG, Sites BD, Shiffrin J. Ultrasound-guided posterior approach for placement of a continuous interscalene catheter. Reg Anesth Pain Med. 2009; 34: 64-8.
[5] Mariano ER, Loland VJ, Ilfeld BM. Interscalene perineural catheter placement using an ultrasound-guided posterior approach. Reg Anesth Pain Med. 2009; 34: 60-3.
[6] Mariano ER, Afra R, Loland NJ, *et al.* Continuous interscalene brachial plexus block *via* an ultrasound-guided posterior approach: A randomized, triple-blinded, placebo-controlled study. Anesth Analg. 2009; 108: 1688-94.
[7] Reina MA, Sala-Blanch X. Cross-sectional microscopic anatomy of the brachial plexus and paraneural sheaths. In: Reina MA, Ed. Atlas of functional anatomy for regional anesthesia and pain medicine. New York: Springer Science and Business Media; 2015: pp. 165.
[8] Soares LG, Brull R, Lai J, Chan VW. Eight ball, corner pocket: The optimal needle position for ultrasound-guided supraclavicular block. Reg Anesth Pain Med. 2007; 32: 94-5.
[9] Boezaart AP, Koorn R, Rosenquist RW. Paravertebral approach to the brachial plexus: An anatomic improvement in technique. Reg Anesth Pain Med. 2003; 28: 241-4.
[10] Boezaart AP, de Beer, JF, Nell ML. Early experience with continuous cervical paravertebral block using a stimulating catheter. Reg Anesth Pain Med. 2003; 28: 406-13.
[11] Boezaart AP, Lucas SD, Elliott CE. Paravertebral block: cervical, thoracic, lumbar and sacral. Curr Opin Anaesthesiol 2009; 22: 637-43.
[12] Boezaart AP, Franco CD. Bocks above the clavicle. In: Boezaart AP, Ed. Anesthesia and orthopaedic surgery. New York: McGraw-Hill; 2006; pp. 291-309.
[13] Boezaart AP. Atlas of peripheral nerve blocks and anatomy for orthopaedic anesthesia. Philadelphia: Saunders Elsevier; 2007: pp. 39-53.
[14] Boezaart AP, Nosovitch MA. Carotid endarterectomy using single injection posterior cervical paravertebral block. Anesth Analg 2005; 101: 1885 - 6
[15] Borgeat A, Ekatodramis G. Brachial plexus block. Current Opinion in Anaesthesiology 2002; 15 (5); 537-542
[16] Boezaart AP, de Beer JF, du Toit C, van Rooyen K. A new technique of continuous interscalene nerve block. Can J Anesth. 1999; 46:275-81.
[17] Winnie AP. Interscalene brachial plexus block. Aneth Analg. 1970; 49: 455-66.
[18] Urmey WF, Talts KH, Sharrock NE. One hundred percent incidence of hemidiaphragmatic paresis associated with interscalene brachial plexus anesthesia as diagnosed by ultrasonography. Anesth Analg. April 1991; 72(4): 498 - 503.

Chapter 4:
Applied Macro- and Microanatomy of the Nerves Below the Clavicle

CHAPTER 4

Applied Macro- and Microanatomy of the Nerves Below the Clavicle

Donald S. Bohannon[1], André P. Boezaart[2,*] and Paul E. Bigeleisen[3]

[1]Department of Anesthesiology, Division of Acute and Perioperative Pain Medicine, University of Florida College of Medicine, Gainesville, Florida, USA; [2]Departments of Anesthesiology and Orthopaedic Surgery and Rehabilitation, Division of Acute and Perioperative Pain Medicine, University of Florida College of Medicine, Gainesville, Florida, USA and [3]Department of Anesthesiology, University of Maryland, Baltimore, Maryland, USA

Abstract: In this chapter, the authors discuss the macro- and microanatomy of the brachial plexus cords below the clavicle. The area below the clavicle is defined, for the purposes of this discussion, as the area from just below the clavicle - the proximal infraclavicular area, to the lateral border of the major pectoral muscle and the deltopectoral groove – the distal infraclavicular area. In the proximal infraclavicular area, the three cords are situated lateral to the axillary artery and vein and all three cords are in a communal circumneural (paraneural) sheath. As the cords track more distally, they spread out around the artery so that the three cords are apart and each is in its own circumneural sheath. The lateral cord is now anterolateral, the medial cord is anteromedial, and the posterior cord is posterior to the axillary artery.

Keywords: Ansa pectoralis, Axillary artery, Axillary vein, Brachial plexus, Brachial plexus sheath, Circumneural sheath, Deltopectoral groove, Epineurium, Infraclavicular block, Lateral cord, Lateral pectoral nerve, Macroanatomy, Major pectoral muscle, Marti-Gruber, Medial cord, Medial pectoral nerve, Microanatomy, Minor pectoral muscle, Paraneural sheath, Posterior cord, Secondary block.

INTRODUCTION

For the purposes of this chapter, the area below the clavicle is the area from the clavicle to the anterior border of the axilla.

As a good understanding of anatomy is essential for performing any regional anesthesia technique or invasive procedure for regional anesthesia or acute pain

***Corresponding author André P. Boezaart:** Departments of Anesthesiology and Orthopaedic Surgery, Division of Acute and Peri-operative Pain Medicine, University of Florida College of Medicine, 1600 SW Archer Road, Gainesville, Florida 32610, USA; Tel: 352-846-0913 (Work); Fax: 352-392-7029;
E-mail: aboezaart@anest.ufl.edu

medical condition, it follows that one must understand the most fundamental principle of successful acute or perioperative pain control by regional anesthesia, namely, Hilton's Law of Anatomy [1]. The principles behind Hilton's Law were first espoused in a series of medical lectures given by John Hilton between 1860 and 1862 [1]. John Hilton (1808–1878) was a British surgeon born in Essex (UK) in 1805. He was appointed demonstrator of anatomy in 1828 at Guy's Hospital and assistant surgeon in 1845; he was appointed surgeon four years later. Ten years later, he became Professor of Anatomy and Surgery at the Royal College of Surgeons. From 1859 to 1862, he presented a series of lectures in the form of a course on "Rest and Pain" [1]. The "Law of Anatomy," which has now reached classical status, was revisited and challenged in 2013 using modern technology [2] and was found to be as sound as it was in 1860.

Hilton's Law of Anatomy states: "The same trunks of nerves whose branches supply the groups of muscles moving a joint furnish also a distribution of nerves to the skin over the insertions of the same muscles; and—what at this moment more especially merits our attention—the interior of the joint receives its nerves from the same source" [2].

Upon reflection, we realize that to move any of the joints of the upper limb, for example, all of the muscles around that specific joint are involved. Furthermore, the skin overlying that joint receives sensory innervation from branches of the brachial plexus. Because of these two facts, we know that to effectively block painful stimuli from any of the joints of the upper limb, we have to block the entire brachial plexus.

A common misunderstanding that also needs to be clarified, at least in our understanding, is that if, for example, 60% of the nerves that supply sensory innervation to a joint are blocked, the pain would be 60% less. Through the lessons we have learned over the years, especially in obstetric anesthesia where we have seen (and our unfortunate patients have experienced) the unpleasant consequences of unblocked segments or hemi-block with epidurals, and many other clinical scenarios, we now realize that blocking 60% of the nerves that innervate a joint or region does not reduce pain by 60%. In fact, it only focuses 100% of the pain into the remaining 40% of the joint, therefore, in fact, worsening the pain and suffering of the patient. Although well intended, it is a probably not true that we are doing anything positive for the patient by blocking "some" of the nerves and therefore removing "some" of the pain. Disbelief in this understanding, however, is based on clinical experience; it has yet to be challenged by formal research.

Simply put, to provide optimal pain relief due to major surgery or trauma to a joint in the upper extremity, the entire brachial plexus must be blocked. Granted, this is not always possible, especially where the plexus is spread out, such as in the distal infraclavicular area. It is most difficult to achieve during a continuous nerve block, where the catheter is placed on one specific part of the plexus; for example, the posterior cord of the brachial plexus during a continuous distal infraclavicular block for pain associated with major wrist or elbow surgery. When the primary block (high-volume and high-concentration initial block) wears off, the secondary block often fails because the other cords are not close enough or are not in the same circumneural (paraneural) space [3] to allow the local anesthetic agent (of too low a volume and concentration) to diffuse to all of the nerve axons of the other two, more distant, cords. Thus, complete coverage of the pain is not achieved (see Microanatomy section).

It is also not always necessary to block all the nerves that innervate a specific joint. Most of the nerves that innervate a joint reach that joint *via* its joint capsule and during or synovectomy surgery, for example, the joint capsule may be destroyed by the surgery, which in effect denervates the joint, making it necessary to block only the nerves that supply sensory innervation to the tissue outside the joint capsule.

MACRO- AND MICROANATOMY

The brachial plexus is formed by the anterior rami of nerves from the 5th cervical root (C5) through to the 1st thoracic root (T1). These roots alternately fuse and bifurcate (Fig. **1** of Chapter 1). The roots combine into three trunks, the superior (upper), middle, and inferior (lower) trunks at the lateral edge of the scalene muscles, and pass over the first rib, where they lie posterior and superior to the subclavian artery. Each trunk then divides into an anterior and posterior division behind the clavicle, and lateral to the 1st rib. The three posterior divisions form the posterior cord, the anterior divisions of the upper and middle trunk form the lateral cord, and the anterior division of the lower trunk forms the medial cord. In the proximal infraclavicular area, the three cords are bundled together in the same circumneural (paraneural) sheath, with each cord is in its own epineurial sheath. This is an important anatomical concept because this position may be the optimal place to block all three cords and assure satisfactory secondary block success. The cords then rearrange and embrace the axillary artery. Inferior to the coracoid process, the cords give off their final terminal branches (Fig. **1** of chapter 1). The medial and lateral cords supply the muscles that cause flexion of the arm, while the posterior cord supplies the muscles that cause extension.

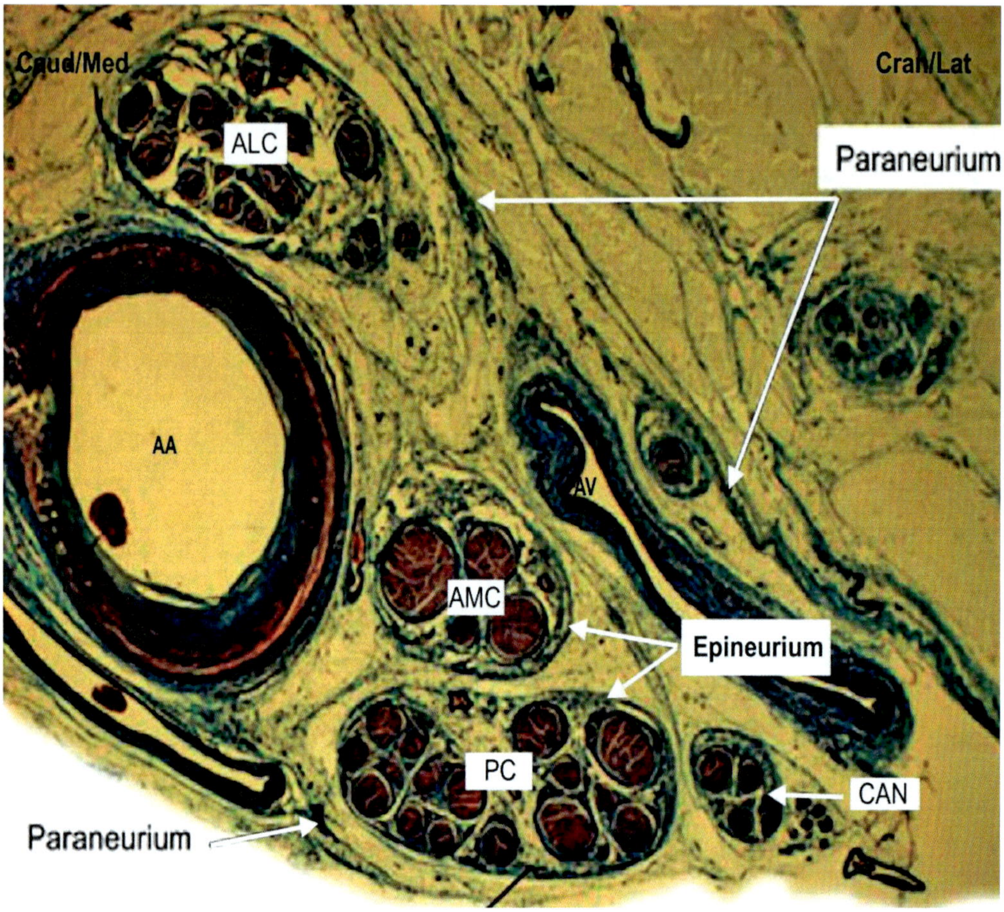

Figure 1: Brachial plexus cords in the proximal infraclavicular area.
Cords are arranged to the lateral side of the axillary artery and vein and in a communal circumneural (paraneural) sheath. Caud/Med = caudal and medial; Cran/Lat = cranial and lateral; AA = axillary artery; AV = branch of axillary vein; ALC = anterolateral cord; AMC = anteromedial cord; PC =posterior cord; CAN = cutaneous antebrachial nerve. (Reprinted from Reina [4] with permission, p. 187).

More lateral or distal, the cords lie around the axillary artery and are named medial, lateral, and posterior cords according to their relation to the second part of the axillary artery, viewed as if the artery descended parallel to the long axis of the body (Fig. **2**). The true position of the axillary artery, however, is at 45 degrees to the long axis of the body, and the lateral cord lies somewhat anterior and cranial to the artery. The medial cord lies anterior and caudal to the artery, while the posterior cord is always posterior to the artery (Fig. **2**).

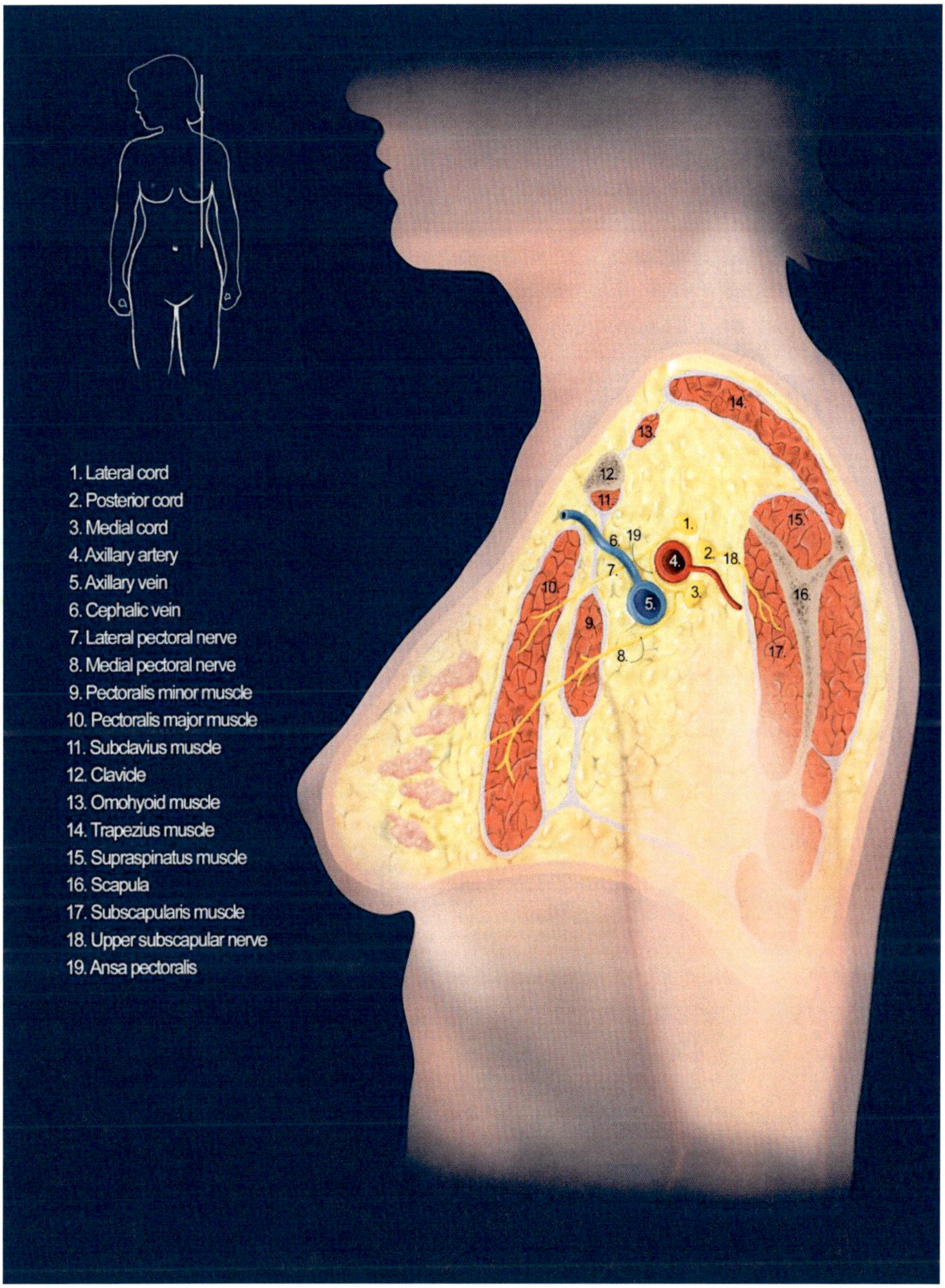

Figure 2: Sagittal macroanatomy through the medial deltopectoral groove.

Note ansa pectoralis communicating branch (19), also sometimes referred to as the Martin-Gruber nerve, between lateral pectoral nerve (7) and medial pectoral nerve (8). The lateral pectoral nerve gives off an articular branch, which is a pure sensory nerve and runs over the coracoid process and supplies the acromioclavicular and subacromial joints with sensory innervation.

The subclavian artery becomes the axillary artery lateral to the first rib, and it is divided into three parts, the first part being medial to, the second part being behind, and the third part being lateral to the minor pectoral muscle near its attachment to the tip of the coracoid process (Fig. **3**).

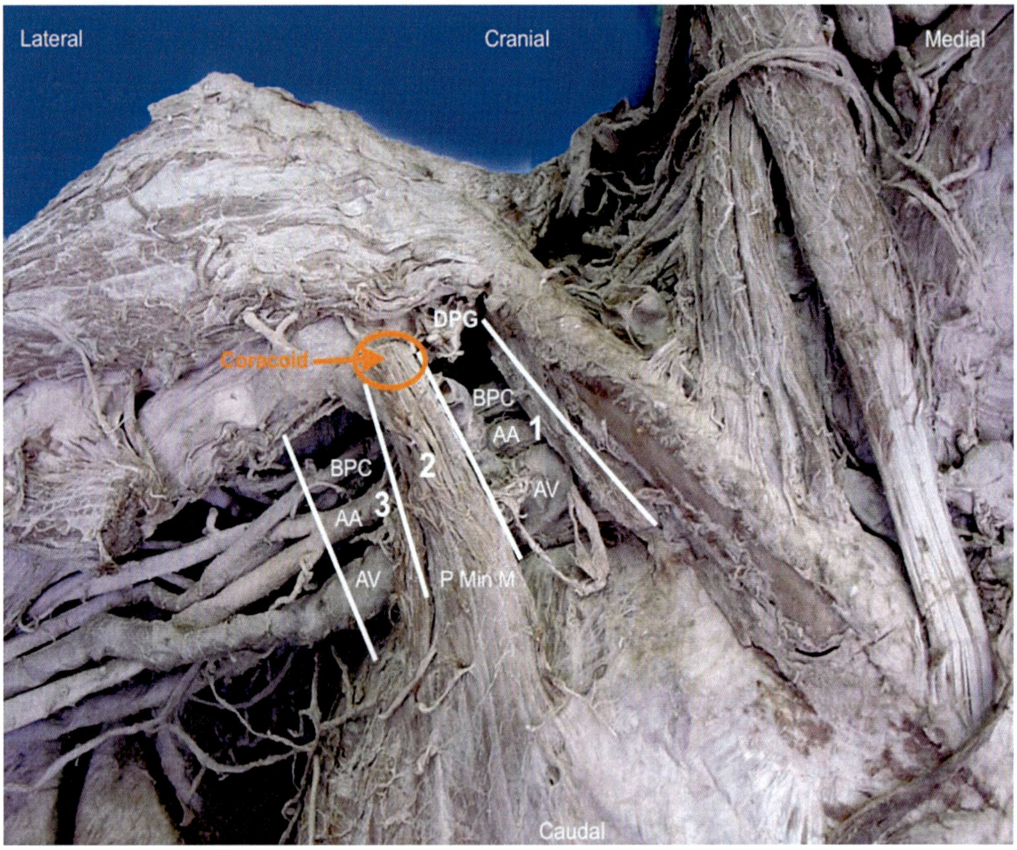

Figure 3a: Macroanatomy of the three parts of the infraclavicular axillary artery.
1 = 1st part of axillary artery; 2 = 2nd part of axillary artery; 3 = 3rd part of axillary artery; AA = axillary artery; AV = axillary vein; BPC = brachial plexus cords; DPG = deltopectoral groove; Coracoid = coracoid process; P Min M = minor pectoral muscle.

The major pectoral muscle had been removed.

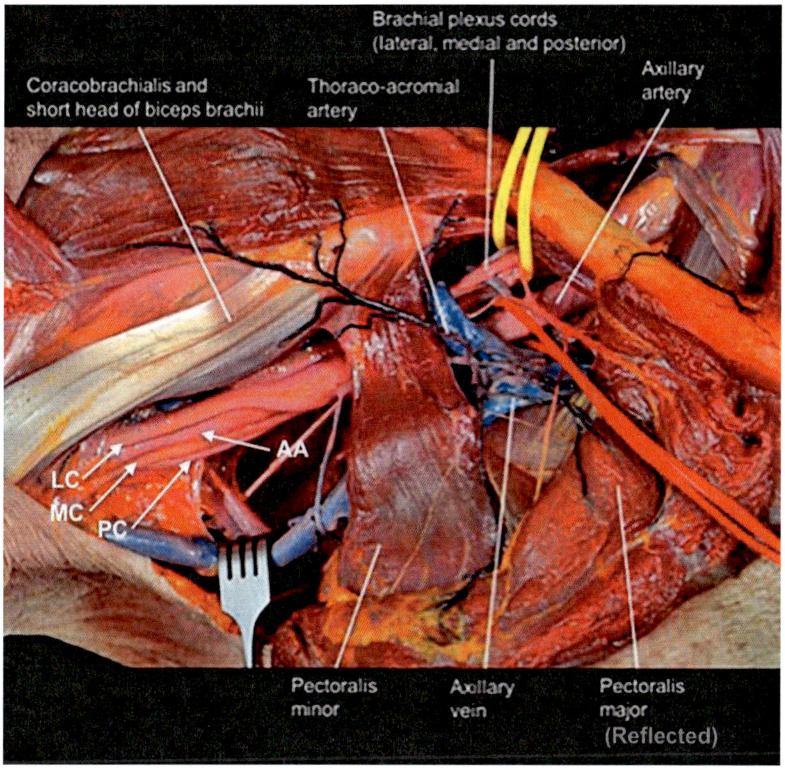

Figure 3b: Macroanatomy of the infraclavicular area showing the brachial plexus cords "rapping around" the axillary artery.
LC = lateral cord; MC = medial cord; PC = posterior cord; AA = axillary artery.

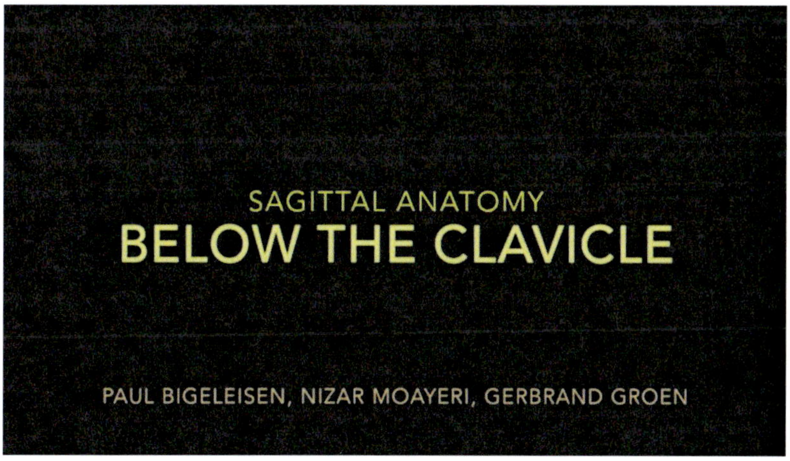

To view this movie click on this link:
https://raeducation.com/ebook

Movie 1: The sagittal anatomy of the brachial plexus below the clavicle.

The medial cord begins behind the first part of the axillary artery and winds inferiorly around the artery to reach its medial position at the second part the axillary artery. The posterior cord at first lies adjacent to the lateral cord in a superoposterior position to the first part of the axillary artery before rotating around to the second part of the artery. The lateral cord is superoposterior and shifts toward its lateral position on the second part of the axillary artery. (There is often anatomical variation in the formation of the cords and their relationship to the second part of the axillary artery, but they generally follow the trend of the described pattern). However, while the posterior cord is always posterior, the lateral and medial cords may rotate in their path toward the second part of the axillary artery.

The pectoral nerves are formed at the level of the trunks or divisions (Fig. **1** of chapter 1), but keep close association with the medial and lateral brachial plexus cords, after which they are respectively named. The pectoral nerves turn anteriorly around and through the minor pectoral muscle and are connected by the Martin-Gruber communicating branch (ansa pectoralis – Fig. **2**) [5].

The important branches of the medial cord are the medial part of the median nerve, which crosses the front of the axillary artery, the terminal ulnar nerve, and the medial cutaneous nerves of the arm and the forearm (Fig. **1**). The important branches of the lateral cord are the musculocutaneous nerve and the lateral part of the median nerve. The posterior cord gives off the axillary nerve posterior, the nerves to the subscapularis muscle, and the latissimus dorsi muscle, and posterior to the axillary artery, the radial nerve. The latter is the largest nerve of the upper limb.

The musculocutaneous nerve branches off from the cord inferior to the coracoid process (Fig. **1**) and deviates superior from the plexus to enter the coracobrachialis muscle 3 to 7 cm inferolateral to the coracoid process.

THE "BRACHIAL PLEXUS SHEATH"

The simple concept of a tubular brachial plexus sheath proposed by Winnie [6] is no longer universally accepted. Thompson [7] convincingly demonstrated that the epineurial septae form partitions that surround components of the brachial plexus (Fig. **4a** and **4b**).

It is of practical importance to understand that the cords lie lateral of the axillary artery in the proximal infraclavicular region (1st part of the axillary artery), where the cords are inside a shared circumneural (paraneural) sheath [4], although each cord lies in its own epineurial sheath [4]. From here, the cords course laterally and caudad more distally in the area of the deltopectoral groove (3rd part of axillary artery) to lie around the axillary artery – each still in its own epineurial sheath, but each also now in its own circumneural sheath [4] (see Movie **1**).

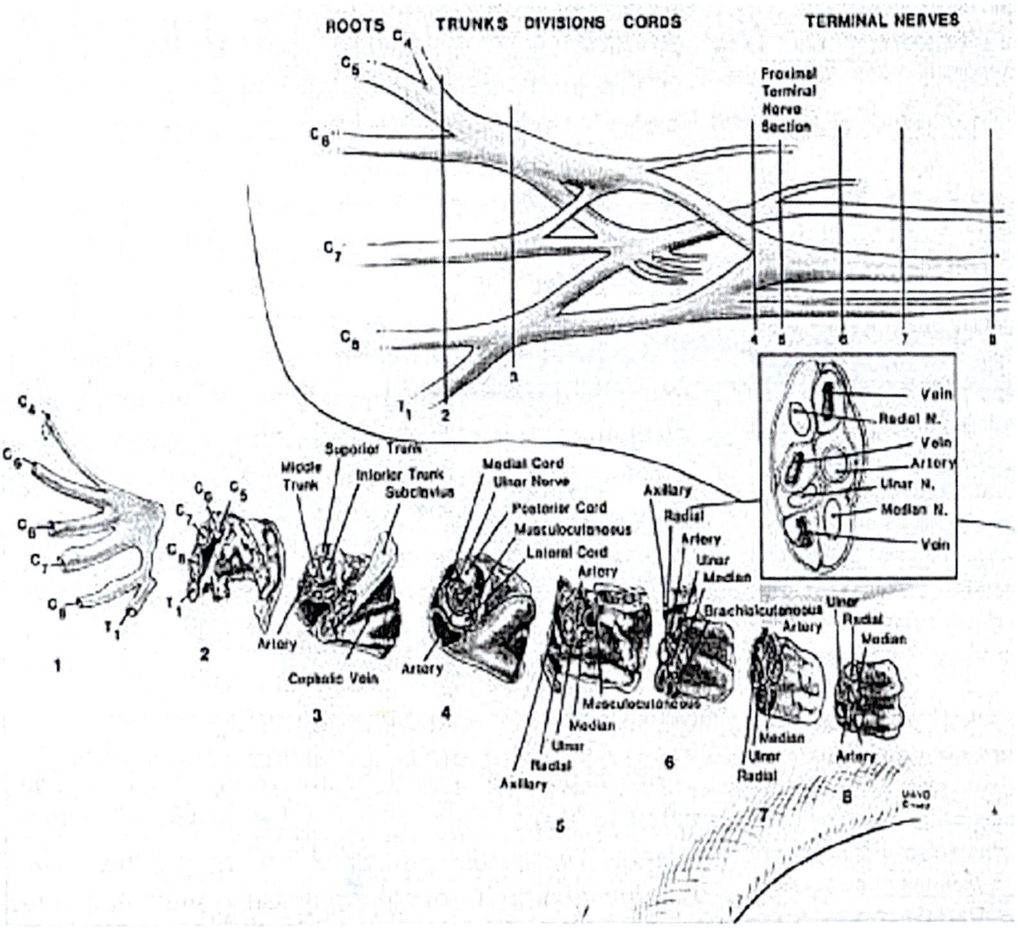

Figure 4a: Brachial plexus sheaths.
To illustrate the brachial plexus sheaths Thompson and Rorie [7] removed the brachial plexus with the surrounding fascial sheath in tact from the left side of a body and transected it at 2-cm intervals. They demonstrated that septa of the same approximate thickness as the fascial sheath extend inward from the sheath to form compartments for the individual nerves. We now know that these compartments are most likely the circumneural spaces (Figs. ***1*** *of chapter 2 and* ***1*** *of chapter 7) [4, 8, 9]. The insert into Fig.* ***(4)*** *shows the fascial compartments containing the nerves, each in its own epineurial sheath, and the relationship of each to the axillary. (Reprinted from Thompson and Rorie [7] with permission.*

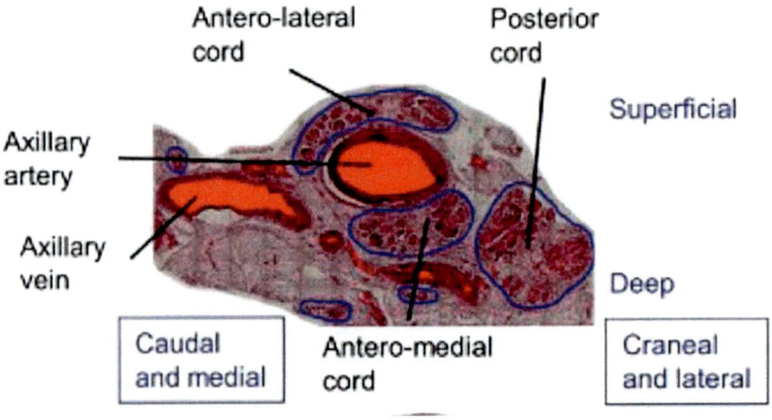

Figure 4b: Sagittal microanatomy of the brachial plexus cords and their relationship to the axillary artery in the second part of the axillary artery behind the coracoid (see Fig. **3a** and **3b**). *(Reprinted from Reina and Sala-Blanch [4] with permission)*

Bigeleisen and his colleagues from the Netherlands have made fine sagittal sections of the neck as depicted in Figs. **5**, **6** and **7** below as well as Movie **1**.

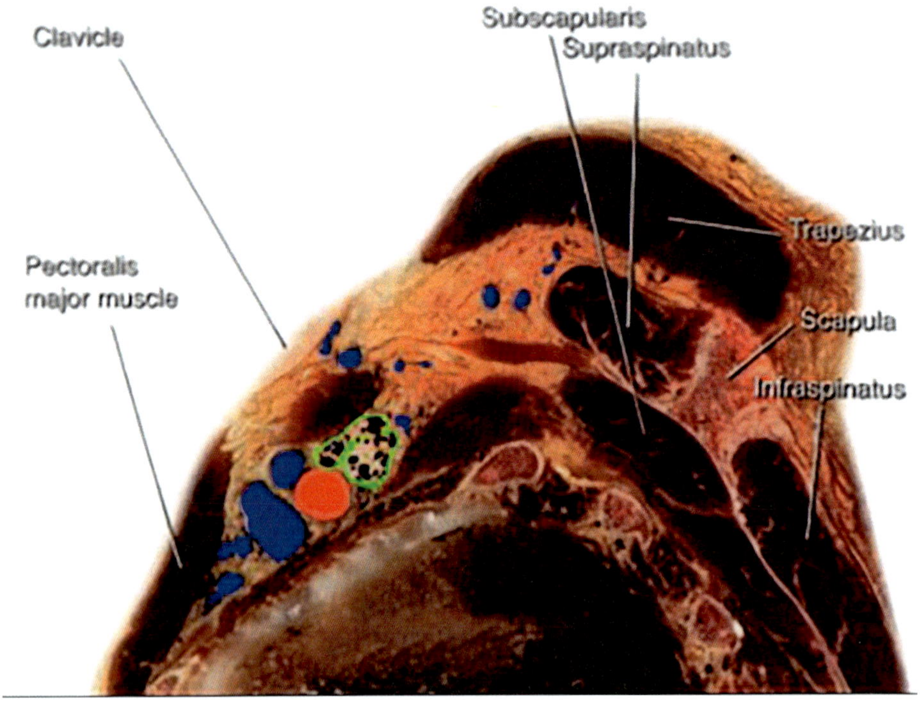

Figure 5: Sagittal anatomy of the brachial plexus cords through the 1st part of the axillary artery: proximal mid-clavicular infraclavicular area.

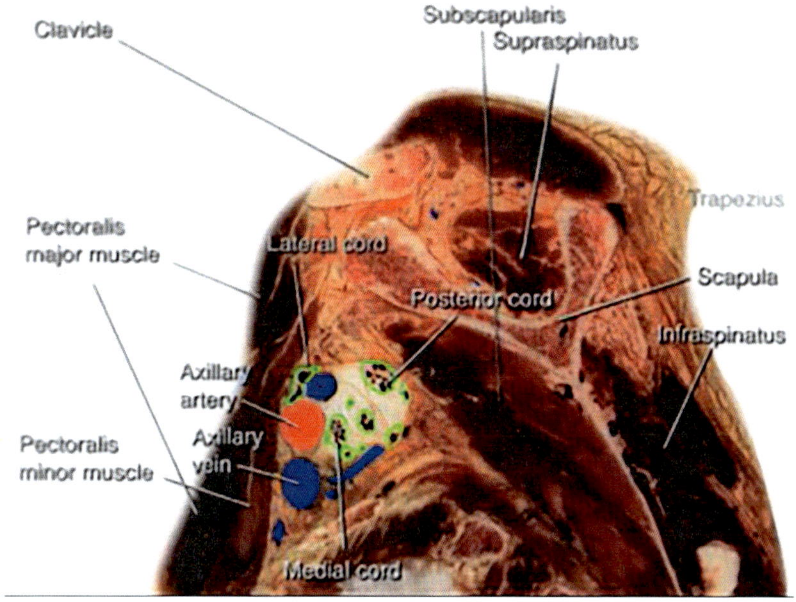

Figure 6: Sagittal anatomy of the brachial plexus cords through the 2nd part of the axillary artery: more distal mid-clavicular infraclavicular area.

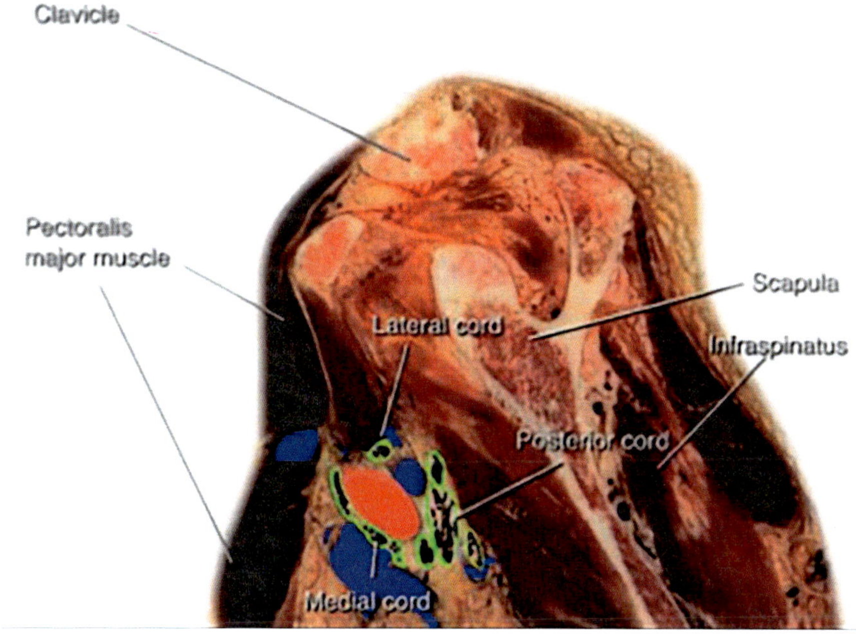

Figure 7: Sagittal anatomy of the brachial plexus cords through the 3rd part of the axillary artery: distal deltopectoral groove infraclavicular area.

ACKNOWLEDGEMENTS

The authors gratefully acknowledge the following people:

- The Head of the Department of Anesthesiology of the College of Medicine of the University of Florida, Dr. Tim Morey and his department for their moral support and continuous encouragement.
- The faculty and fellows of the Division of acute and perioperative pain medicine for affording the authors the time to produce this work by covering their clinical duties.
- Corey Astrom of the Department of Anesthesiology of the College of Medicine of the University of Florida for her professional and high quality text editing.
- Mary K Bryson for her illustration of Fig. (**2**).
- Professors Gerbrand Groen and Paul Bigeleisen and Dr. Nizar Moayeri from the University Medical College in Utrecht, The Netherlands for their production of Movie **1** and providing Figs. (**5-7**).
- Raeducation.com LLC for their financial support.

CONFLICT OF INTEREST

The authors confirm that this chapter contents have no conflict of Interest.

ABBREVIATIONS

AA	= axillary artery
ALC	= anterolateral cord
AMC	= anteromedial cord
AV	= axillary vein
AV	= branch of axillary vein
BPC	= brachial plexus cords

CAN	=	cutaneous antebrachial nerve
Caud/Med	=	caudal and medial
Coracoid	=	coracoid process
Cran/Lat	=	cranial and lateral
DPG	=	deltopectoral groove
LC	=	lateral cord
MC	=	medial cord
P Min M	=	minor pectoral muscle
PC	=	posterior cord

REFERENCES

[1] Hilton, J. On Rest and Pain: A Course of Lectures on the Influence of Mechanical and Physiological Rest in the Treatment of Accidents and Surgical Diseases, and the Diagnostic Value of Pain, delivered at the Royal College of Surgeons of England in the years 1860, 1861, 1862 and 1863.

[2] Hébert-Blouin M-N, Tubbs RS, Carmichael SW, Spinner RJ. Hilton's Law revisited. Clin Anat 2014; 27: 548-55.

[3] Reina MA, Sala-Blanch X. Cross-sectional microscopic anatomy of the brachial plexus and paraneural sheaths. In: Reina MA, Ed. Atlas of functional anatomy for regional anesthesia and pain medicine. New York: Springer Science and Business Media, 2015: pp. 185.

[4] Reina MA, Sala-Blanch X. Cross-sectional microscopic anatomy of the brachial plexus and paraneural sheaths. In: Reina MA, Ed. Atlas of functional anatomy for regional anesthesia and pain medicine. New York: Springer Science and Business Media, 2015: pp. 187.

[5] Shu HS, Chantelot C, Oberlin C, *et al.* Martin-Gruber communicating branch: Anatomical and histological study. Surg Radiol Anat 1992; 21: 115-8.

[6] Winnie AP. Plexus anesthesia, Volume 1. Copenhagen: Schultz Medical Information, 1983: pp. 49-51.

[7] Thompson GE, Rorie DK. Functional anatomy of the brachial plexus. Anesthesiology 1983; 59: 117-22.

[8] Boezaart AP, Zasimovich Y, Parvataneni HK. Long-acting local anesthetic agents and additives: Snake oil, voodoo or the real deal? Pain Med 2015; 16: 13-7.

[9] Andrerson HL, Anderson SL, Tranun-Jensen J. Injecting inside the paraneural sheath or the sciatic nerve: Direct comparison among ultrasound imaging, macroscopic anatomy and histologic analysis. Reg Anesth Pain Med 2012; 37: 410-4.

Chapter 5:
Sonoanatomy of the Nerves Below the Clavicle

CHAPTER 5

Sonoanatomy of the Nerves Below the Clavicle

André P. Boezaart[1,*], Barys V. Ihnatsenka[2] and Yury Zasimovich[2]

[1]*Departments of Anesthesiology and Orthopaedic Surgery and Rehabilitation, Division of Acute and Perioperative Pain Medicine, University of Florida College of Medicine, Gainesville, Florida, USA and* [2]*Department of Anesthesiology, Division of Acute and Perioperative Pain Medicine, University of Florida College of Medicine, Gainesville, Florida, USA*

Abstract: The area below the clavicle is where an infraclavicular block is typically performed. Although a very popular and useful approach for single injection nerve blocks for regional anesthesia, infraclavicular blocks have been met with disappointment as far as continuous nerve blocks are concerned. The most likely reason is probably because infraclavicular blocks are usually performed in the area of the deltopectoral groove, where the three cords are arranged around the axillary artery and are relatively far apart. A better option for continuous nerve block catheter placement would probably be more proximal, directly under the clavicle, where all three the cords are together just after crossing the first rib with the vein most medial, the artery more lateral, and the bundle of brachial plexus cords most lateral (very similar to the femoral nerve). This chapter outlines these differences ultrasonographically. The ultrasound-assisted approach to the lateral and medial pectoral nerves, the so-called "PEC 1" block," is also discussed. The proximal and distal infraclavicular nerves, as well as the pectoralis approach to the lateral and medial pectoral muscles, are discussed in this chapter with the help static images and video productions.

Keywords: Acute pain medicine, Axillary artery, Axillary vein, Brachial plexus, Brachial plexus cords, Continuous infraclavicular block, Continuous nerve blocks, Deltopectoral groove, Distal infraclavicular nerve, Dynamic ultrasound, First rib, Infraclavicular block, Lateral cord, Lateral pectoral nerve, Medial cord, Medial pectoral nerve, PEC 1 block, Pectoralis approach, Posterior cord, Proximal infraclavicular nerves, Regional anesthesia, Static ultrasound.

INTRODUCTION

Ultrasound is a dynamic process whereby structures can and should be followed to their origins and destinations for optimal identification [1]. Because of this, it is not

***Corresponding author André P Boezaart:** Departments of Anesthesiology and Orthopaedic Surgery, Division of Acute and Peri-operative Pain Medicine, University of Florida College of Medicine, 1600 SW Archer Road, Gainesville, Florida 32610, USA; Tel: 352-846-0913 (Work); Fax: 352-392-7029; E-mail: aboezaart@anest.ufl.edu

always satisfactory to study static ultrasound images. When studying the sonoanatomy of the infraclavicular area, the authors strongly advise readers to first study the macroanatomy and then to view the accompanying video recording (Movie **1**) and sagittal sectional anatomy video recording (Movie **2**) that illustrates the dynamic and static sonoanatomy of the brachial plexus below the clavicle.

PROXIMAL INFRACLAVICULAR BRACHIAL PLEXUS CORDS

To obtain the ultrasound images of the infraclavicular brachial plexus described in this chapter, the model was positioned in the supine position with her upper body slightly elevated to ensure that her veins were collapsed. At times, the subject was requested to perform the Valsalva maneuver to ensure expansion of the axillary vein for demonstration purposes. The shoulder joint was elevated and the arm adducted. We placed the ultrasound probe on the clavicle and slid it down just off of the clavicle to obtain the proximal infraclavicular view (Fig. **1**) (Movie **1**).

The ultrasound probe used for all images in this chapter was a 6- to 13-MHz linear probe with a 38-cm footprint (HFL - 38, SonoSite Fujifilm, Bothell, WA, USA) [1].

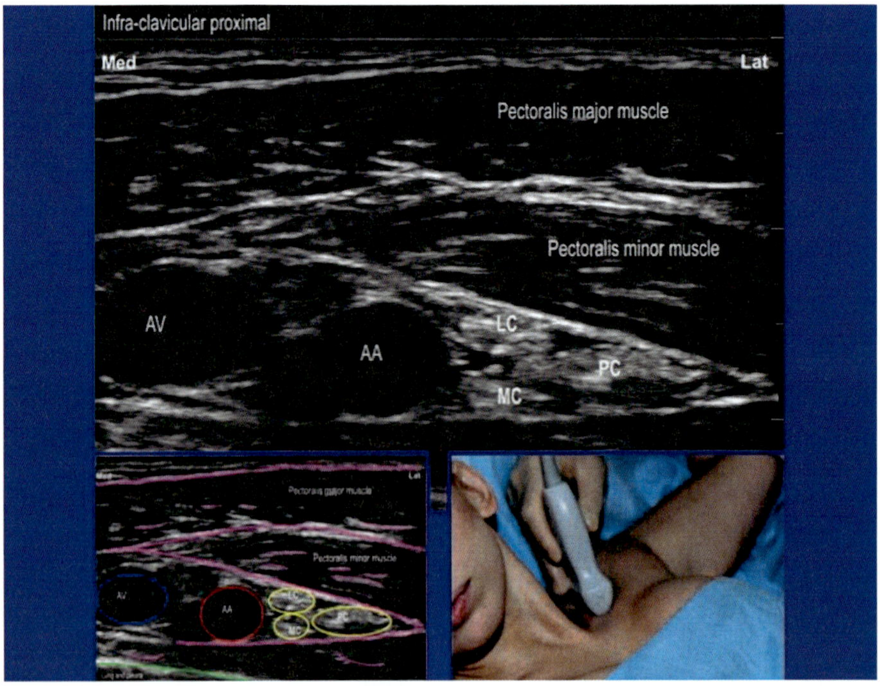

Figure 1: Sonoanatomy of the proximal brachial plexus below the clavicle.
Med = medial; Lat = lateral; AA = axillary artery; AV = axillary vein; LC = lateral cord of the brachial plexus; MC = median cord of the brachial plexus; PC = posterior cord of the brachial plexus.

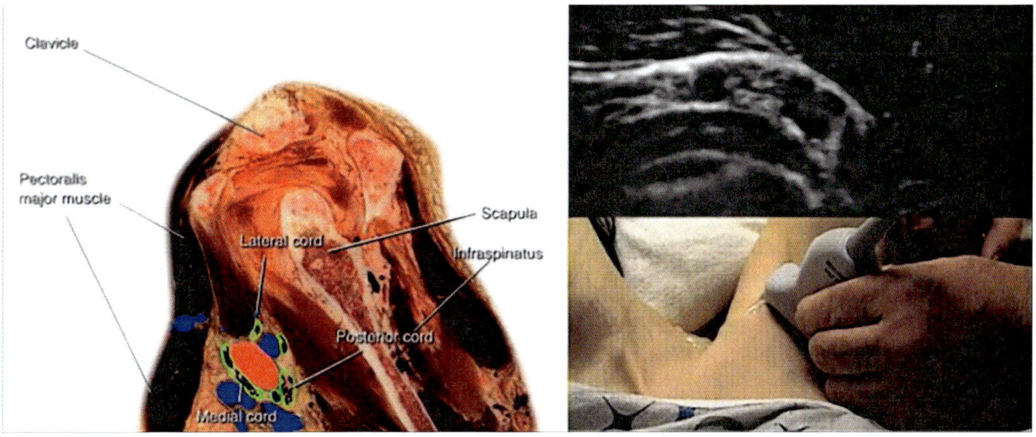

Figure 4: Sagittal section view of the distal brachial plexus cords, the positioning of the ultrasound probe and the resulting ultrasound image.

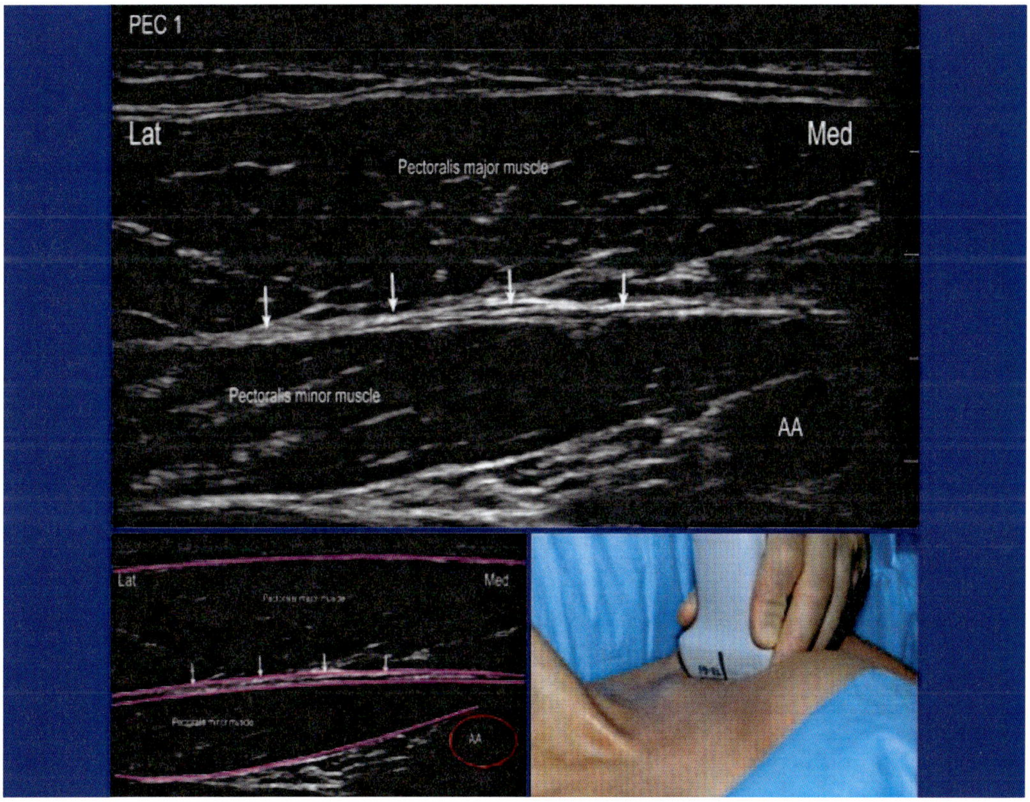

Figure 5: Sonoanatomy of the fascial plane between the major and minor pectoral muscles.
Lat = lateral; Med = medial; AA = axillary artery. Arrows indicate the pectoralis fascia plane where the medial and lateral pectoral nerves are situated.

VIEW OF PECTORALIS FASCIA: THE LATERAL AND MEDIAL PECTORAL NERVES

The ultrasound probe is placed in the deltopectoral groove as in the previous section and is then moved medially and slightly rotated to obtain the best view of the major and minor pectoral muscles (Fig. **3** and Movie **2**). The medial and lateral pectoral nerves are situated between the two fascia layers that engulf these two muscles. The fascia layers are split with local anesthetic agent injected in this fascial space to block these two nerves for breast surgery. This is the so-called "PEC 1 block." (See also Movie **3**).

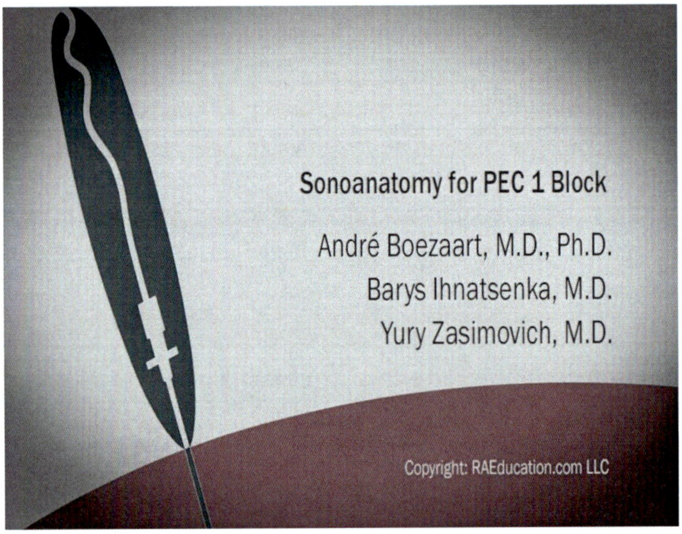

To view this movie click on this link:
https://raeducation.com/ebook

Movie 3: Dynamic sonoanatomy of the pectoralis fascia (PEC 1).

ACKNOWLEDGEMENTS

The authors gratefully acknowledge the following people:

- The Head of the Department of Anesthesiology of the College of Medicine of the University of Florida, Dr. Tim Morey, and his department for their moral support and continuous encouragement.

- The faculty and fellows of the Division of acute and perioperative pain medicine for affording the authors the time to produce this work by covering their clinical duties.

- Corey Astrom of the Department of Anesthesiology of the College of Medicine of the University of Florida for her professional and high quality text editing.

- Nancy Hagen of the Iowa Public Radio for the narration of the movies.

- Dr. Anastacia Munro for her help with the preparation of the chapter and ultrasound images.

- Raeducation.com LLC for their financial support.

- Professors Gerbrand Groen and Paul Bigeleisen and Dr. Nizar Moayeri from the University Medical College in Utrecht, The Netherlands for their making of Movie 2 and providing Figs. (**2** and **4**).

CONFLICT OF INTEREST

The authors confirm that this chapter contents have no conflict of Interest

ABBREVIATIONS

AA	=	axillary artery
AV	=	axillary vein
Caud	=	caudad
Ceph	=	cephalad
Lat	=	lateral
LC	=	lateral cord of the brachial plexus
MC	=	median cord of the brachial plexus
Med	=	medial
PC	=	posterior cord of the brachial plexus.

REFERENCES

[1] Ihnatsenka BV, Boezaart AP. Ultrasound: Basic understanding and learning the language. Int J Shoulder Surg. 2010;4:55-62.

[2] Reina MA, Sala-Blanch X. Cross-sectional microscopic anatomy of the brachial plexus and paraneural sheaths. In: Reina MA, ed. Atlas of functional anatomy for regional anesthesia and pain medicine. New York: Springer Science and Business Media; 2015: pp. 187.

[3] Karmakar MK, Shariat AN, Pangthipampai P, Chen J. High-definition ultrasound imaging defines the paraneural sheath and the fascial compartments surrounding the sciatic nerve at the popliteal fossa. Reg Anesth Pain Med 2013; 38: 447-51.

CHAPTER 6

Macroanatomy of the Nerves in the Axilla, and at the Elbow and Wrist

André P. Boezaart*

Departments of Anesthesiology and Orthopaedic Surgery and Rehabilitation, Division of Acute and Perioperative Pain Medicine, University of Florida College of Medicine, Gainesville, Florida, USA

Abstract: Counting the axillary nerve, which is not truly in the axilla, there are seven peripheral nerves in the axilla that arise from the brachial plexus. These are the medial cutaneous nerves to the arm and the forearm, the ulnar nerve, which arises from the medial cord, the median nerve, which comes from the medial and lateral cords, the radial nerve, which arises from the posterior cord, and the musculocutaneous nerve, which originates from the lateral cord. These nerves and their areas of sensory distributions are discussed in this chapter. The intercostobrachial nerve, which does not originate from the brachial plexus, arises from the first and second thoracic spinal root and innervates the skin in the medial upper arm and axilla. The motor functions of these nerves are discussed in Chapter 9.

Keywords: Acute pain medicine, Axilla, Axilla borders, Axillary artery, Axillary nerve, Brachial artery, Brachial plexus, Brachial vein, Intercostobrachial nerve, Lateral cord, Medial cord, Medial cutaneous nerve of the forearm, Medial cutaneous nerves of the arm, Median nerve, Musculocutaneous nerve, Posterior cord, Radial nerve, Regional anesthesia, Second thoracic spinal root, Ulnar nerve.

INTRODUCTION

The brachial plexus enters the axilla as the lateral, medial and posterior cords (Fig. **1** of chapter 1, 2, 5 and 8 of chapter 4). The axilla is a fat-filled pyramidal cavity between the upper thorax and the arm. It has an apex, a base and four "walls": lateral, medial, anterior and posterior. The apex of the axilla projects into the neck as the cervico-axillary canal through which the axillary blood vessels and brachial plexus cords pass. The first rib, the superior border of the scapula, the posterior border of the clavicle, and the medial aspect of the coracoid process form this canal. The skin and axillary fascia between pectoralis major and latissimus dorsi muscles

***Corresponding author André P. Boezaart:** Departments of Anesthesiology and Orthopaedic Surgery, Division of Acute and Peri-operative Pain Medicine, University of Florida College of Medicine, 1600 SW Archer Road, Gainesville, Florida 32610, USA; Tel: 352-846-0913 (Work); Fax: 352-392-7029;
E-mail: aboezaart@anest.ufl.edu

form the base of the axilla. It is convex, thus conforming to the shape of the armpit, and narrows from the lateral wall of the chest into the arm.

The anterior and posterior walls are easily palpable between forefinger and thumb. The pectoralis muscles form the anterior wall, with a small contribution at the superior part by the covering of the clavipectoral fascia. The posterior wall is slightly lower than the anterior, and is formed mainly by teres major muscle, with subscapularis above and latissimus dorsi below. The anterior and posterior walls converge laterally onto the palpable humeral intertubercular sulcus, the narrow lateral wall. The medial wall is formed by the first four ribs and their respective intercostal muscles, and the upper part of the serratus anterior muscle.

MACROANATOMY

Nerves in the Axilla

The axilla contains the axillary vessels, the infraclavicular part of the brachial plexus and its branches (Fig. **1** of chapter 1), lateral branches of some intercostal nerves, many lymph nodes and vessels, loose adipose tissue and often the "tail" of the breast. The axillary artery is a continuation of the subclavian artery and represents that part of the vessel between the outer border of the first rib and the inferior border of the teres major muscle, where its name changes from axillary artery to brachial artery. It is important to note that its direction changes with the position of the arm: it is almost straight when the arm is in abduction at 90 degrees, and becomes more concave as the arm is raised or convex as the arm is lowered to alongside the chest. The axillary vein, like the artery, is defined superiorly by the first rib and clavicle. Above the first rib, the subclavian vein does not lie within the neurovascular bundle as it is forming between the scalene muscles, but rather is separated from the artery by the insertion of the anterior scalene muscle. However, as it passes over the first rib and under the clavicle, the subclavian vein in becoming the axillary vein does join the neurovascular bundle. Thus, parts of the plexus are sandwiched between artery and vein.

The passage of the subclavian artery under the clavicle, becoming the axillary artery, sees a significant change in the relationship between the artery and the brachial plexus. While the subclavian artery lies anterior and close to the trunks of the plexus, and distal to the clavicle, the axillary artery lies more central to the three cords of the plexus. The first part of the artery is medial to the lateral and posterior cords and anterior to the medial cord! *En route* to the axilla, the cords rotate around the artery, and as they pass behind the pectoralis minor muscle their positions become truly medial, lateral and posterior as their names suggest.

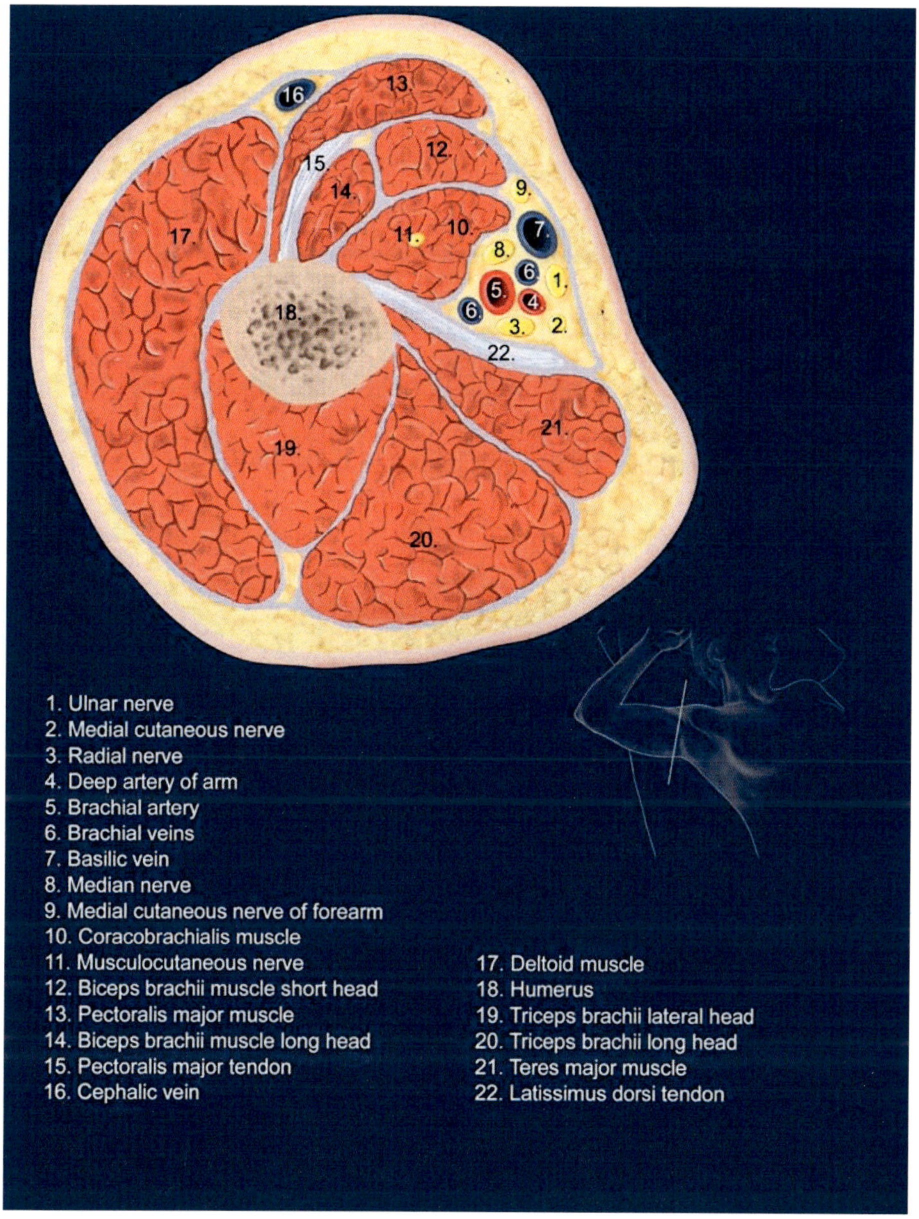

Figure 1: Cross section through the axilla

In the axilla, the musculocutaneous nerve lies between the biceps (12,14) and coracobrachialis(13) muscles, but more proximal it lies in the coracobrachialis muscle. The medial cutaneous nerve of the forearm (9) lies anterior and superficially in the neurovascular bundle, usually anterolateral to the basilica vein, while the ulnar nerve lies anterior to the brachial artery and vein and inferomedial to the basilic vein (7). The median nerve (8) is situated anterolateral to the brachial artery (5), while the radial nerve (3) and median cutaneous nerve of the arm (2) are posteromedial Nerves in the mid-humeral area.

Around the lateral edge of the pectoralis minor muscle the cords give rise to the terminal nerves of the plexus. It is only the median, radial, ulnar, and medial antebrachial cutaneous nerves that will continue with the artery and vein within the axillary sheath. The musculocutaneous and axillary nerves, two of the major terminal nerves, are not in the sheath at this level. They have left under cover of the pectoralis minor muscle at the level of the coracoid process. The musculocutaneous nerve enters the coracobrachialis muscle and continues down the arm within it, (essentially parallel to the sheath). The axillary nerve leaves the sheath almost immediately after arising from the posterior cord.

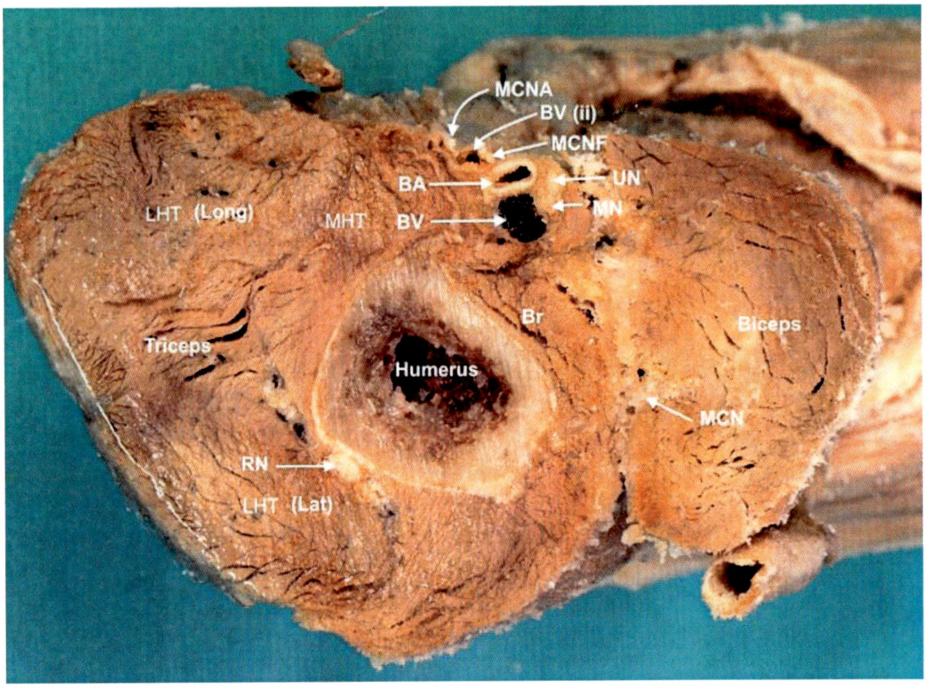

Figure 2: Anatomic section through mid-humeral area.
Triceps = triceps brachii muscle; MHT = medial head of triceps; LHT (Long) = long head of triceps; LHT (Lat) = lateral head of triceps; Biceps = biceps brachii muscle; Br = brachialis muscle; BA = brachial artery; BV = brachial vein; BV (ii) = basilica vein; RN = radial nerve; MCN = musculocutaneous nerve; MN = median nerve; UN = ulnar nerve; MCNA = medial cutaneous nerve of the arm; MCNF = medial cutaneous nerve of the forearm.

Nerves at the Elbow

The ***radial** (musculo-spiral)* ***nerve*** is the largest branch of the brachial plexus, and arises from the posterior cord (Fig. **1** of chapter 1). In the axilla it passes down in front of the tendons of the latissimus dorsi and teres major muscles. Passing over the inner to outer side of the humerus, it winds round it in the musculo-spiral groove with the profunda artery. It passes from the inner to the outer side of the bone, between the internal and external heads of the triceps muscle and pierces the external intermuscular septum and descends between the brachialis (anticus) and supinator longus to the front of the external condyle, where it divides into the radial and posterior interosseous nerves (Fig. **2**) (see Chapter 8). The radial nerve has 4 branches; the muscular, which innervates the muscles of the back of the arm and forearm, a cutaneous branch (Figs. **3** and **4** of chapter 1), the radial nerve and the posterior interosseous nerve (See Chapter 8).

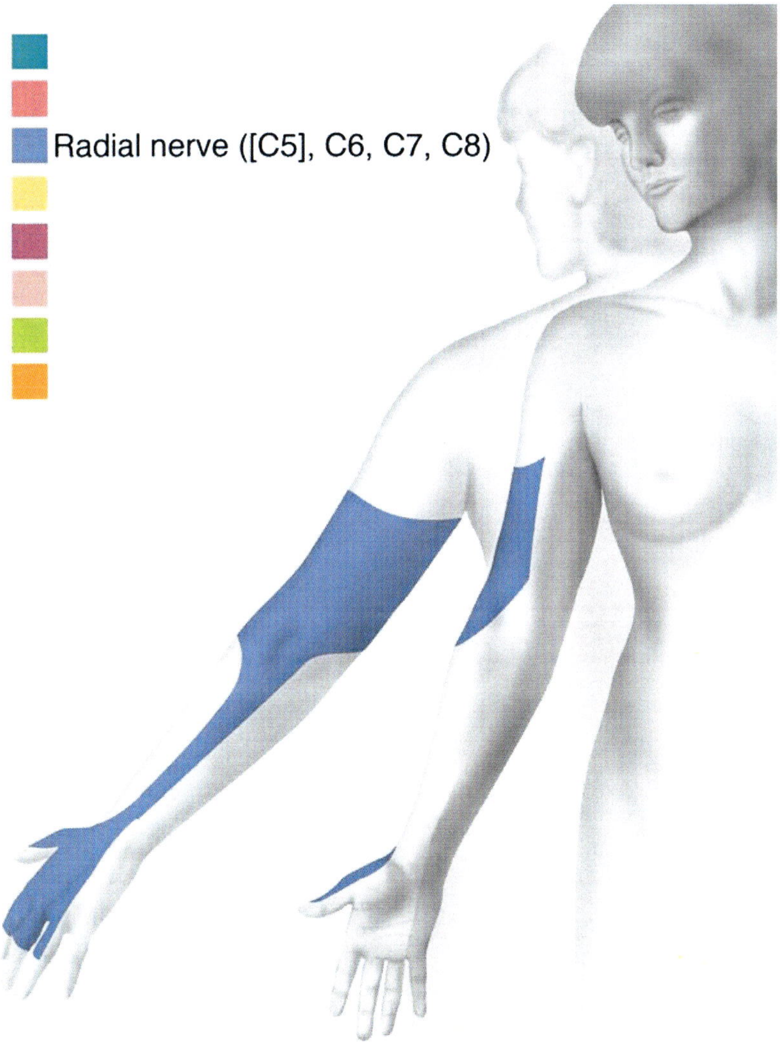

Figure 3: Neurotomes of the radial nerve (with its corresponding dermatomal origins).

The ***musculocutaneous nerve*** arises from the posterior cord of the brachial plexus and innervates the biceps brachii, coracobrachialis and greater part of the brachialis anticus muscles. It perforates the coracobrachialis muscle and passes obliquely between the biceps and brachialis muscles to the outer side of the arm. A little below the elbow it winds around the outer border of the tendon of the biceps, perforating the deep fascia and becomes cutaneous. When it passes behind the median cephalic vein it divides into an anterior and posterior branch (See Chapter 8). For dermatomal innervation see Fig. (**4**). Also see Fig. (**4**) of chapter 1.

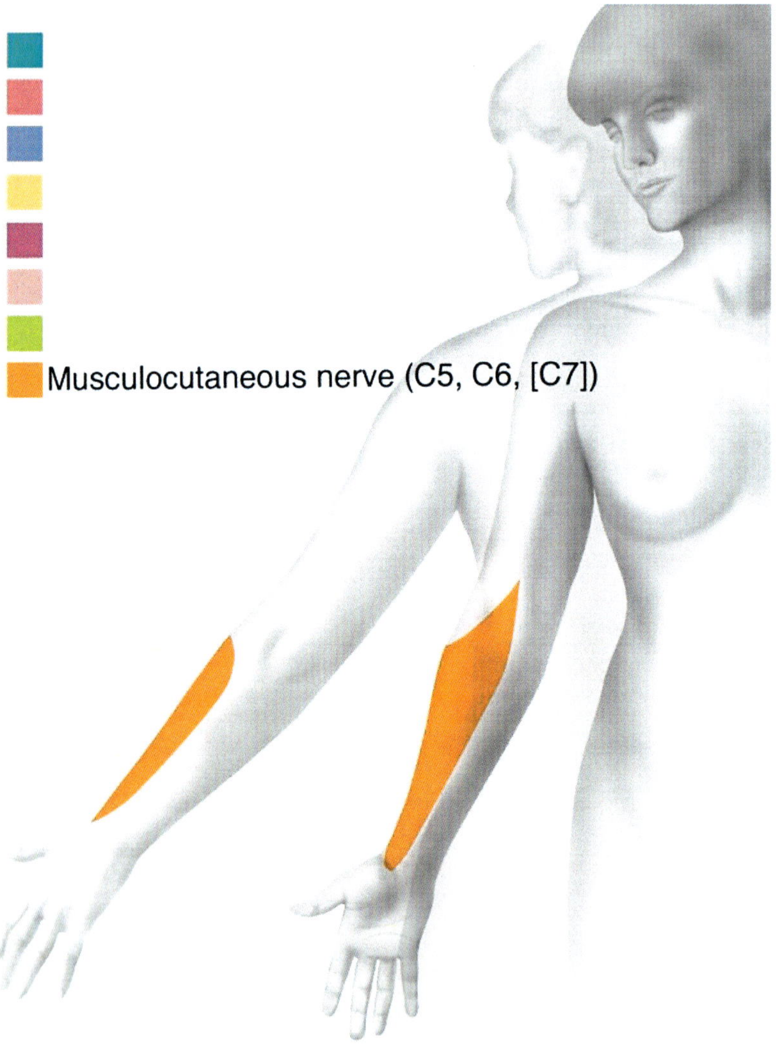

Figure 4: Neurotomes of the musculocutaneous nerve (with its corresponding neurotomal origins).

The ***median nerve*** arises from the lateral and medial cords of the brachial plexus and unites in front of the axillary artery. As it descends through the arm it lies in front of the outer side of the brachial artery and lies on the inner side to the bend in the elbow, below the biceps fascia. It is separated from the elbow joint by the brachialis muscle. In the forearm it passes beneath the flexor digitorum profundus and superficialis muscles after giving off an anterior interosseous branch. At the wrist the median nerve lies between the tendons of the flexor digitorum superficialis and flexor polices longus muscles and deep to the tendon of the palmaris longus muscle. This nerves gives off no branches in the arm except a nerve to the pronator teres muscle. In the forearm it gives off the anterior interosseous branch and muscular branches, and two articular branches to the elbow joint (See Chapter 8). For dermatomal innervation see Fig. (**5**). Also see Fig. (**4**) of chapter 1.

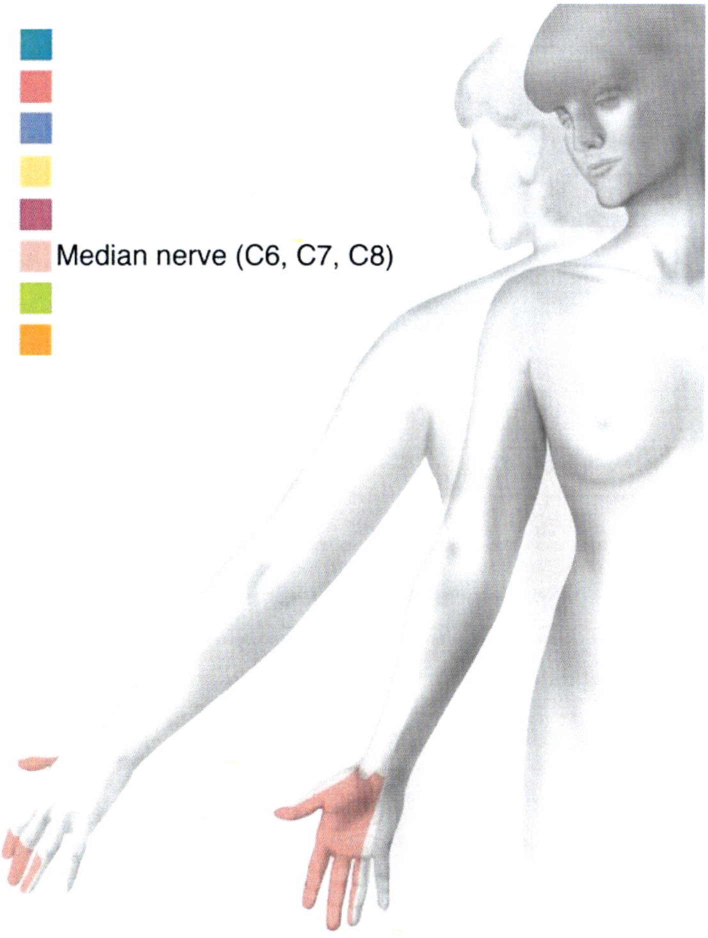

Figure 5: Neurotomes of the median nerve (with its corresponding dermatomal origins).

The ***ulnar nerve*** arises from the medial cord of the brachial plexus. It courses to the inner side of the axillary artery and holds that relation to the brachial artery to the middle of the arm. From there it runs obliquely across the medial head of the triceps brachii muscle, pierces the intermuscular septum, and descends to the ulnar groove between the medial condyle of the humerus and the olecranon of the ulna. The inferior profunda artery accompanies it. In the forearm it descends between the flexor profundus and the flexor carpi ulnaris in its upper half. For its lower half it lies on the flexor digitorum profundus with the flexor carpi ulnaris on its medial side. In the upper arm the ulnar nerve does not give off any branches, while in the forearm it gives off articular branches to the elbow, two muscular branches to the flexor carpi ulnaris and flexor profundus digitorum, a cutaneous branch, a dorsal cutaneous nerve and an articular branch to the wrist joint. In the hand it gives off deep and superficial palmar branches (See chapter 8). For dermatomal innervation see Fig. (**7**). Also see Fig. (**4**) of chapter 1.

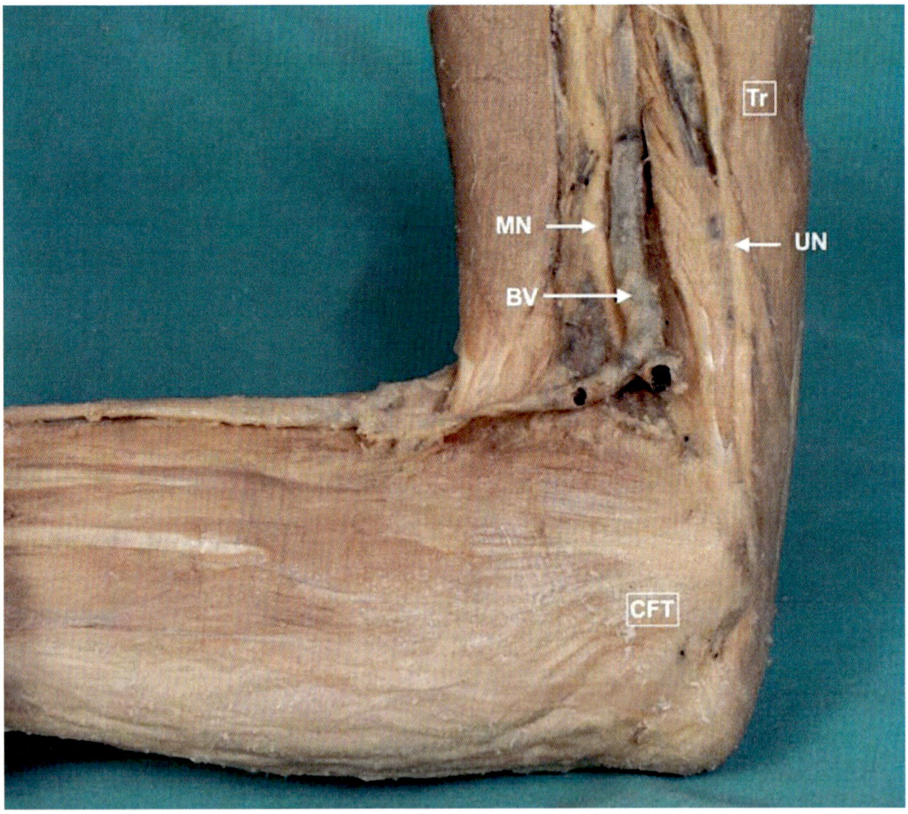

Figure 6: Anatomy of the ulnar and median nerves.
Tr = triceps brachii muscle; CFT = common flexor tendon; BV = basilic vein; MN = median nerve; UN = ulnar nerve.

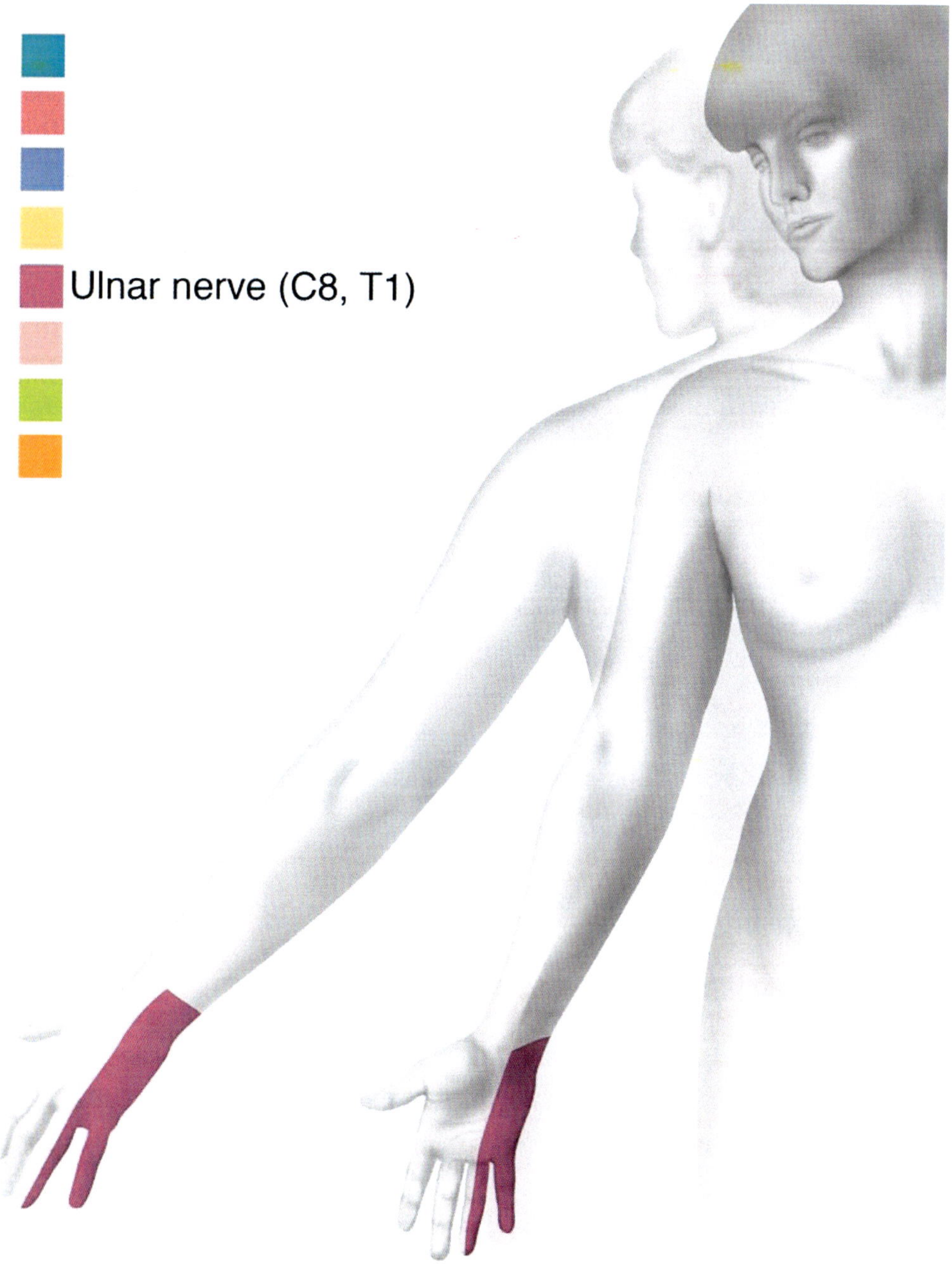

Figure 7: Neurotomes of the ulnar nerve (with its corresponding dermatomal origins).

The ***median cutaneous nerves*** of the arm and forearm originate from the medial cord (Fig. **1** of chapter 1).

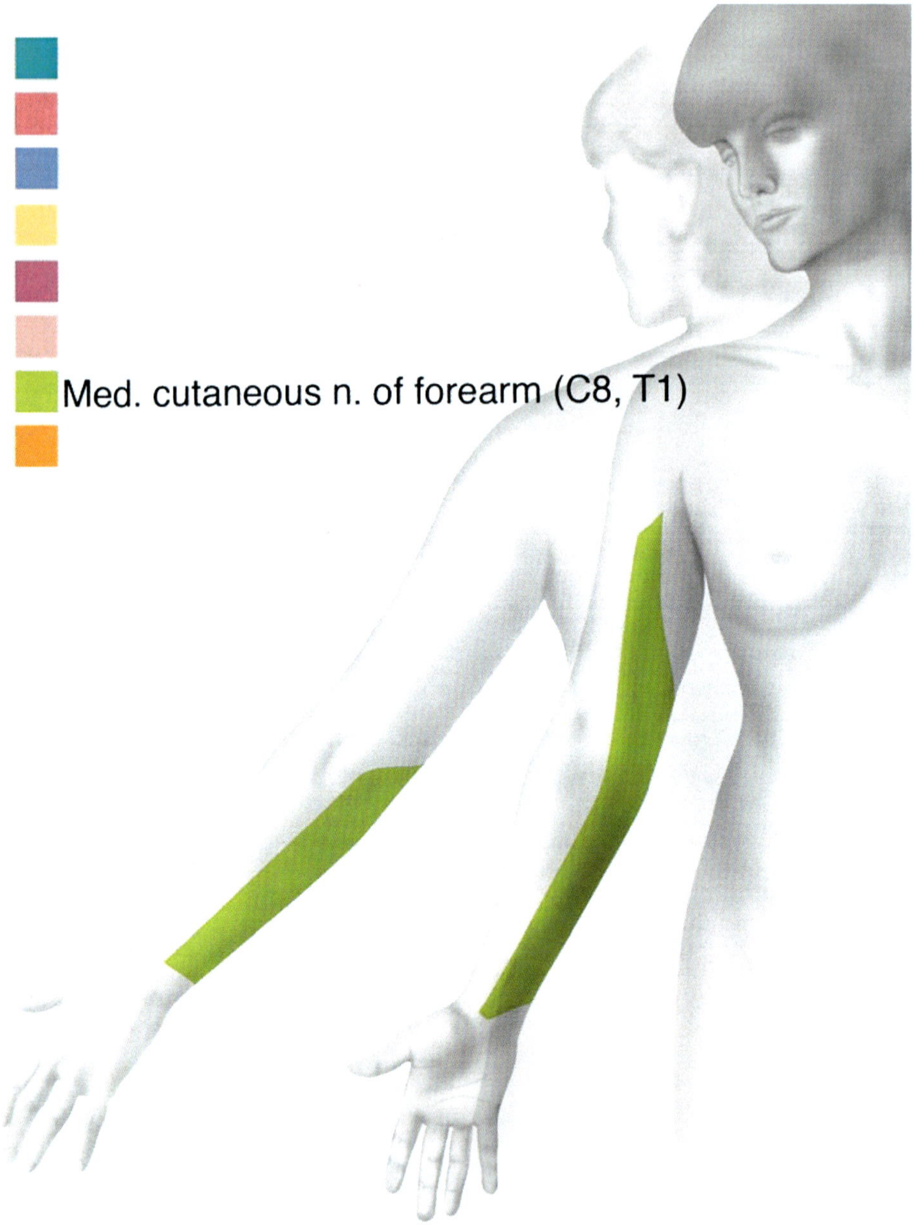

Figure 8: Neurotomes of the median cutaneous nerve of the forearm (with its corresponding dermatomal origins).

The ***superficial cervical plexus***, ***axillary nerve*** and ***intercosto-brachial nerve*** supply sensory innervation to the arm as depicted in Fig. (**9**), while the ***axillary nerve*** supply motor innervation to the deltoid muscle.

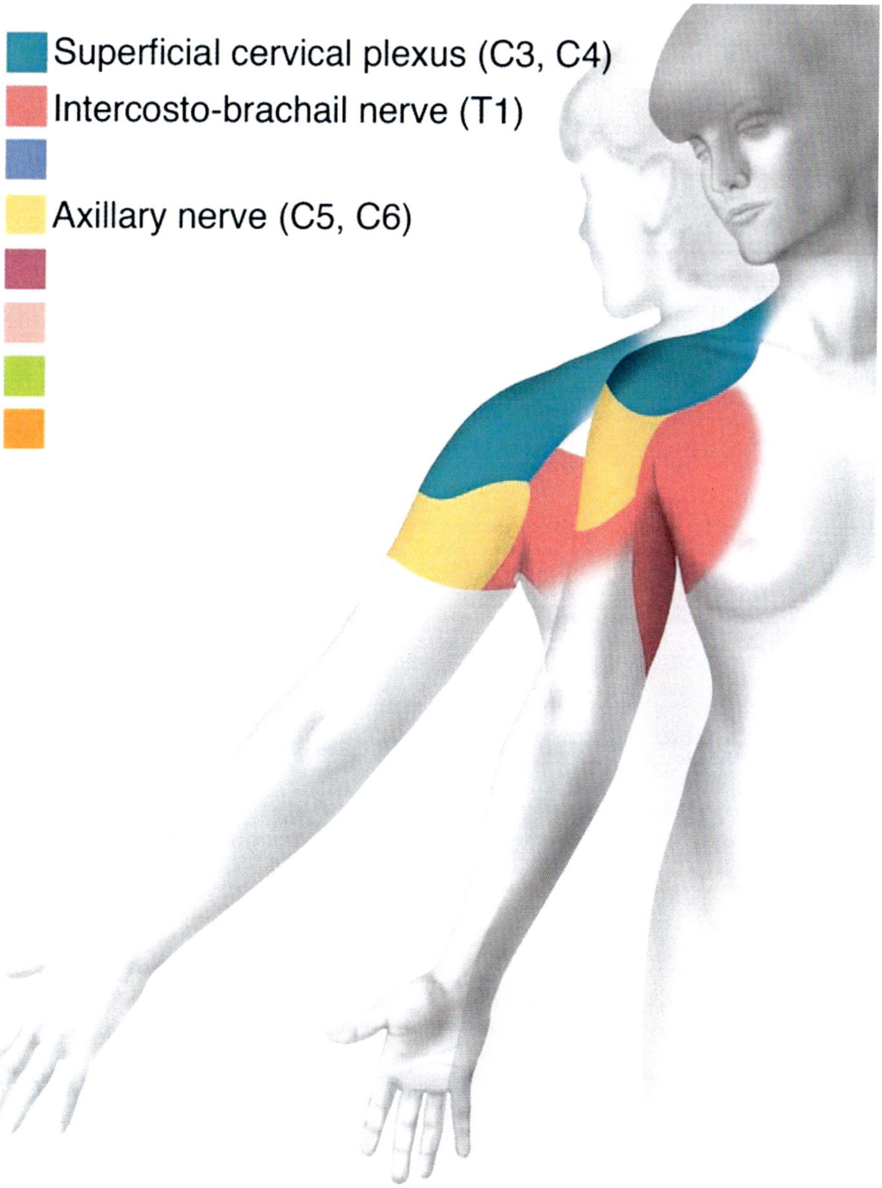

Figure 9: Neurotomes of the superficial cervical plexus, the axillary nerve and the intercosto-brachial nerve (with their corresponding dermatomal origins).

SURFACE ANATOMY

The landmarks for the axillary brachial plexus block are easily identified With the patient positioned supine and the upper arm externally rotated and abducted to 90 degrees, and with the elbow flexed to 90 degrees, the following can be palpated to assist placement of the stimulating needle:

- The groove between biceps brachialis and coracobrachialis muscles in front and the triceps muscle behind
- The inferior border of the pectoralis major muscle
- The pulsation of the axillary artery felt against the humerus.

ACKNOWLEDGEMENTS

The author gratefully acknowledge the following people:

- The Head of the Department of Anesthesiology of the College of Medicine of the University of Florida, Dr. Tim Morey, and his department for their moral support and continuous encouragement.
- The faculty and fellows of the Division of acute and perioperative pain medicine for affording the author the time to produce this work by covering his clinical duties.
- Corey Astrom of the Department of Anesthesiology of the College of Medicine of the University of Florida for her professional and high quality text editing.
- Mary K Bryson for her illustrations of Figs. (**1**, **3**, **5**, **7** and **9**).
- Raeducation.com LLC for their financial support.

CONFLICT OF INTEREST

The author confirms that this chapter contents have no conflict of Interest.

ABBREVIATIONS

BA	=	brachial artery
Biceps	=	biceps brachii muscle
Br	=	brachialis muscle

BV (ii)	=	basilica vein
BV	=	brachial vein
CFT	=	common flexor tendon
LHT (Lat)	=	lateral head of triceps
LHT (Long)	=	long head of triceps
MCN	=	musculocutaneous nerve
MCNA	=	medial cutaneous nerve of the arm
MCNF	=	medial cutaneous nerve of the forearm
MHT	=	medial head of triceps
MN	=	median nerve
RN	=	radial nerve
Tr	=	triceps brachii muscle
Triceps	=	triceps brachii muscle
UN	=	ulnar nerve

SUGGESTED FURTHER READING

[1] Hilton, J. On Rest and Pain: a Course of Lectures on the Influence of Mechanical and Physiological Rest in the Treatment of Accidents and Surgical Diseases, and the Diagnostic Value of Pain, delivered at the Royal College of Surgeons of England in the years 1860, 1861, 1862 and 1863.

[2] Hébert-Blouin M-N, Tubbs RS, Carmichael SW, Spinner RJ. Hilton's Law revisited. Clin Anat. 2014; 27: 548-55.

Chapter 7:
Microanatomy of the Nerves in the Axilla

CHAPTER 7

Microanatomy of the Nerves in the Axilla

André P. Boezaart*

Departments of Anesthesiology and Orthopaedic Surgery and Rehabilitation, Division of Acute and Perioperative Pain Medicine, University of Florida College of Medicine, Gainesville, Florida, USA

Abstract: In this chapter, the author combines the established views of the microstructure of the ulnar nerve as an example of a singe peripheral nerve, with some newer concepts that have emerged only recently. The position and importance of the circumneural (paraneural) sheath and subcircumneural (subparaneural) space are discussed, as well as the other membranes and compartments surrounding this peripheral nerve, namely, the endoneurium, perineurium, epineurium, and epimysium. The subepimyseal space is discussed in the context of peripheral nerve block.

Keywords: Acute pain medicine, Axon, Circumneural sheath, Continuous peripheral nerve block, Endoneurium, Epimysium, Fascia, Fascicles, Gliding apparatus, Microanatomy, Nerve axon, Paraneural sheath, Perineurium Epineurium, Peripheral nerve block, Regional anesthesia, Single peripheral nerve, Subcircumneural space, Subepimyseal space, Subparaneural space, Ulnar nerve, Ultrastructure.

MICROANATOMY OF THE ULNAR NERVE

The microstructure of all the nerves in the axilla is similar. We consider the ulnar nerve here as an example of a nerve in the axilla. Like any other mixed peripheral nerve, the ulnar nerve is composed of numerous fasciculi; each surrounded by a dense perineurium and held together by a looser epineurium [1-3].

The ***endoneurium*** (Fig. **1**, No. 12) is a fine cylindrical lamina that encloses groups of axons with their respective Schwann cells. The axons consist of different axon fiber types, depending of the type of nerve in question (see Table **1** of Chapter 2). Both myelinated and unmyelinated axons are surrounded by collagen fibers of the endoneurium, but the endoneurium is permeable and thus does not interfere with molecule passage through it. The single-layered

***Corresponding author André P. Boezaart:** Departments of Anesthesiology and Orthopaedic Surgery, Division of Acute and Peri-operative Pain Medicine, University of Florida College of Medicine, 1600 SW Archer Road, Gainesville, Florida 32610, USA; Tel: 352-846-0913 (Work); Fax: 352-392-7029;
E-mail: aboezaart@anest.ufl.edu

endothelial cells of the capillaries in the endoneurium contribute to the blood-nerve barrier [3]. The term endoneurium is sometimes incorrectly used to denote the intrafascicular compartment of the nerve. Its use should be restricted to refer to intrafascicular connective tissue, excluding the perineurial partitions that may subdivide fascicles [1]. Approximately 40% to 50% of the intrafascicular space is occupied by non-neural elements and anywhere from 20% to 30% of this is endoneurial fluid (CSF) and connective matrix – the endoneurium [1, 3].

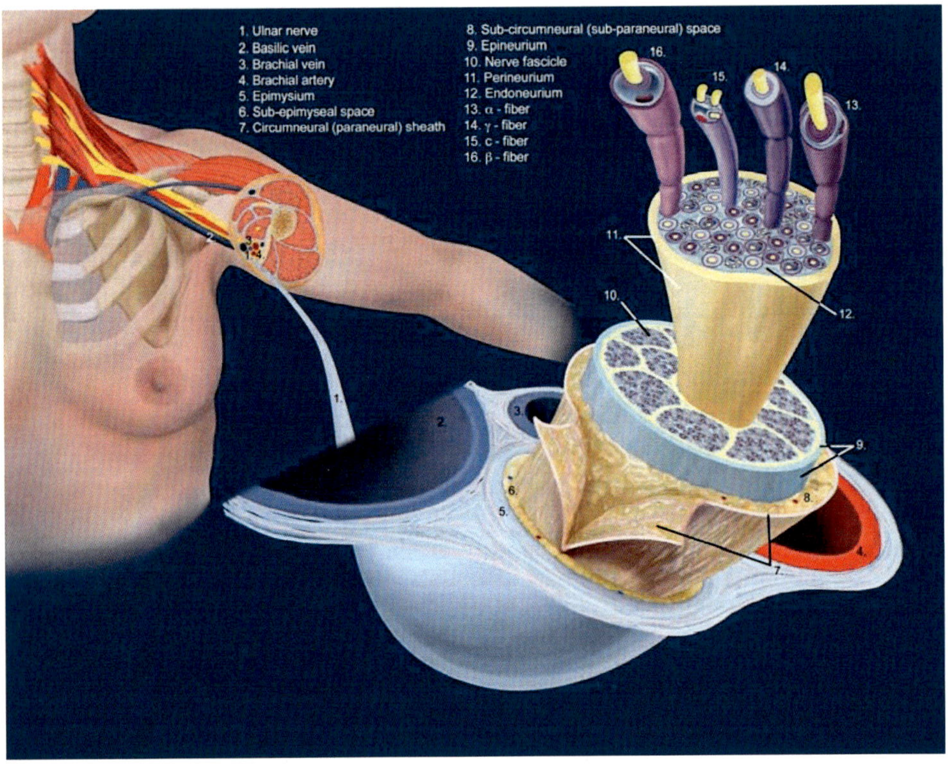

Figure 1: Ultrastructure of the ulnar nerve.

1. *The ulnar nerve, like all the peripheral nerves in the axilla, lies in its own circumneural sheath (7).*
2. *Outside the circumneural sheath is the subepimyseal space (6), which is surrounded by the epimysium (5), which is the fascia that surrounds the nerves, muscles, and blood vessels.*
3. *Deep to the circumneural sheath (7) (also called the paraneural sheath) is the subcircumneural space, which is thought to be the ideal space for the needle in catheter placement for single injection or continuous nerve blocks.*
4. *The next layer, which engulfs the nerve fascicle bundle, is the epineurium (9).*
5. *Each fascicle is surrounded by its own perineurium (11).*
6. *Inside the perineurium are the endoneurium and nerve axons (13-16) (Table **1** of Chapter 2).*

The ***perineurium*** (Fig. **1**, No. 11) comprises multiple single-cell layers that enclose individual nerve fascicles [3]. They become progressively thinner as the number of fascicles increase. As Key and Retzius [1] describe, the essential structure of the perineurium is a lamellated arrangement of flattened cells separated by layers of collagenous connective tissue that provides an ensheathment for both the somatic and peripheral autonomic nerves and their ganglia. The cellular lamellae are composed of concentric sleeves of flattened polygonal cells that are equipped to function as a metabolically active diffusion barrier, although they do not have the morphologic features of a true epithelium.

The ***epineurium*** (Fig. **1**, No. 9) consists of a condensation of areolar connective tissue that surrounds the perineurial ensheathment of the fascicles of uni- and multifascicular nerves [3, 4]. The attachment of the epineurium to surrounding connective tissue is loose, allowing the nerve to be relatively mobile except where tethered by entering blood vessels or branches [4]. Greater amounts of connective tissue are normally present where nerves cross over joints. In general, the more fascicles there are, the greater the quantity of epineurium.

Variable quantities of adipose tissue are also present in the epineurium, particularly in the larger nerves. After studying the distribution of fat in human nerves and finding predominance in the sciatic nerve, researchers feel that this tissue probably has a protective function in cushioning the fascicles against injury by compression. The susceptibility to compression injury is likely to be less in large multifascicular nerves with considerable quantities of epineurium and fat than in smaller and unifascicular nerves.

The ***vasa nervorum*** enter the epineurium, where they communicate with a longitudinal anastomotic network of arterioles and venules [4]. The epineurium also contains lymphatic vessels, which are not present within the fascicles. These lymphatic channels accompany the arteries of the peripheral nerves and pass into the regional lymph nodes [5].

Anderson and colleagues [6] recently demonstrated the ***circumneural (paraneural) sheath*** [7] in dissections, while Karmakar and his colleagues [8] described the appearance of the circumneural sheath with high-definition ultrasound. In neurosurgical texts, it has been known as the "gliding apparatus" of the nerve [9]. We now know that injection of a local anesthetic agent or catheter placement in the subcircumneural space (subparaneural space) is ideal for single-injection and continuous nerve block, respectively [9]. Reina and colleagues stained sections through the brachial plexus and peripheral nerves with Masson's trichrome staining to convincingly demonstrate the microscopic ultrastructure of the circumneural (paraneural) sheaths [3] (See Figs. **7**, **8** and **9** of chapter 2).

ACKNOWLEDGEMENTS

The author gratefully acknowledge the following people:

- The Head of the Department of Anesthesiology of the College of Medicine of the University of Florida, Dr. Tim Morey, and his department for their moral support and continuous encouragement.

- The faculty and fellows of the Division of Acute and Perioperative Pain Medicine of the above Department of Anesthesiology for affording the author the time to produce this work by covering his clinical duties.

- Corey Astrom of the Department of Anesthesiology of the College of Medicine of the University of Florida for her professional and high quality text editing.

- Mary K Bryson for her illustrations of Fig. (**1**).

- Raeducation.com LLC for their financial support.

CONFLICT OF INTEREST

The author invented the "stimulating catheter and receives royalties from TeleFlex for its sales.

DISCLOSURE

Parts of this work have been previously published in Boezaart AP. Microanatomy of the peripheral nervous system revisited, and its implications for paravertebral (para-neuraxial) blocks. Proceedings of the 10th Annual pre-ASA Meeting, Orthopedic Anesthesia Pain Rehabilitation Society (www.OAPRS.org); 2013 October 11; San Francisco, California. United States of America [10].

REFERENCES

[1] Key A, Retzius G. Studies in the anatomy of the nervous system and connective tissue. Stockholm: Samson and Wallin, circa 1876.

[2] Horster H, Whitman L. The method of intraneural injection. [Die Methode der intraneuralen Injektion]. Z Hygiene 1931; 113: 113.

[3] Reina MA, Ed. Atlas of functional anatomy for regional anesthesia and pain medicine. New York: Springer, 2015; pp. 3-126.

[4] French JD, Strain WH, Jones GE. Mode of extension of contrast substances injected into peripheral nerves. J Neuropathol Exp Neurlogy 1948; 7: 47-58.

[5] Moore DC, Hain RF Ward A, Bridenbaugh LD. Importance of the perineural spaces in nerve blocking. JAMA 1954; 156: 1050-5.

[6] Andrerson HL, Anderson SL, Tranun-Jensen J. Injecting inside the paraneural sheath or the sciatic nerve: Direct comparison among ultrasound imaging, macroscopic anatomy and histologic analysis. Reg Anesth Pain Med 2012; 37: 410-4.

[7] Karmakar MK, Shariat AN, Pangthipampai P, Chen J. High-definition ultrasound imaging defines the paraneural sheath and the fascial compartments surrounding the sciatic nerve at the popliteal fossa. Reg Anesth Pain Med 2013; 38: 447-51.

[8] Millesi H, Zoch G, Rath T. The gliding apparatus of peripheral nerve and its clinical significance. Ann Chir Main Memb Super 1990; 9: 87-97.

[9] Boezaart AP. The Sweet Spot of the Nerve: Is the "paraneural sheath" named correctly, and does it matter? Reg Anesth Pain Med 2014; 39: 557-8.

[10] Boezaart AP. Microanatomy of the peripheral nervous system revisited, and its implications for paravertebral (para-neuraxial) blocks. Proceedings of the 10th Annual pre-ASA Meeting, Orthopedic Anesthesia Pain Rehabilitation Society (www.OAPRS.org); 2013 October 11; San Francisco, California. United States of America.

Chapter 8:
Sonoanatomy of the Nerves in the Axilla, and Around the Elbow and Wrist Joints

CHAPTER 8

Sonoanatomy of the Nerves in the Axilla, and Around the Elbow and Wrist Joints

Barys V. Ihnatsenka[1], André P. Boezaart[2,*] and Yury Zasimovich[1]

[1]Department of Anesthesiology, Division of Acute and Perioperative Pain Medicine, University of Florida College of Medicine, Gainesville, Florida, USA and [2]Departments of Anesthesiology and Orthopaedic Surgery and Rehabilitation, Division of Acute and Perioperative Pain Medicine, University of Florida College of Medicine, Gainesville, Florida, USA

Abstract: Ultrasound is a dynamic process whereby structures can and should be followed to their origins and destinations for optimal identification. Because of this, it is not always satisfactory to study static ultrasound images. When studying sonoanatomy, the authors strongly advise readers to first study the macro- and microanatomy and then to view the accompanying video production that illustrates the dynamic sonoanatomy (Movie **1**). In this chapter, the authors explain the static sonoanatomy of the axilla and the rest of the arm, and with the aid of a video production, the dynamic sonoanatomy of these structures and areas.

Keywords: Acute pain medicine, Axilla, Axilla borders, Axillary artery, Axillary nerve, Brachial artery, Brachial plexus, Brachial vein, Dynamic ultrasound, Intercostobrachial nerve, Lateral cord, Medial cord, Medial cutaneous nerve of the forearm, Medial cutaneous nerves of the arm, Median nerve, Musculocutaneous nerve, Posterior cord, Radial nerve, Regional anesthesia, Second thoracic spinal root, Ulnar nerve, Ultrasound.

SONOANATOMY

Nerves in the Axilla

Nerve blocks in the axilla may somewhat have fallen out popularity in some institutions, probably because of the realization that it should be easier to block three cords that are relatively close together instead of seven peripheral nerves that are further apart. With the introduction of ultrasound practitioners have also become more willing to attempt supra- or infraclavicular block, that previously carried a perhaps higher risk of pneumothorax. Furthermore, the use of continuous

***Corresponding author André P. Boezaart:** Departments of Anesthesiology and Orthopaedic Surgery, Division of Acute and Peri-operative Pain Medicine, University of Florida College of Medicine, 1600 SW Archer Road, Gainesville, Florida 32610, USA; Tel: 352-846-0913 (Work); Fax: 352-392-7029; E-mail: aboezaart@anest.ufl.edu

nerve blocks in the axilla was not met with enthusiasm because of the high incidence of secondary block failure, again because these peripheral nerves are relatively far apart and in their own circumneural (paraneural) sheath, making it difficult to achieve satisfactory results with a continuous axillary block. The coming of age of ultrasound-guided nerve blocks may have reversed this trend - at least for as far as single-injection blocks are concerned. It is now possible to identify each nerve individually in the axilla and block whichever nerve or nerves are the most appropriate for the surgical situation.

When obtaining the images for this section (Figs. **1**-**8**), we positioned the model in the supine position with her arm abducted. Ultrasound scanning took place with a 6- to 13-MHz linear probe with a 38-cm footprint (HFL - 38, SonoSite Fujifilm, Bothell, WA, USA) and started high in the axilla just posterior to the tendon of the major pectoral muscle (Fig. **1**). All nerves in the axilla can and should be followed further down the arm, making their individual recognition easier (Figs. **1** and **2**).

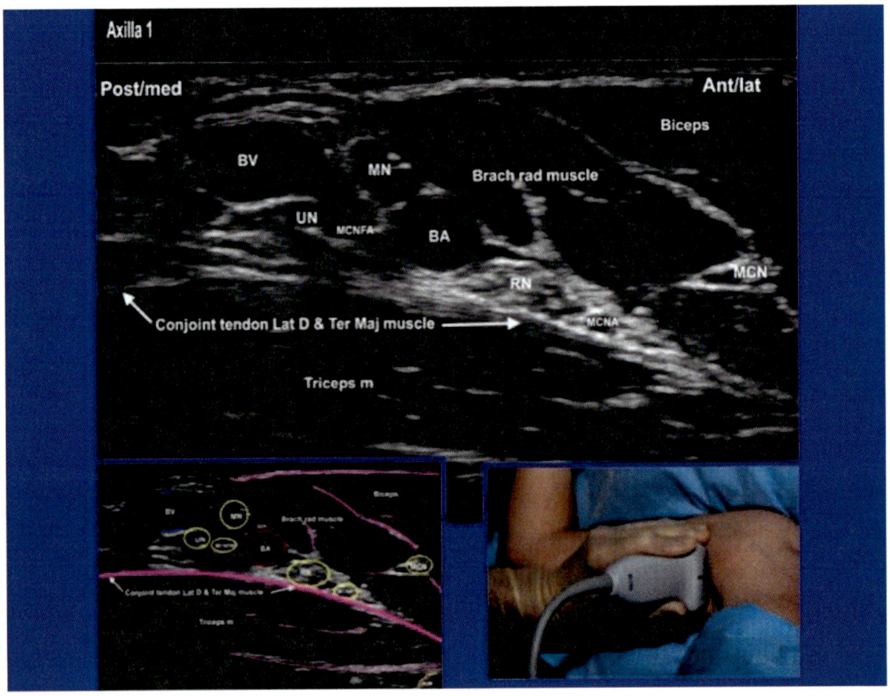

Figure 1: Sonoanatomy of the nerves in the axilla.
Post/med = posteromedial; Ant/lat = anterolateral; Biceps = biceps brachii muscle; Brach rad muscle = brachioradial muscle; BA = brachial artery; BV = brachial vein; Lat D = latissimus dorsi muscle; Ter Maj muscle = teres major muscle; Triceps m = triceps brachii muscle; UN = ulnar nerve; MCNFA = medial cutaneous nerve of the forearm; RN = radial nerve; MCNA = medial cutaneous nerve of the arm; MCN = musculocutaneous nerve.

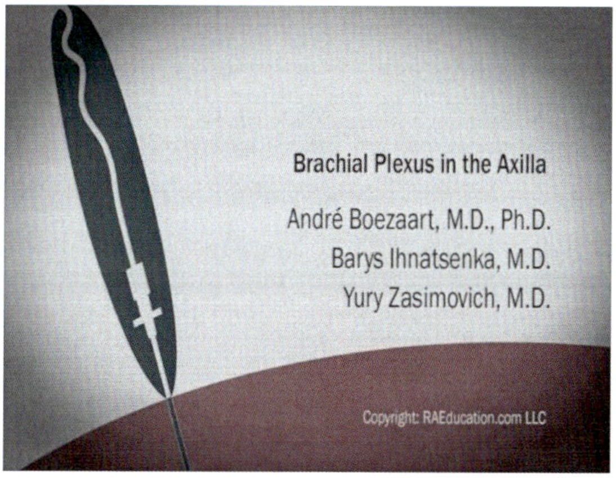

To view this movie click on this link:
https://raeducation.com/ebook

Movie 1: Dynamic sonoanatomy of the nerves in the axilla.

The radial nerve can now be followed down and can be seen splitting away from the other nerves posteriorly to where it joins the deep artery of the arm, which later splits into the radial collateral and middle collateral arteries, as it courses around the humerus *via* the spiral radial groove.

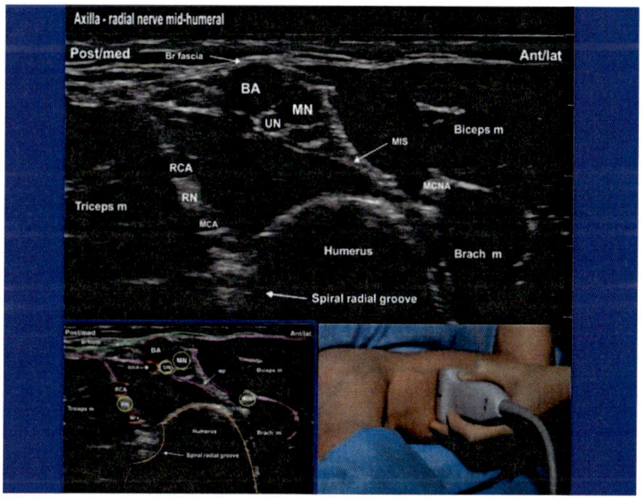

Figure 2: Sonoanatomy of the radial nerve as it courses around the humerus through the spiral radial groove.
Post/med = posteromedial; Ant/lat = anterolateral; br fascia =brachial fascia; BA = brachial artery; Biceps m = biceps brachii muscle; Brach m = brachialis muscle; Triceps m = triceps brachii muscle; UN = ulnar nerve; MN = median nerve; MIS = medial intermuscular septum; MCNA = medial cutaneous nerve of the arm; RCA = radial collateral artery; MCA = middle collateral artery; RN = radial nerve.

Note that the deep artery of the arm usually accompanies the radial nerve through the spiral radial groove around the humerus, but in some subjects, as in this model, it was seen to split earlier into its two branches (Fig. **2**).

Nerves Around the Elbow

Each one of the nerves in the axilla can be followed down to the elbow, where they can individually be blocked should the need arise or the clinical situation demand it. Nerve blocks around the elbow are usually regarded as "rescue" blocks and are usually not primary blocks [3].

The median nerve is a large nerve, and when followed distally, runs with the median cutaneous nerve of the forearm for some distance before it moves more anterior (Fig. **3**).

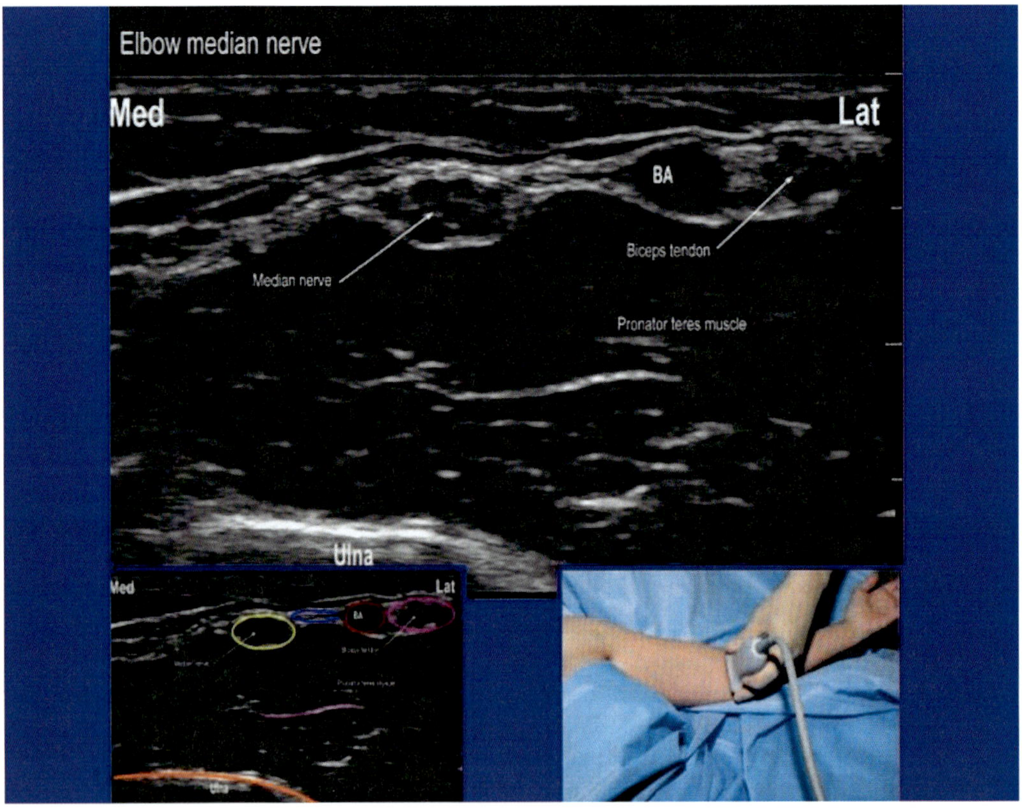

Figure 3: The median nerve at the elbow.
Med = medial; Lat = lateral; BA = brachial artery.

Note that the brachial vein, situated in this image between the brachial artery and the median nerve, has been compressed by the external pressure of the ultrasound probe.

Above the elbow, the radial nerve is usually a solitary nerve that splits into a deep and a superficial branch at or below the elbow (Fig. **4**).

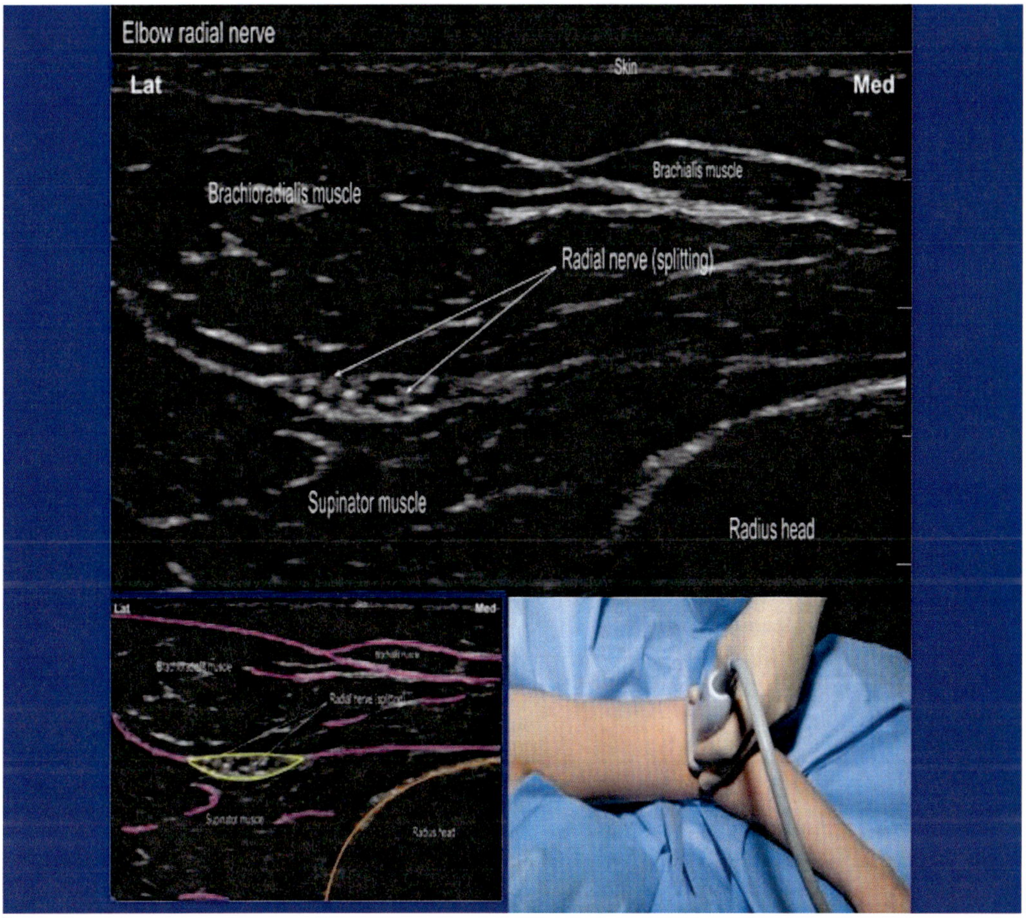

Figure 4: Radial nerve at the elbow.
Lat = lateral; Med = medial.

Note that in this image, the radial nerve is in the process of splitting (Fig. **4**). Each branch can be followed further distally.

The ulnar nerve, when followed down from the axilla, courses distally, accompanied by the superior ulnar collateral artery on the anterior border of the triceps brachii muscle. The superior ulnar collateral artery joins the posterior ulnar recurrent artery before it and the ulnar nerve pass behind the ulna through the sulcus ulnaris between the medial epicondyle of the humerus and the olecranon of the ulna (Fig. **5**).

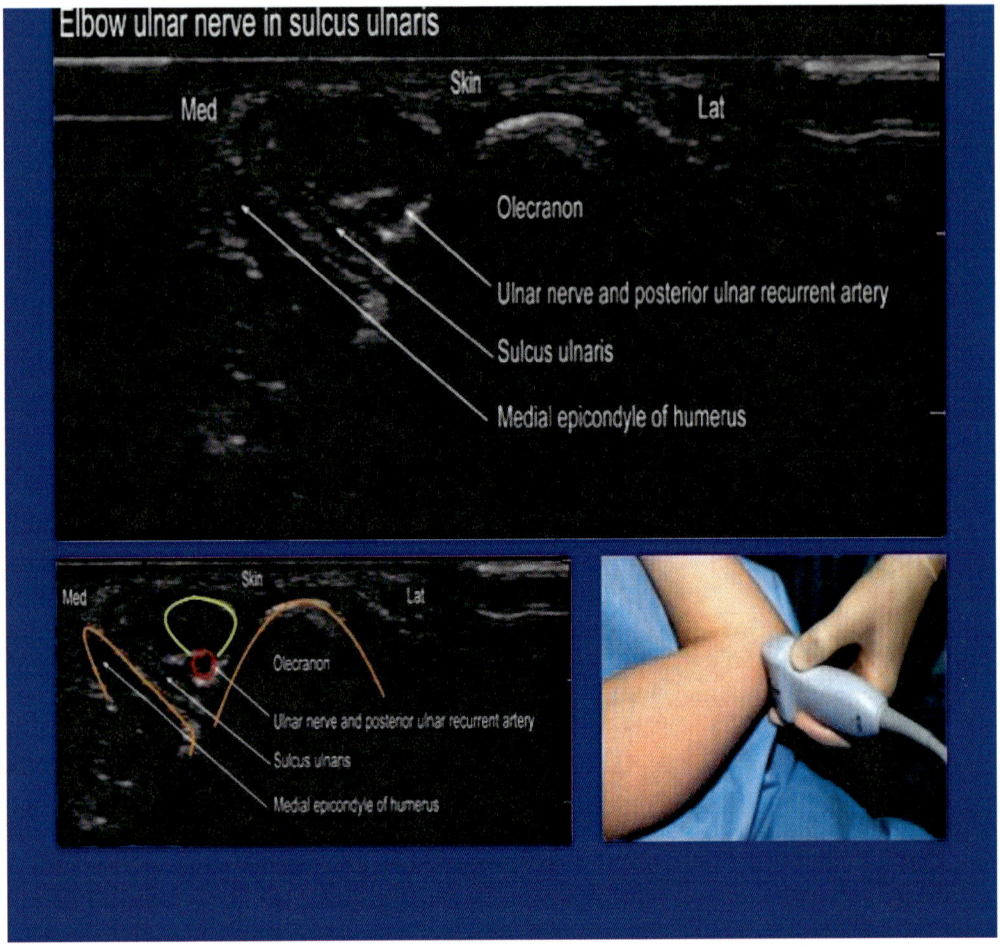

Figure 5: The ulnar nerve and posterior ulnar recurrent artery in the sulcus ulnaris behind the elbow.
Med = medial; Lat = lateral.

Note that the nerve is in a tight compartment and does not lend itself to safe nerve block (Fig. **5**).

Most likely the best place to find the musculocutaneous nerve is just above the elbow (Fig. **6**). After supplying the biceps brachii and brachialis muscles with motor innervation, it emerges below the elbow between the biceps brachii and brachialis muscles as the pure sensory lateral cutaneous nerve of the forearm (Fig. **6**).

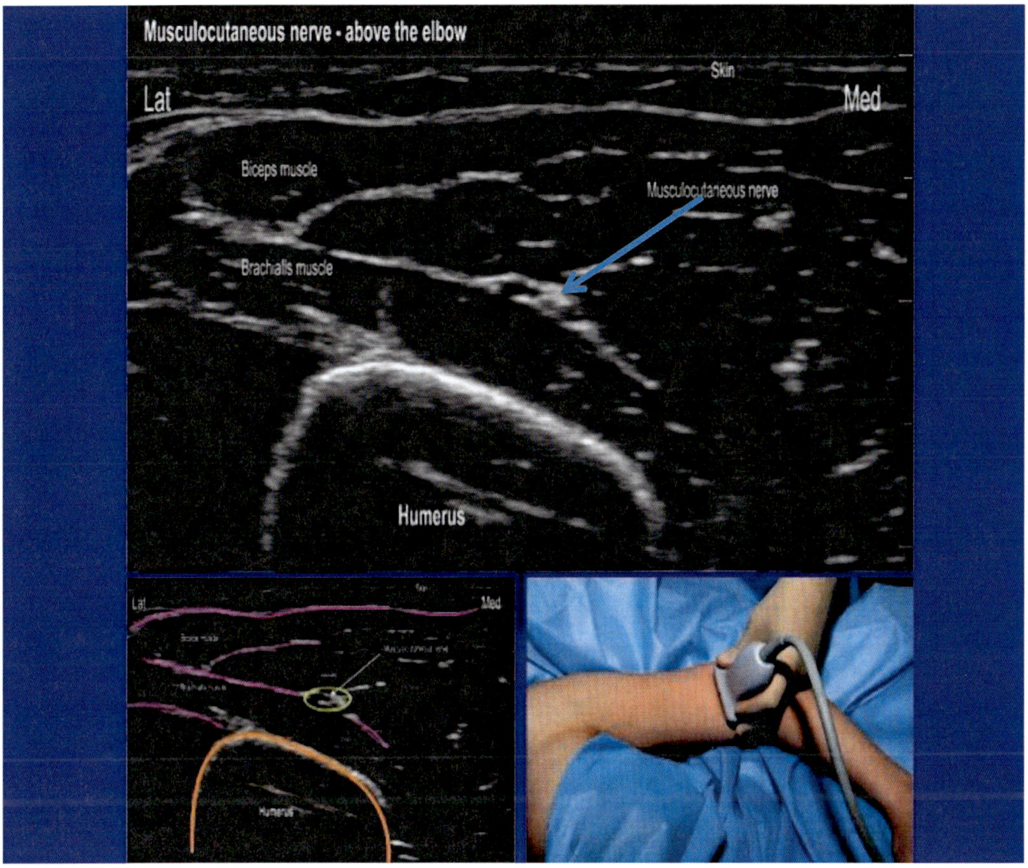

Figure 6: Musculocutaneous nerve in the distal upper arm just above the elbow.
Lat = lateral; Med = medial.

Nerves at the Wrist

Nerve blocks at the wrist are almost always "rescue" blocks and are very rarely primary blocks for surgery. All of the nerves at the wrist can be visualized with ultrasound, but only the median (Fig. **7**) and ulnar nerves (Fig. **8**) are truly practical possibilities

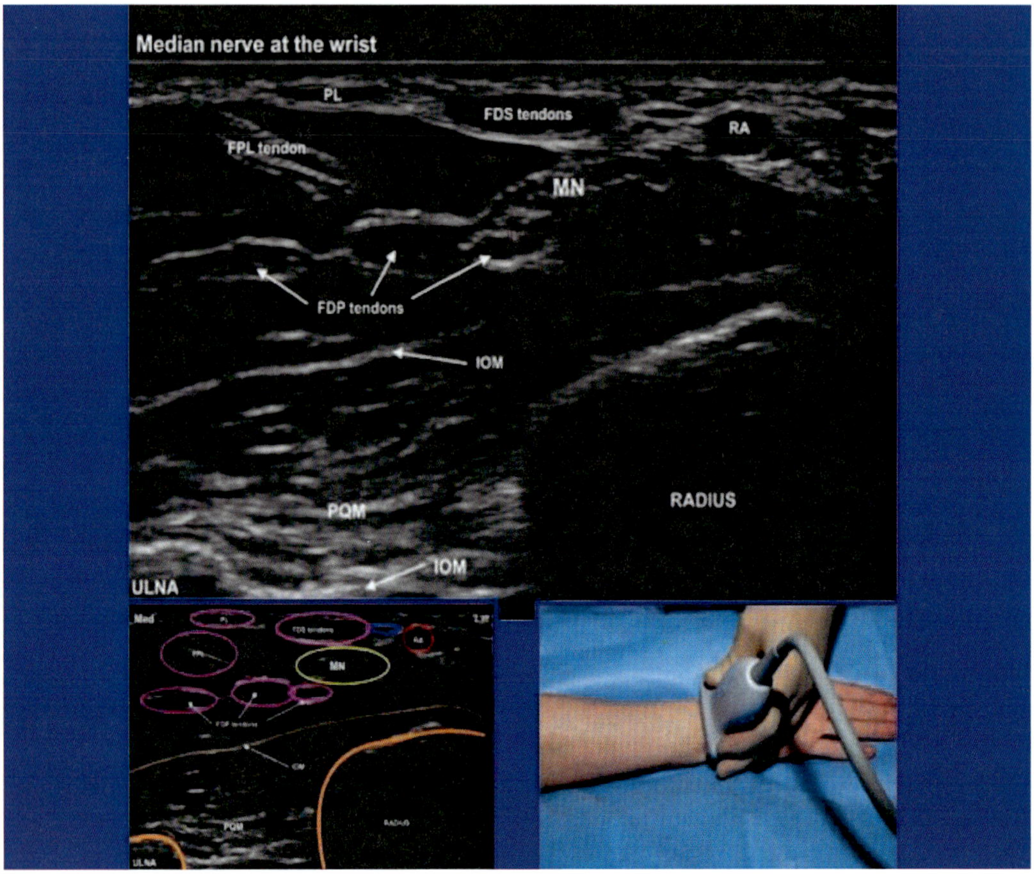

Figure 7: Sonoanatomy of the median nerve at the wrist.
Med = medial; Lat = lateral; Pl = palmaris longus muscle; FDS tendons = flexor digitorum superficialis tendon; RA = radial artery; FPL = flexor pollicis longus muscle; FDP = flexor digitorum profundus muscle and tendons; IOM = interosseous membrane; PQM = pronator quadratus muscle; MN = median nerve.

If the median nerve is followed further distally, it goes under the thick transverse carpal ligament or flexor retinaculum.

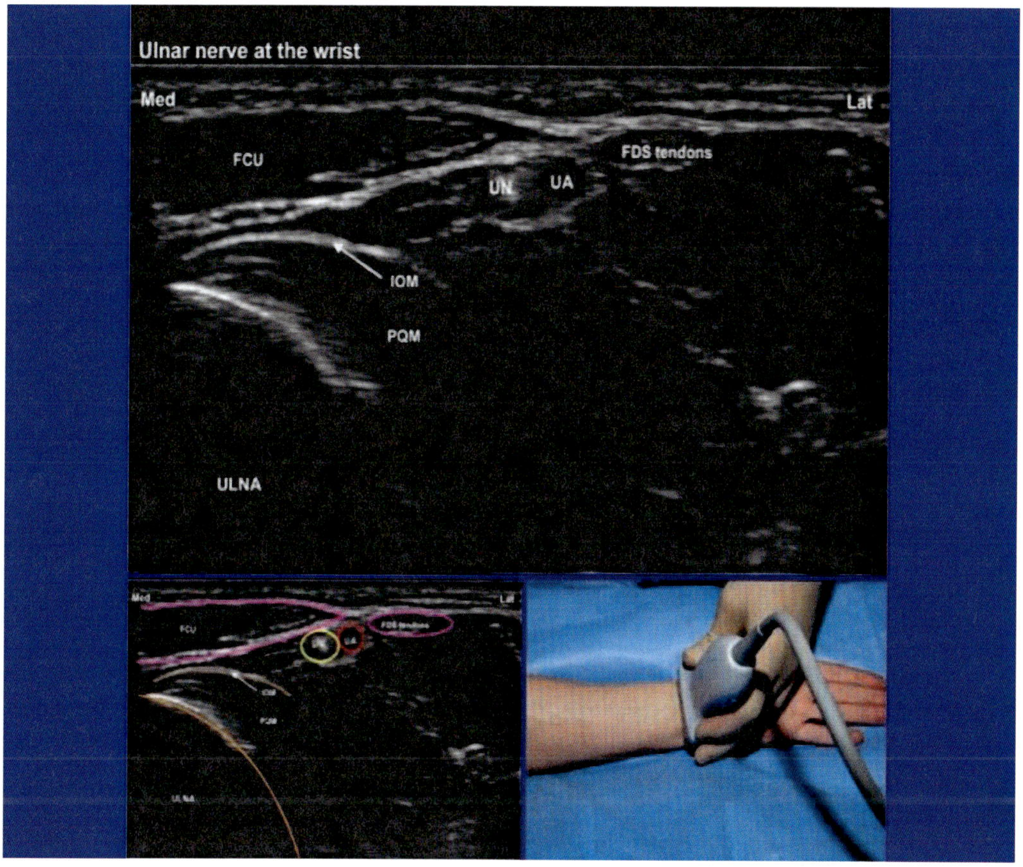

Figure 8: Sonoanatomy of the ulnar nerve at the wrist.
Med = medial; Lat = lateral; FCU = flexor carpi ulnaris tendon; FDS = flexor digitorum superficialis tendons; IOM = interosseous membrane; PQM = pronator quadratus muscle; UA = ulnar artery; UN = ulnar nerve.

ACKNOWLEDGEMENTS

The authors gratefully acknowledge the following people:

- The Head of the Department of Anesthesiology of the College of Medicine of the University of Florida, Dr. Tim Morey, and his department for their moral support and continuous encouragement.

- The faculty and fellows of the Division of Acute and Perioperative Pain Medicine of the above Department of Anesthesiology for affording the authors the time to produce this work by covering their clinical duties.

- Corey Astrom of the Department of Anesthesiology of the College of Medicine of the University of Florida for her professional and high quality text editing.

- Nancy Hagen of the Iowa Public Radio for her narration of the movies.

- Dr. Anastacia Munro for her help with the preparation of the chapter and ultrasound images.

- Raeducation.com LLC for their financial support.

CONFLICT OF INTEREST

The authors confirm that this chapter contents have no conflict of Interest

ABBREVIATIONS

Ant/lat	=	anterolateral
BA	=	brachial artery
Biceps	=	biceps brachii muscle
Biceps m	=	biceps brachii muscle
br fascia	=	brachial fascia
Brach m	=	brachialis muscle
Brach rad muscle	=	brachioradial muscle
BV	=	brachial vein
FCU	=	flexor carpi ulnaris tendon
FDP	=	flexor digitorum profundus muscle and tendons
FDS	=	flexor digitorum superficialis tendons
FDS tendons	=	flexor digitorum superficialis tendon

FPL	=	flexor pollicis longus muscle
IOM	=	interosseous membrane
Lat	=	lateral
Lat D	=	latissimus dorsi muscle
MCA	=	middle collateral artery
RN	=	radial nerve
MCN	=	musculocutaneous nerve
MCNA	=	medial cutaneous nerve of the arm
MCNFA	=	medial cutaneous nerve of the forearm
Med	=	medial
MIS	=	medial intermuscular septum
MN	=	median nerve
Pl	=	palmaris longus muscle
Post/med	=	posteromedial
PQM	=	pronator quadratus muscle
RA	=	radial artery
RCA	=	radial collateral artery
RN	=	radial nerve
Ter Maj musce	=	teres major muscle
Triceps m	=	triceps brachii muscle
UA	=	ulnar artery
UN	=	ulnar nerve

SUGGESTED FURTHER READING

[1] Ihnatsenka BV, Boezaart AP. Ultrasound: Basic understanding and learning the language. Int J Shoulder Surg. 2010;4:55-62.

[2] Steel AC, Harrop-Griffiths W. Nerve blocks in the axilla. In: Boezaart AP, Ed. Anesthesia and orthopaedic surgery, New York: McGraw-Hill, 2006; pp. 321-30.

[3] Boezaart AP. Atlas of peripheral nerve blocks and anatomy for orthopaedic anesthesia, Philadelphia, PA: Saunders Elsevier, 2008: pp. 89-124.

CHAPTER 9

Functional Anatomy of the Nerves of the Upper Extremity

André P. Boezaart*

Departments of Anesthesiology and Orthopaedic Surgery and Rehabilitation, Division of Acute and Perioperative Pain Medicine, University of Florida College of Medicine, Gainesville, Florida, USA

Abstract: All or most of the nerves of interest to regional anesthesiologists or acute pain physicians are mixed nerves with autonomic, sensory, motor, and proprioception functions. Each function is conducted by a specific type of nerve axon. We have provided an overview of these axons and their functions in Chapter 2 (Table **1** of Chapter 2). For the purposes of this chapter, the authors focus on the sensory and motor functions of each of the nerves. To create the video productions that accompany this chapter, Mary Bryson painted the muscles and nerves on a model and we used percutaneous nerve mapping as described by Bösenberg and his colleagues to illustrate the motor function of each nerve (Movies **1** to **11**). With the aid of a peripheral nerve stimulator, the path of many superficial peripheral nerves can be "mapped" prior to skin penetration by stimulating the motor component of the peripheral nerve percutaneously with 1.5- to 2.5-mA current output.

Keywords: Accessory nerve, Acute pain medicine, Autonomic function, Axillary nerve, Body painting, Brachial plexus cords, Brachial plexus roots, Brachial plexus trunks, Dorsal scapular nerve, Long thoracic nerve, Median nerve, Mixed nerves, Motor function, Musculocutaneous nerve, Nerve axon, Percutaneous nerve mapping, Percutaneous nerve stimulation, Peripheral nerve stimulator, Phrenic nerve, Proprioception function, Radial nerve, Regional anesthesia, Sensory function, Suprascaplular nerve, Ulnar nerve.

THE BRACHIAL PLEXUS ROOTS

The brachial plexus is formed by the union of the 5th, 6th, 7th and 8th cervical spinal roots (C5-C8) and the 1st thoracic spinal root (T1). Contribution to the plexus from the 4th cervical spinal root (C4) and 2nd thoracic spinal root (T2) vary. In the most common arrangement, the C5 and C6 rami unite at the lateral

***Corresponding author André P. Boezaart:** Departments of Anesthesiology and Orthopaedic Surgery, Division of Acute and Peri-operative Pain Medicine, University of Florida College of Medicine, 1600 SW Archer Road, Gainesville, Florida 32610, USA; Tel: 352-846-0913 (Work); Fax: 352-392-7029;
E-mail: aboezaart@anest.ufl.edu

border of the middle scalene muscle to form the upper (superior) trunk, C7 continues as the middle trunk, and C8 and T1 join behind the anterior scalene muscle to form the lower (inferior) trunk (see Chapter 1).

THE C5 AND C6 SPINAL ROOT AND UPPER TRUNK

The C5 and C6 spinal roots join to form the upper trunk, and further distal, the upper trunk gives rise to the lateral cord, from which the nerves to the scalene muscles, long thoracic, lateral pectoral, musculocutaneous, and median and anterior interosseous nerves arise. The motor responses evoked from stimulation of the C5 and C6 spinal roots or upper trunk therefore would be [1, 2]:

1. Bending of the cervical spine forward and ipsilaterally, with slight rotation of the neck to the other side.
2. Protraction (forward drawing) of the scapula (Movie **1**).
3. Glenohumeral extension.
4. Glenohumeral adduction.
5. Elbow flexion (Movie **2**).
6. Pronation of the forearm.
7. Wrist flexion.
8. Flexion of the fingers [metacarpophalangeal (MP) and proximal interphalangeal (PIP) joints].
9. Extension of the PIP and distal interphalangeal (DIP) finger joints.
10. Abduction and rotation of the thumb.
11. Opposition of the thumb.
12. Flexion of the interphalangeal (IP) joint of the thumb.

Of all these possible motor responses, the one most prevalent and obvious during C5, C6, or upper trunk stimulation during cervical paravertebral or high interscalene block is flexion of the elbow joint - a biceps brachii motor response. (For dermatomes and osteotomes of brachial plexus spinal roots, see Figs. **2** and **3** of chapter 1).

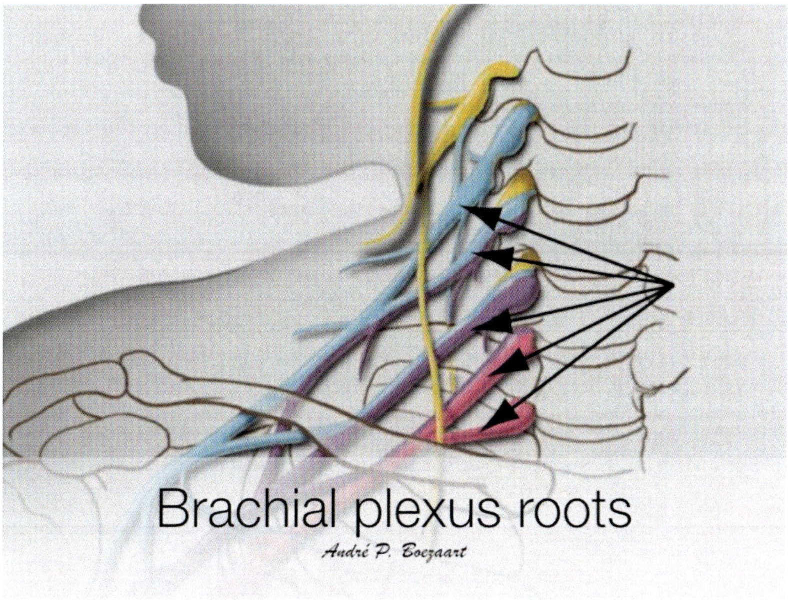

To view this movie click on this link:
https://raeducation.com/ebook

Movie 1: Direct electrical stimulation of the C5/6 nerve root during cervical paravertebral block.

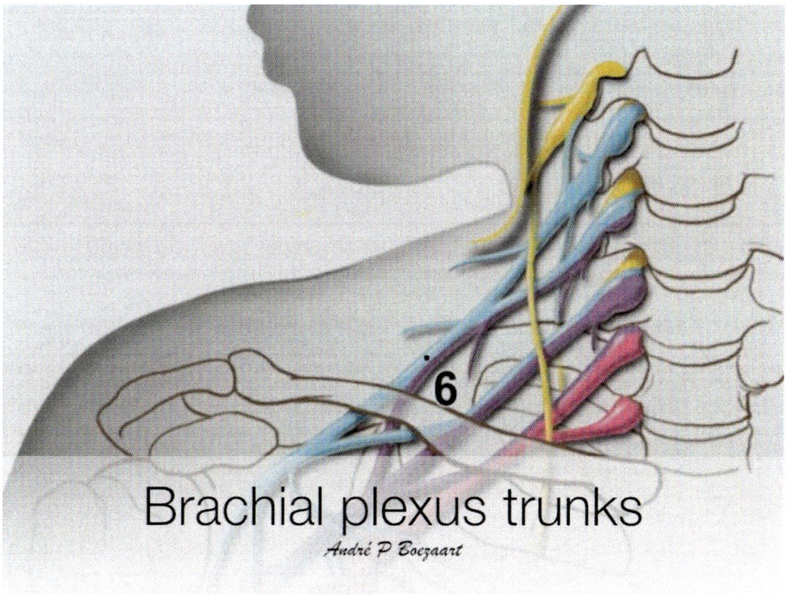

To view this movie click on this link:
https://raeducation.com/ebook

Movie 2: Percutaneous electrical stimulation of the upper trunk of the brachial plexus.

THE C7 SPINAL ROOT AND MIDDLE TRUNK

The C7 spinal root continues as the middle trunk and more distally to the posterior cord of the brachial plexus. The nerve to the longus colli and all five of the scalene muscles, the axillary and radial nerves, and all of the nerves to the extensor muscles of the arm and forearm arise from the posterior cord of the brachial plexus. The motor responses evoked from stimulation of the C7 spinal root or middle trunk therefore would be [1]:

Forward flexion of the neck.

Bending of the cervical spine forward and ipsilaterally, with sight slight rotation to the other side.

Glenohumeral flexion, horizontal abduction, and medial rotation of the humerus.

Glenohumeral extension.

Glenohumeral vertical extension.

Elbow extension.

Wrist extension.

Extension of all the MP, PIP, and DIP of the fingers.

Abduction of the thumb.

Of all these possible motor responses, the one most prevalent and obvious during C7 or middle trunk stimulation during cervical paravertebral or high interscalene block is extension of the elbow joint - a triceps brachii motor response.

THE C8 AND T1 SPINAL ROOTS AND LOWER TRUNK

The spinal roots of C8 and T1 join behind the anterior scalene muscle to continue as the lower trunk on the cervical parietal pleura of the dome (cupula) of the lung. The C8 fibers join to form the posterior cord, while the T1 fibers, for the most part, form the medial cord. The nerves derived from the posterior cord have been highlighted in the previous section. A nerve to the scalene muscles, the medial pectoral, median, and ulnar nerves arises from the medial cord. The motor responses evoked from stimulation of the C8 and T1 spinal roots or lower trunk therefore would be [1]:

- All the motor responses mentioned for the posterior cord of the brachial plexus in the previous section.
- Pronation of the forearm.
- Wrist flexion and abduction.
- Flexion fingers (MP and PIP joints).
- Extension of the PIP and DIP joints.
- Abduction of the fingers.
- Abduction and rotation of the thumb.
- Opposition of the thumb.

Of all these possible motor responses, the one most prevalent and obvious during C8, T1, or lower trunk stimulation during cervical paravertebral block is flexion of the finger joints.

THE LONG THORACIC NERVE

The long thoracic nerve arises from spinal roots C5, C6, and C7. The branches from the upper two roots (C5 and C6) run between the ventral and dorsal parts of the middle scalene muscles (see Chapters 1 and 3), unite with the muscles, and are then joined by a branch from the C7 root, which runs anterior to the middle scalene muscle. The long thoracic nerve then crosses the outer border of the first rib and descends further along the outer thoracic wall on the surface of the serratus anterior muscle. The motor responses evoked from stimulation of long thoracic nerve therefore would be [4]:

- Forward flexion of the arm and contraction of the serratus anterior muscle that can be palpated on the lateral chest wall.

THE BRACHIAL PLEXUS CORDS

Borene *et al.* [3] simplified the interpretation of upper limb motor responses to stimulation by pointing out that the pinkie (fifth digit) moves toward the cord being stimulated with the following phrase, “At the cords the pinkie towards.” The anatomy of the brachial plexus is complex and it is difficult to remember all of the terminal nerves and the muscles supplied by each nerve. Borene *et al.* proposed a simple way to identify the cord being stimulated: When applying an electrical current (*e.g.*, 1.0-1.5 mA) to evoke an action potential in the entire lateral cord, the pinkie will move laterally from the anatomical position (pronation) (Fig. **1**). Posterior movement of the pinkie (extension) indicates posterior cord stimulation (Fig. **2**), whereas its medial movement (fifth finger flexion and ulnar deviation) indicates medial cord stimulation (Fig. **3**). This is best observed by using higher stimulating currents to ensure that all the motor fascicles of a cord are stimulated.

It is clear that finger flexion can differ according to which part of the cord forming the median nerve is stimulated. The lateral part of the median nerves controls the flexor muscles of the thumb and fingers two and three, whereas the medial portion of the median nerve controls the flexor muscles of fingers four and five.

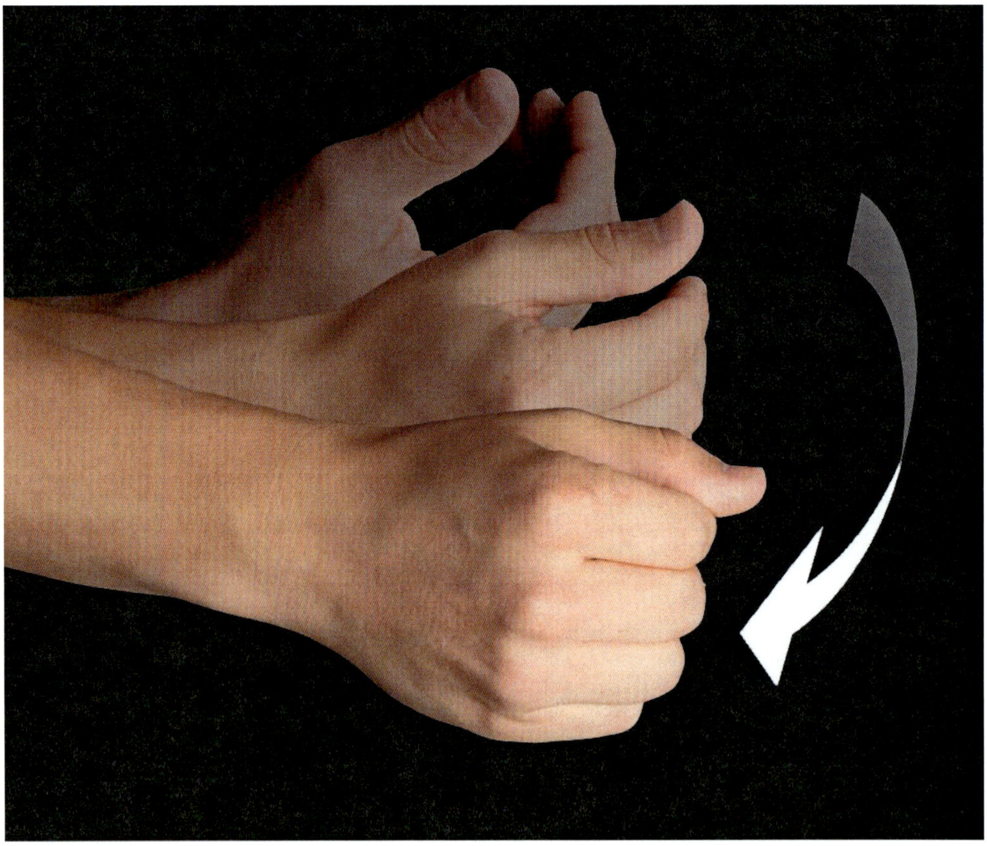

Figure 1: Electrical stimulation of the lateral cord of the brachial plexus - the pinkie moves lateral.

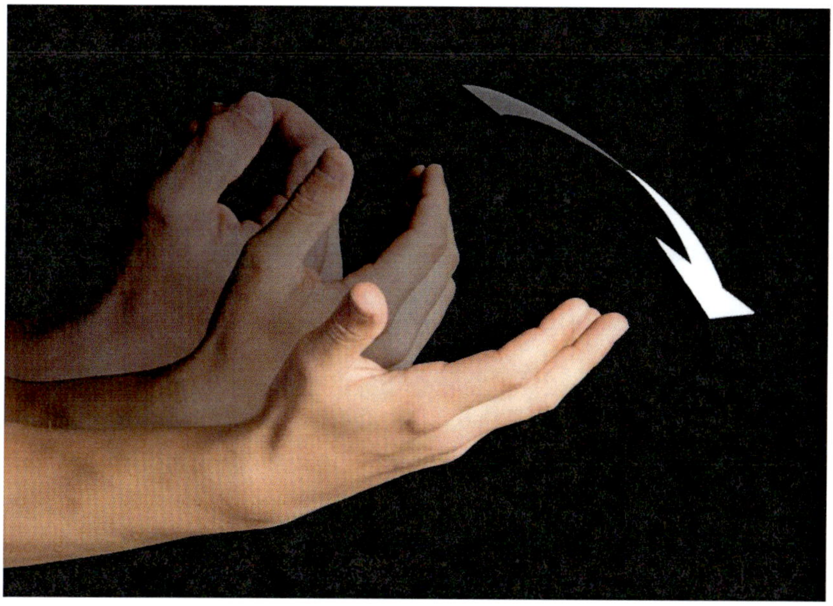

Figure 2: Electrical stimulation of the posterior cord of the brachial plexus - the pinkie moves posterior.

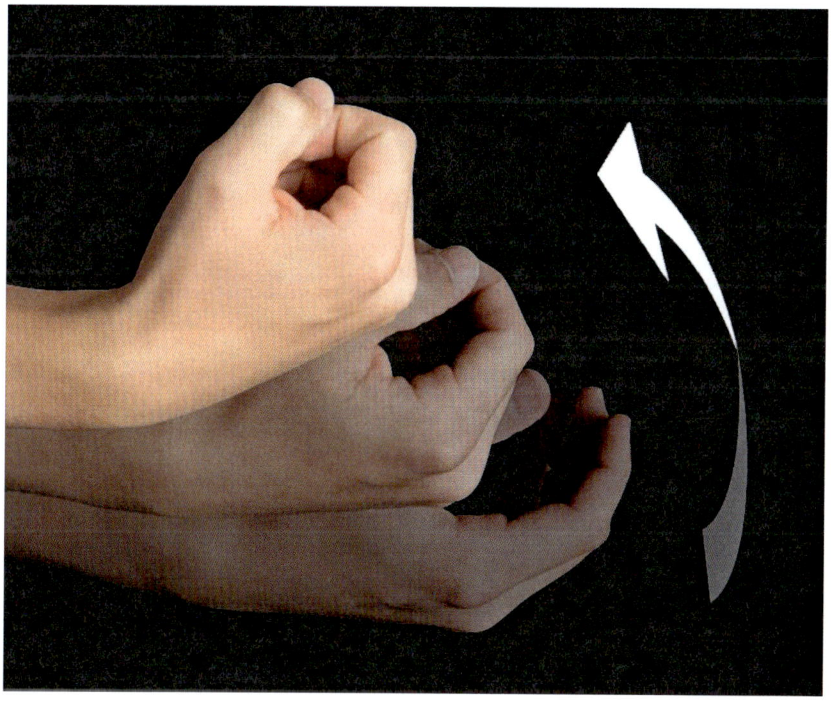

Figure 3: Electrical stimulation of the medial cord of the brachial plexus - the pinkie moves medial.

THE CERVICAL PLEXUS

The cervical plexus is formed by the ventral rami of the upper four cervical spinal roots. It lies deep to the sternocleidomastoid and levator scapulae muscles and its branches can be divided into deep and superficial groups (see Chapter 23). The superficial branches provide cutaneous innervation to the head, neck, and chest, whereas the deep branches are largely motor nerves to the deep muscles of the neck, which include the anterior recti, and rectus capitis lateralis and middle scalene muscles. The branches also supply motor innervation to the sternocleidomastoid (C2 and C3), trapezius (C3 and C4), and levator scapulae (C3 and C4) muscles and the diaphragm *via* the phrenic nerve. The phrenic nerve arises from the 3rd, 4th, and 5th spinal roots. The nerves to the sternocleidomastoid (C2 and C3) and trapezius muscles (C3 and C4) communicate with the cervical accessory nerve, which is a cranial nerve that also innervates these muscles. The motor responses evoked from stimulation of the cervical plexus spinal roots therefore would be [4]:

- Rotation of the head in the opposite direction (sternocleidomastoid muscle).
- Elevation of the shoulder - upper fibers of trapezius muscle, retraction of the scapula - middle fibers of trapezius muscle and rotation of the scapula - lower fibers of trapezius muscle (*via* spinal accessory nerve) (Movie **3**).
- Elevation of the scapula (levator scapulae muscle *via* dorsal scapular nerve).
- Abdominal twitches (diaphragm *via* phrenic nerve).

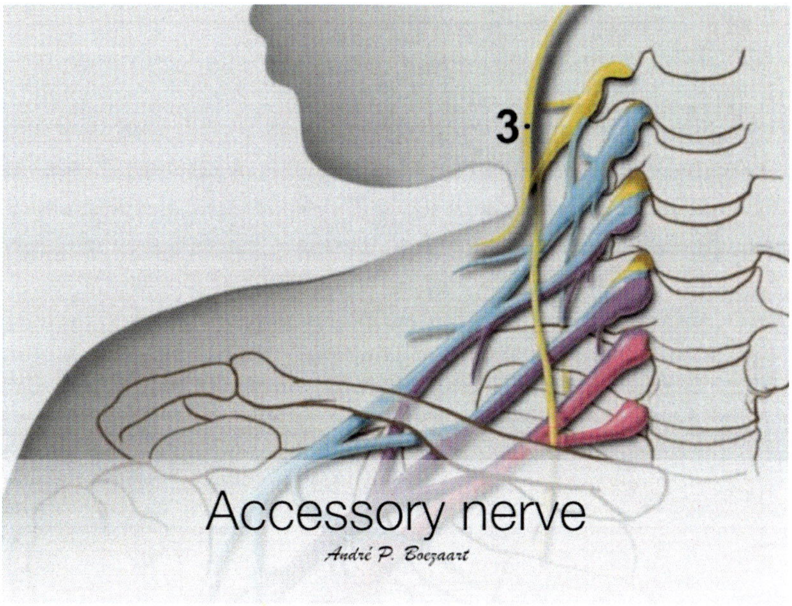

To view this movie click on this link:
https://raeducation.com/ebook

Movie 3: Percutaneous electrical stimulation of the cervical accessory nerve.

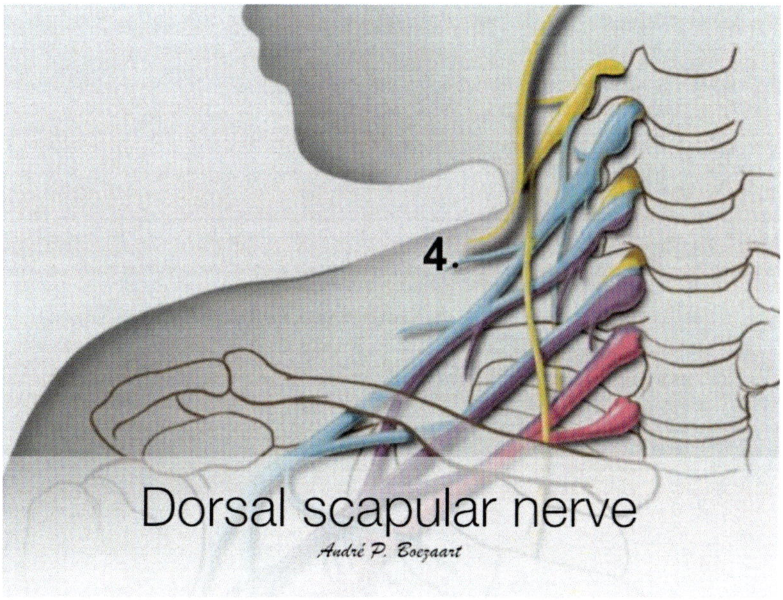

To view this movie click on this link:
https://raeducation.com/ebook

Movie 4: Percutaneous electrical stimulation of the dorsal scapular nerve.

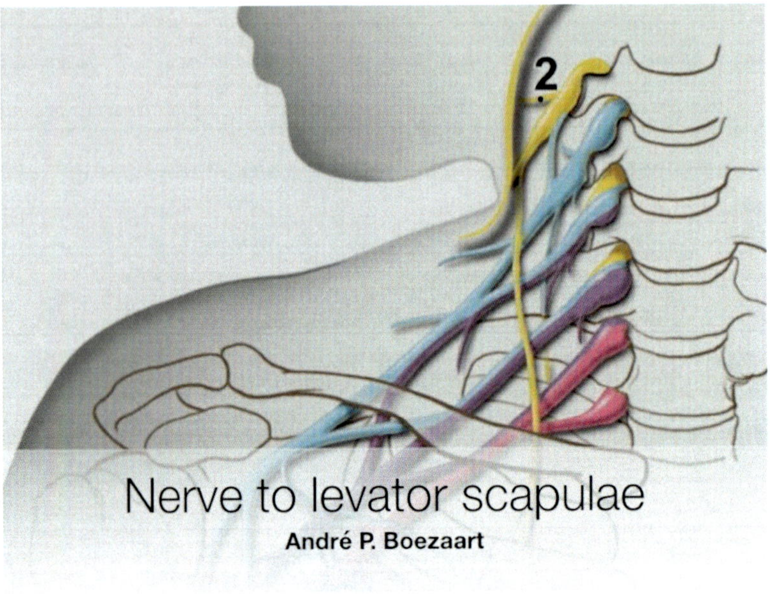

To view this movie click on this link:
https://raeducation.com/ebook

Movie 5: Percutaneous electrical stimulation of the nerve to levator scapulae.

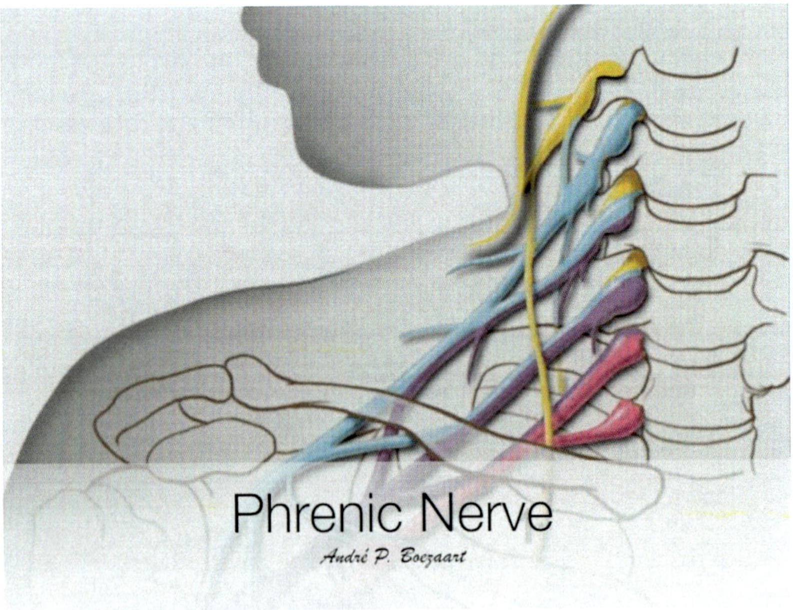

To view this movie click on this link:
https://raeducation.com/ebook

Movie 6: Percutaneous electrical stimulation of the phrenic nerve.

THE SUPRASCAPULAR NERVE

Fibers to the suprascapular nerve are derived from the 5th and 6th cervical roots, and occasionally from C4; the nerve arises from the upper trunk of the brachial plexus. It passes obliquely outward beneath the trapezius and omohyoid muscles to reach the suprascapular notch of the scapula. It innervates the supraspinatus, infraspinatus, subscapularis, and teres major muscles - the rotator cuff of the shoulder muscles. Electrical stimulation of the suprascapular nerve causes rotation of the arm [1] (Movie **7**).

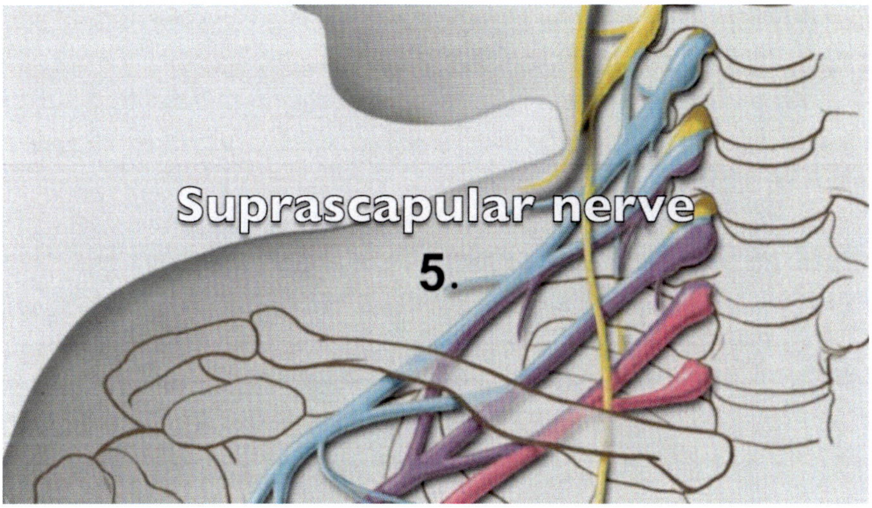

To view this movie click on this link:
https://raeducation.com/ebook

Movie 7: Percutaneous electrical stimulation of the suprascapular nerve.

THE AXILLARY NERVE

The axillary nerve arises in the axilla as the smaller of the two terminal divisions of the posterior cord of the brachial plexus (C5 and C6). It descends posterior to the axillary artery and anterior to the subscapularis muscle. It curves posteriorly through the quadrangular space, with the capsule of the shoulder joint above it, the surgical neck of the humerus laterally, the long head of triceps brachii medially, and the teres major below. The axillary nerve innervates the deltoid and teres minor muscles. Electrical stimulation, typically during infraclavicular or axillary nerve block, results in a motor response of these two muscles, most prominently and visibly of the deltoid muscle [1]. The sensory neurotome innervated by the axillary nerve is depicted in Fig. (**4**).

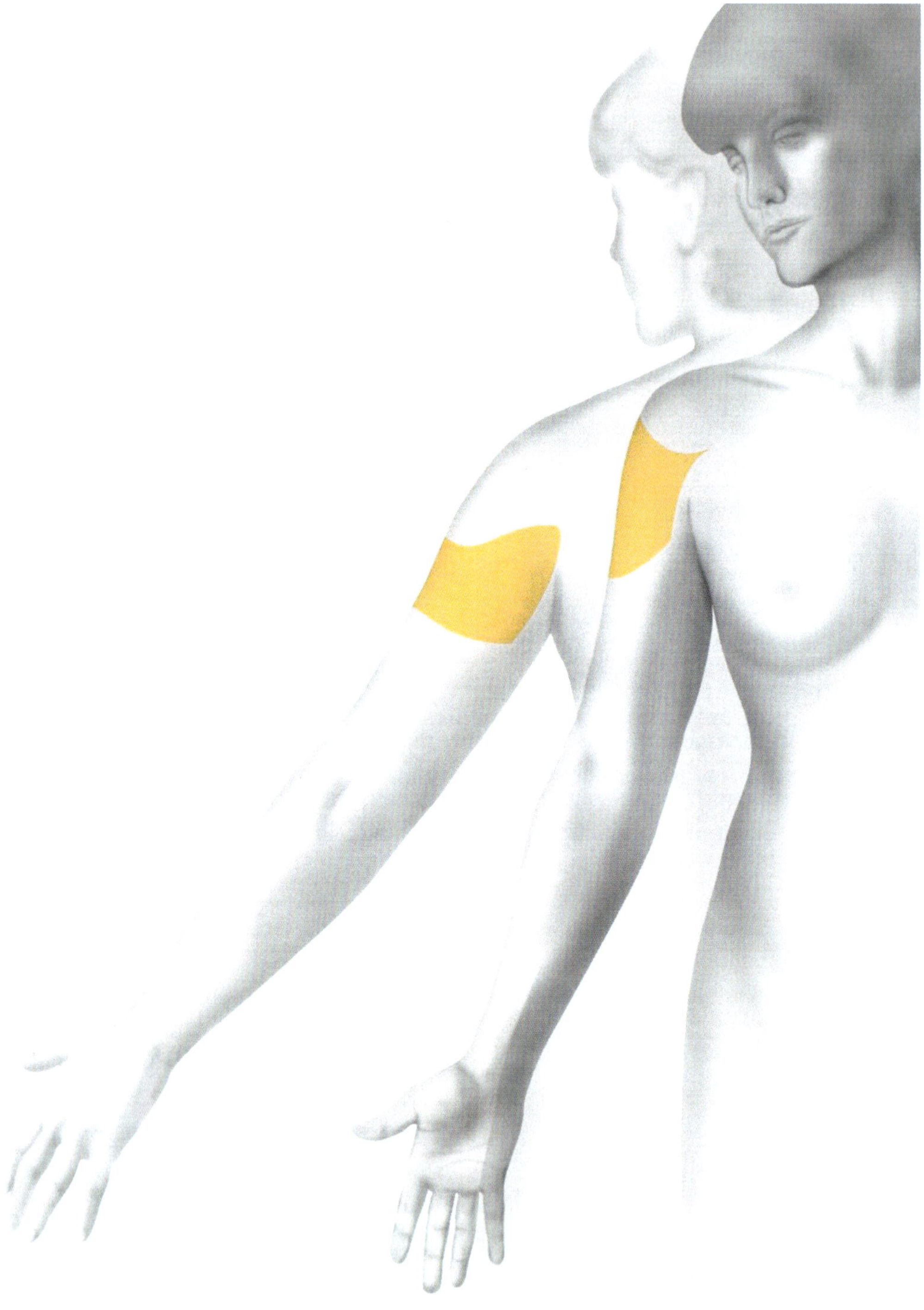

Figure 4: Sensory neurotomal innervation of the axillary nerve: the so-called "sergeant's patch."

THE RADIAL NERVE

The radial nerve is the largest terminal branch of the brachial plexus and arises from the posterior cord (C5, C6, C7, and C8). From its origin on the posterior axillary wall, it descends behind the axillary artery to enter the axilla (see Chapters 6 and 8). The motor innervations of this nerve are depicted in Fig. (**5**) and electrical stimulation of this nerve, typically during infraclavicular or axillary nerve block, causes motor responses in the extensor muscles of the arm and forearm [1] (Movie **8**). The sensory neurotomal innervation of the radial nerve is depicted in Fig. (**6**).

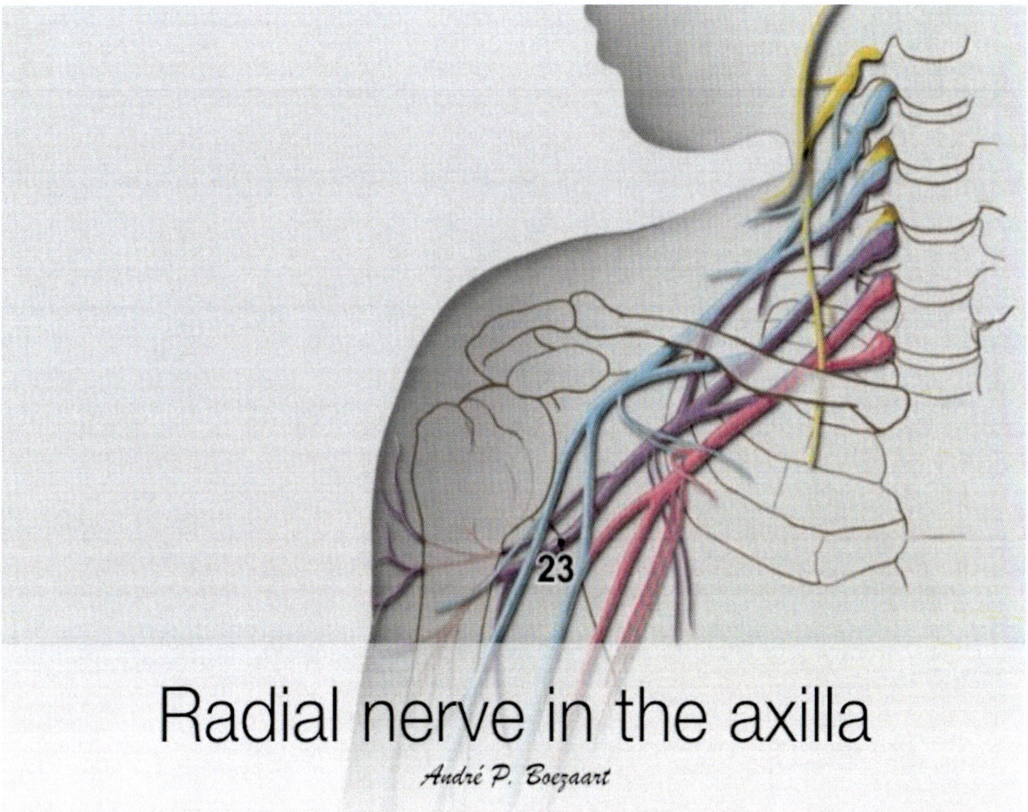

To view this movie click on this link:
https://raeducation.com/ebook

Movie 8: Percutaneous electrical stimulation of the radial nerve.

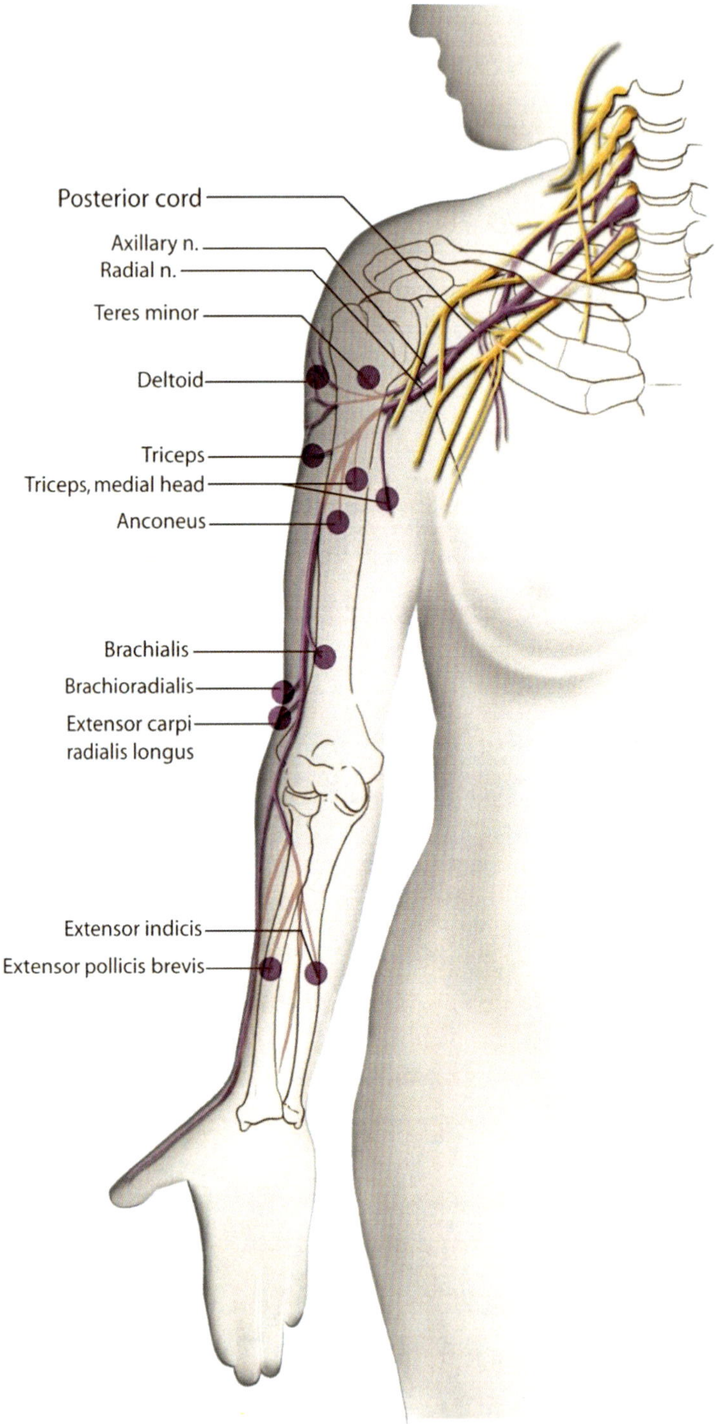

Figure 5: Schematic representation of the muscles innervated by the radial nerve.

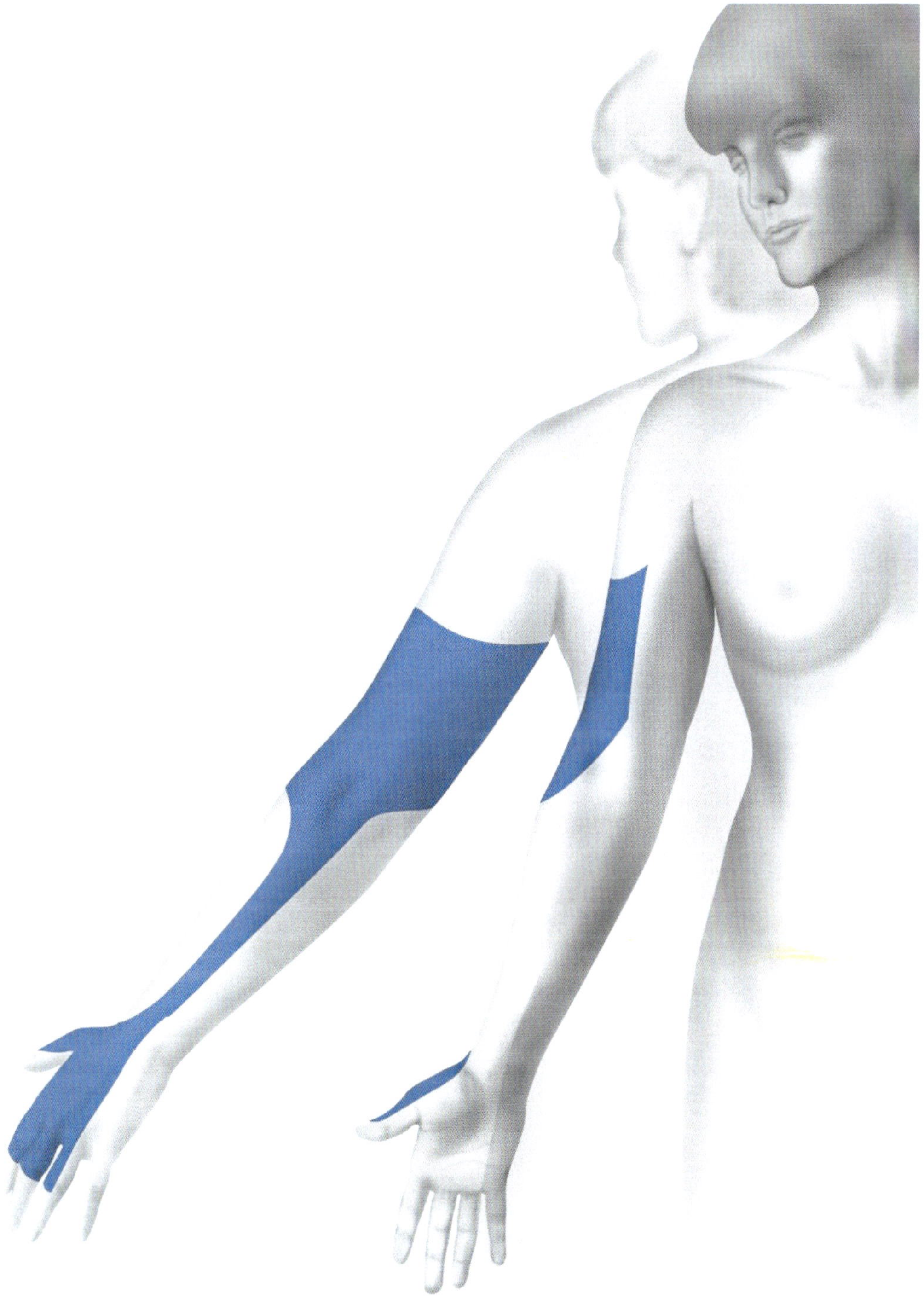

Figure 6: Sensory neurotomal innervation of the radial nerve.

THE ULNAR NERVE

The ulnar nerve is derived from the median cord of the brachial plexus (C8 and T1). In the axilla, it courses between the axillary artery and vein and remains between the brachial artery and vein (see Chapters 6 and 8). The motor innervations of the ulnar nerve are limited to the hand and are depicted in Fig. **7**, while the sensory neurotomal innervation is depicted in Fig. (**8**). Electrical stimulation of the ulnar nerve as typically seen during axillary nerve block would be flexion of the fingers [1] (Movie **9**).

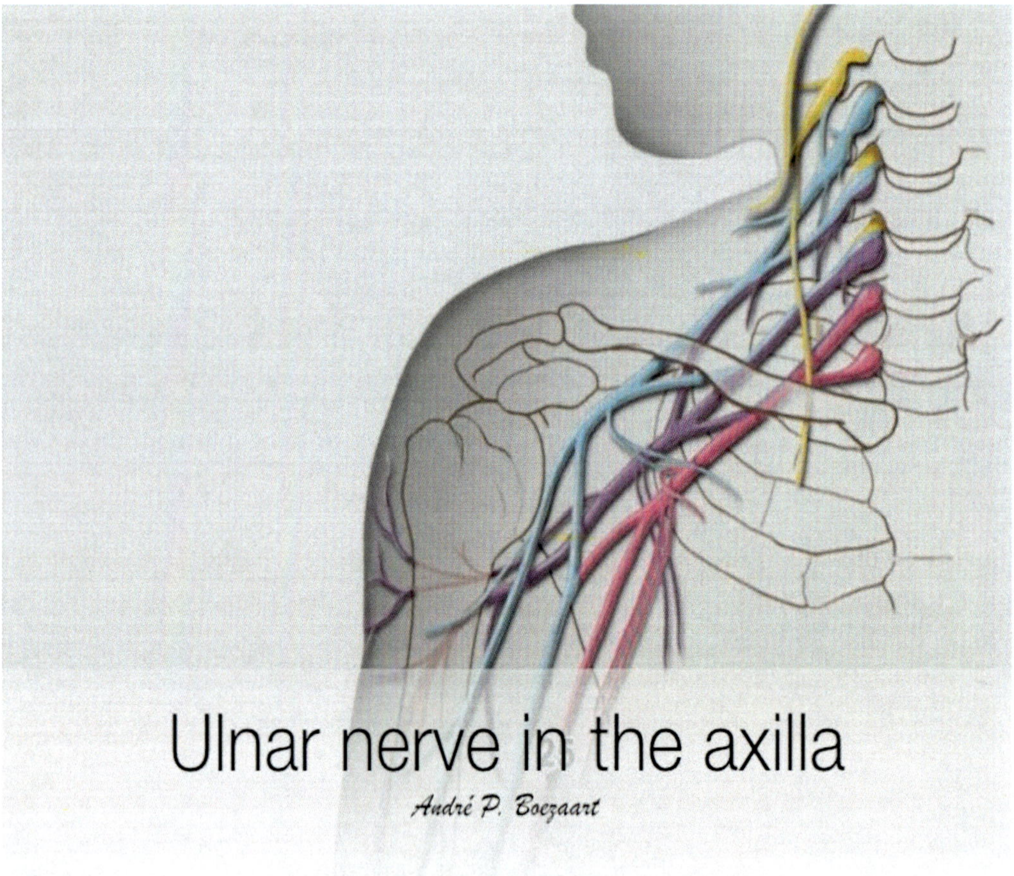

To view this movie click on this link:
https://raeducation.com/ebook

Movie 9: Percutaneous electrical stimulation of the ulnar nerve.

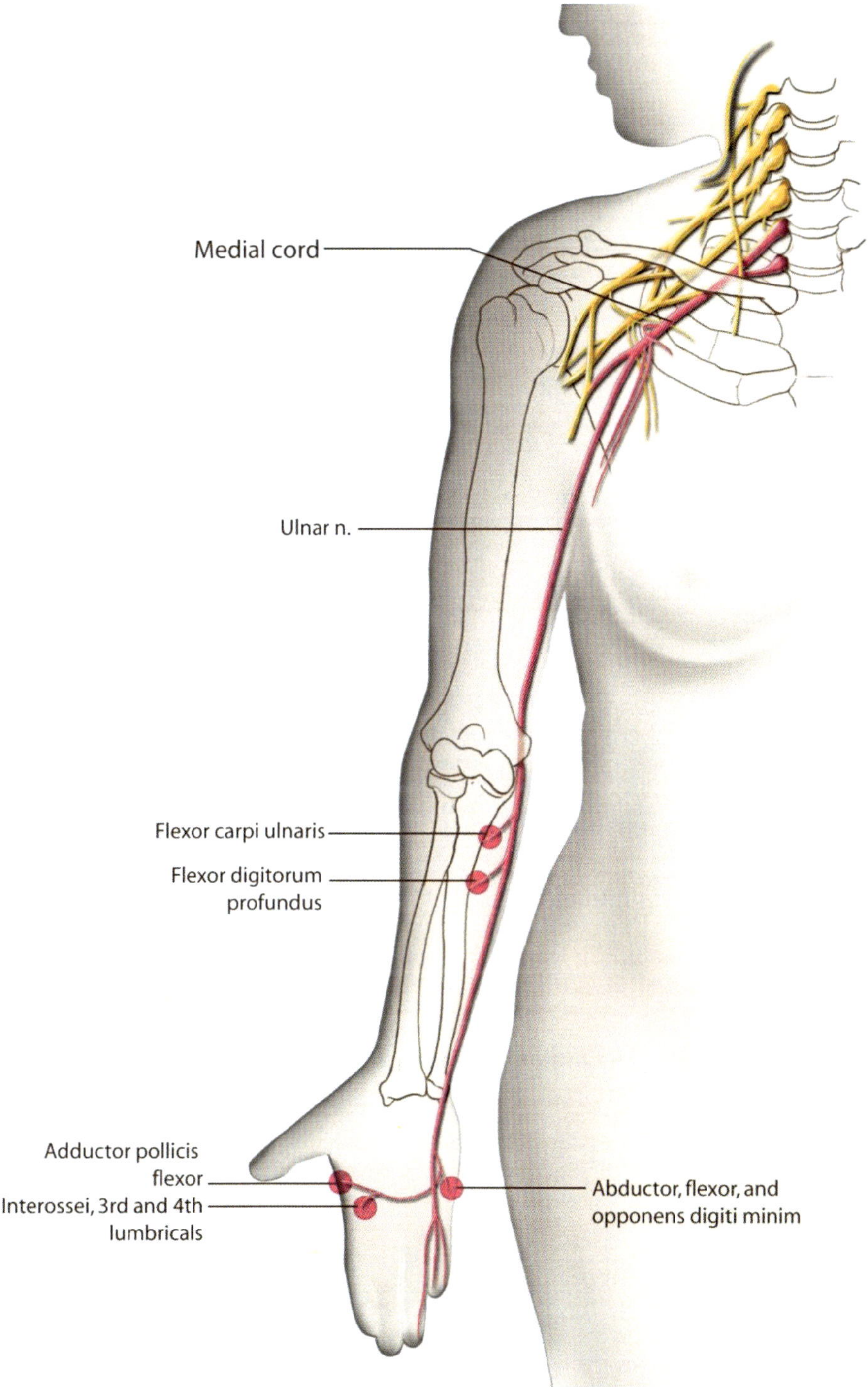

Figure 7: Schematic representation of the muscles innervated by the ulnar nerve.

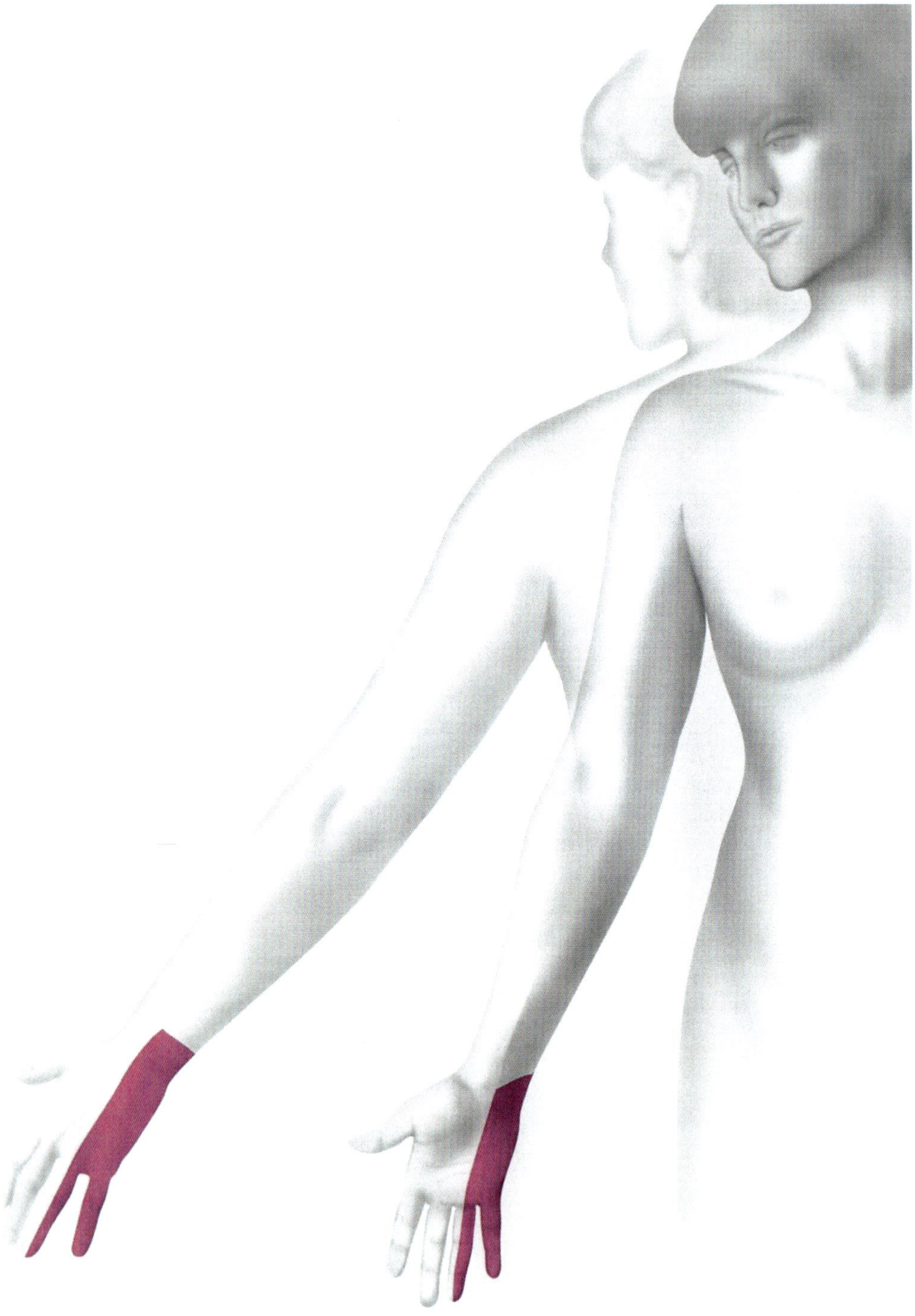

Figure 8: Sensory neurotomal innervation of the ulnar nerve.

THE MEDIAN NERVE

The median nerve is formed in the axilla from the medial (C8 and T1) and lateral cords (C5, C6, and C7) of the brachial plexus. The median nerve innervates muscles in the forearm and hand, as depicted in Fig. (**9**), and the sensory neurotomes are shown in Fig (**10**). Electrical stimulation of the median nerve as is typically seen during axillary nerve block would be pronation of the forearm and flexion of the wrist and fingers *via* the deep flexors of the fingers and flexion and abduction and opposition of the thumb [1] (Movie **10**).

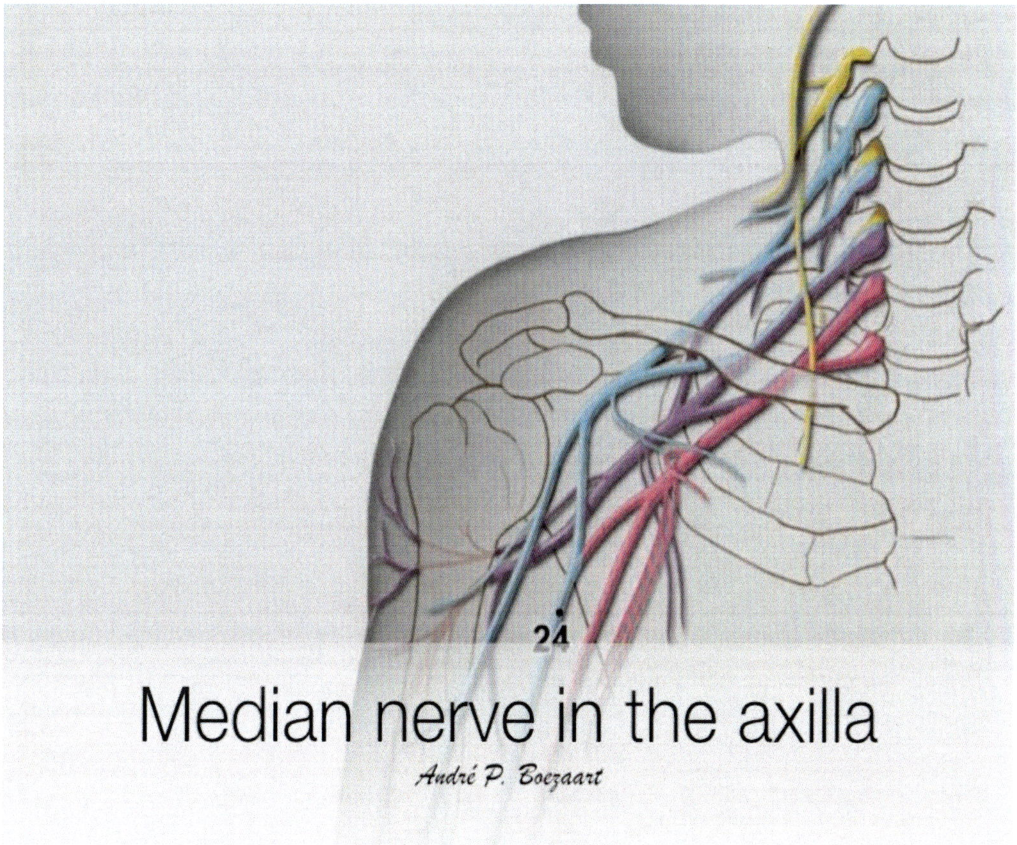

To view this movie click on this link:
https://raeducation.com/ebook

Movie 10: Percutaneous electrical stimulation of the median nerve.

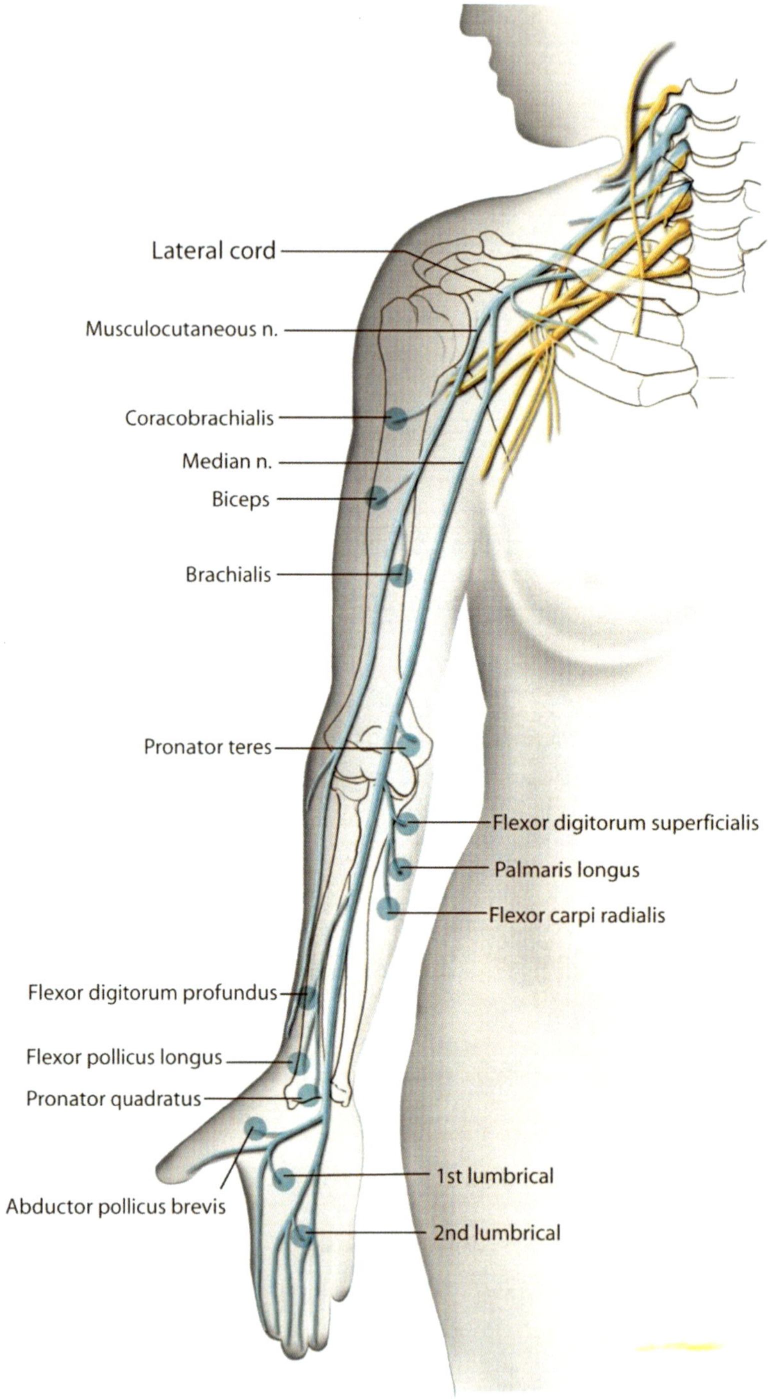

Figure 9: Schematic representation of the muscles innervated by the median and musculocutaneous nerves.

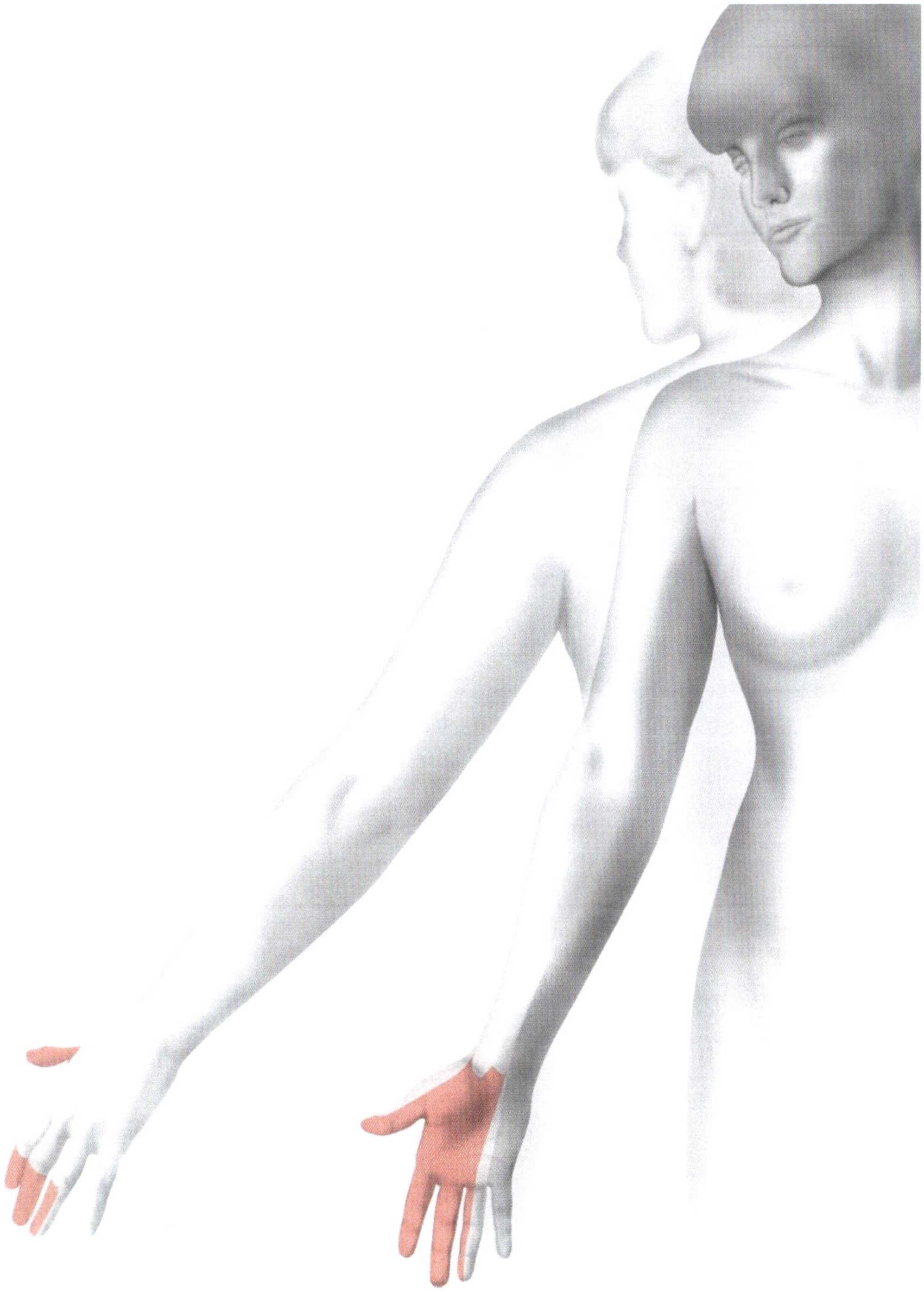

Figure 10: Sensory neurotomal innervation of the median nerve.

THE MUSCULOCUTANEOUS NERVE

The musculocutaneous nerve arises from the lateral cord of the brachial plexus (C5, C6, and occasionally C7). It comes off the lateral cord near the lower border of the major pectoral muscle and pierces the coracobrachialis muscle, which it innervates, to reach the interval between the brachialis and biceps muscles. It also innervates the latter muscle [1] (Movie **11**). Below the elbow, it pierces the deep fascia lateral to the tendon of the biceps brachii muscle and from there it continues as the posterior cutaneous nerve of the forearm. The sensory neurotomal innervation of the musculocutaneous nerve is shown in Fig. (**11**).

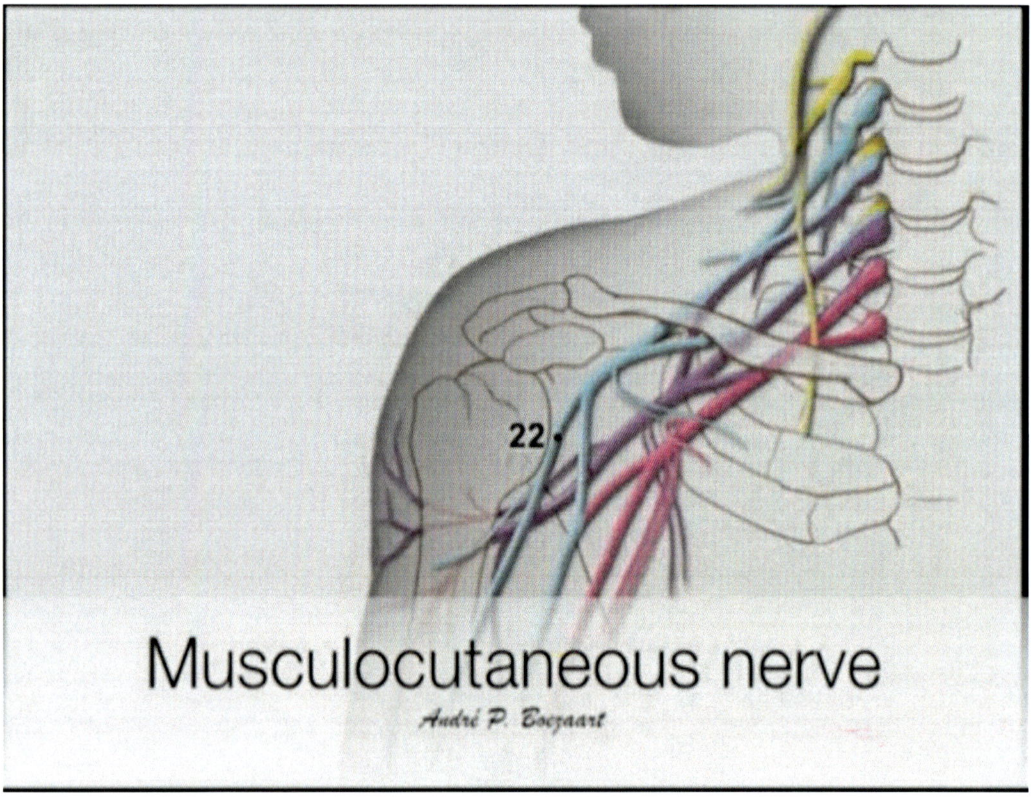

To view this movie click on this link:
https://raeducation.com/ebook

Movie 11: Percutaneous electrical stimulation of the musculocutaneous nerve.

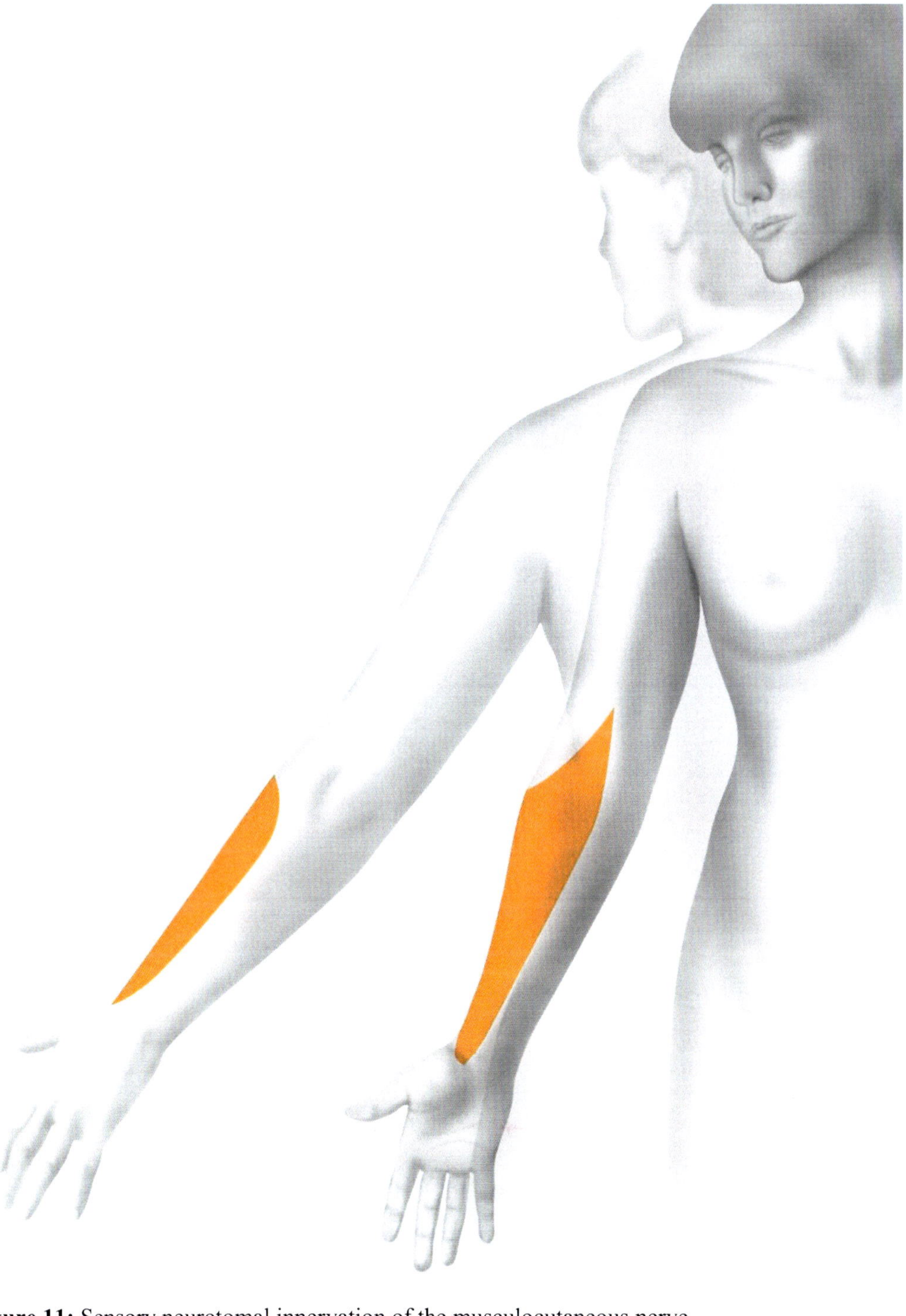

Figure 11: Sensory neurotomal innervation of the musculocutaneous nerve.

ACKNOWLEDGEMENTS

The author gratefully acknowledge the following people:

- The Head of the Department of Anesthesiology of the College of Medicine of the University of Florida, Dr. Tim Morey, and his department for their moral support and continuous encouragement.
- The faculty and fellows of the Division of Acute and Perioperative Pain Medicine of the above Department of Anesthesiology for affording the author the time to produce this work by covering his clinical duties.
- Corey Astrom of the Department of Anesthesiology of the College of Medicine of the University of Florida for her professional and high quality text editing.
- Mary K. Bryson for the body painting of the model, Kathy Fear CRNA (Iowa City).
- Nancy Hagen of the Iowa Public Radio for her narration of the movies.
- Raeducation.com LLC for their financial support.

CONFLICT OF INTEREST

The author confirms that this chapter contents have no conflict of Interest.

ABBREVIATIONS

MP = metacarpophalangeal

PIP = proximal interphalangeal

DIP = distal interphalangeal

IP = interphalangeal

REFERENCES

[1] Boezaart AP, Franco CD. Blocks above the clavicle. In: Boezaart AP, Ed. Anesthesia and orthopaedic surgery. New York: McGraw-Hill, 2006; pp. 291-309.
[2] Bösenberg AT, Raw R, Boezaart AP. Surface mapping of peripheral nerves in children with a nerve stimulator. Paediatr Anaesth 2002; 12: 398-403.
[3] Borene SC, Rosenquist RW, Koorn R, Haider N, Boezaart AP. An indication for continuous cervical paravertebral block (posterior approach to the interscalene space). Anesth Analg 2003; 97: 898-900.
[4] Leis AA, Trapani VC. Atlas of electromyography. Cambridge, UK: Oxford University Press, 2000; pp. 95-105.

Chapter 10:
Applied Macroanatomy of the Anterior Thigh

CHAPTER 10

Applied Macroanatomy of the Anterior Thigh

André P. Boezaart*

Departments of Anesthesiology and Orthopaedic Surgery and Rehabilitation, Division of Acute and Perioperative Pain Medicine, University of Florida College of Medicine, Gainesville, Florida, USA

Abstract: There are four areas of interest to the regional anesthesiologist and acute pain physician in the anterior thigh. These include three nerves and their branches and one specific area. These nerves are the femoral nerve with its seven branches, the obturator nerve with its two branches, and the lateral cutaneous nerve of the thigh. The adductor canal is the anatomical area of interest, as an adductor canal block, although much debated and its true value questioned, has been popularized in recent years. These nerves and their areas of sensory distributions and the adductor canal are discussed in this chapter. A fourth nerve, the genitofemoral nerve, and more specifically, its femoral branch, also features in this area and is discussed in this chapter.

Keywords: Acute pain medicine, Adductor canal, Adductor canal block, Adductor muscles, Anterior thigh, Femoral nerve, Genitofemoral nerve., Lateral cutaneous nerve of the thigh, Nerve to sartorius, Obturator nerve, Quadriceps muscles, Rectus femoris, Regional anesthesiologist, Saphenous nerve, Sartorius muscle, Subsartorial plexus, Subsartorial space, Vastus intermedius, Vastus lateralis, Vastus medialis.

INTRODUCTION

In this chapter, we will discuss the macroanatomy of the femoral, the obturator and saphenous nerves, and the lateral cutaneous nerve of the thigh. The anatomy of the adductor canal and sensory innervation of the knee and hip joint will also be discussed.

As a good understanding of anatomy is essential for performing any regional anesthesia technique or invasive procedure for regional anesthesia or acute pain medical condition, it follows that one must understand the most fundamental principle of successful acute or perioperative pain control by regional anesthesia,

***Corresponding author André P. Boezaart:** Departments of Anesthesiology and Orthopaedic Surgery, Division of Acute and Peri-operative Pain Medicine, University of Florida College of Medicine, 1600 SW Archer Road, Gainesville, Florida 32610, USA; Tel: 352-846-0913 (Work); Fax: 352-392-7029; E-mail: aboezaart@anest.ufl.edu

namely, Hilton's Law of Anatomy [1]. The principles behind Hilton's Law were first espoused in a series of medical lectures given by John Hilton between 1860 and 1862 [1]. John Hilton (1808-1878) was a British surgeon born in Essex (UK) in 1805. He was appointed demonstrator of anatomy in 1828 at Guy's Hospital and assistant surgeon in 1845; he was appointed surgeon four years later. Ten years later, he became Professor of Anatomy and Surgery at the Royal College of Surgeons. From 1859 to 1862, he presented a series of lectures in the form of a course on "Rest and Pain" [1]. The "Law of Anatomy," which has now reached classical status, was revisited and challenged in 2013 using modern technology [2] and was found to be as sound as it was in 1860.

Hilton's Law of Anatomy states: "The same trunks of nerves whose branches supply the groups of muscles moving a joint furnish also a distribution of nerves to the skin over the insertions of the same muscles; and—what at this moment more especially merits our attention—the interior of the joint receives its nerves from the same source" [2].

Upon reflection, we realize that to move any of the joints of the lower limb, all of the muscles around that specific joint are involved. Furthermore, the skin overlying that area receives sensory innervation from branches of the lumbosacral plexus. Because of these two facts, we know that to effectively block painful stimuli from any of the joints of the lower limb, we have to block the entire lumbosacral plexus. In their paper on revisiting Hilton's Law of Anatomy, Marie-Noëlle Hébert-Blouin and colleagues [2] pointed out certain exceptions to this rule, of which the rectus femoris is the most glaring example. While the rectus femoris forms part of the quadriceps group of muscles that move the knee joint, the branch of the femoral nerve that supplies motor innervation to this muscle does not supply sensory innervation to the knee joint, but only to the hip joint, which the rectus femoris muscle also moves. In defense of Hilton's Law, if one reads the law carefully, it does not say "muscle" but "group of muscles." Therefore, the Law remains applicable because the quadriceps group of muscles moves the knee joint, and to provide analgesia to the knee joint, all the nerves to the quadriceps group of muscles must be blocked.

A common misunderstanding that needs our attention is that if, for example, 60% of the nerves that supply sensory innervation to a joint are blocked, the pain generated from that joint would be 60% less. Through the lessons we have learned over the years, especially in obstetric anesthesia where we have seen (and our unfortunate patients have experienced) the unpleasant consequences of unblocked segments or hemi-block with epidurals, and many other clinical scenarios, we now realize that blocking 60% of the nerves that innervate a joint does not reduce pain by 60%. In fact, it only focuses 100% of the pain into the remaining 40% of the joint, therefore, in fact, worsening the pain and suffering of the patient. Although well intended, it is probably not true that we are doing anything positive for the patient by blocking "some" of the nerves and therefore removing "some" of the pain. Disbelief in this misunderstanding, however, is based on clinical experience; it has yet to be challenged by formal research.

Simply put, to provide optimal pain relief due to major surgery or trauma to a joint in the lower extremity, the entire lumbosacral plexus must be blocked. Granted, this is not always possible, especially where the plexus is spread out, as is the case with the lumbosacral plexus. It is especially difficult to achieve during a continuous nerve block, where the catheter is placed on one specific part of the plexus; for example, the lumbar plexus during a continuous lumbar plexus block for pain associated with major knee surgery. When the primary block (high-volume and high-concentration initial block) wears off, the secondary block often fails because the other roots are not close enough or are not in the same circumneural (paraneural) space [3] (see Chapter 2, Fig. **1**) to allow the local anesthetic agent (of too low a volume and concentration) to diffuse to all of the nerve axons of the other more distant roots. Thus, complete coverage of the pain is not achieved (see Microanatomy, Chapters 2, 11, and 14).

It is also not always necessary to block all the nerves that innervate a specific joint. Most of the nerves that innervate a joint reach that joint *via* its joint capsule and during hip replacement surgery or perhaps synovectomy, for example, the joint capsule is destroyed by the surgery, which in effect denervates the joint, making it necessary to block only the nerves that supply sensory innervation to the tissue outside the joint capsule.

MACROANATOMY

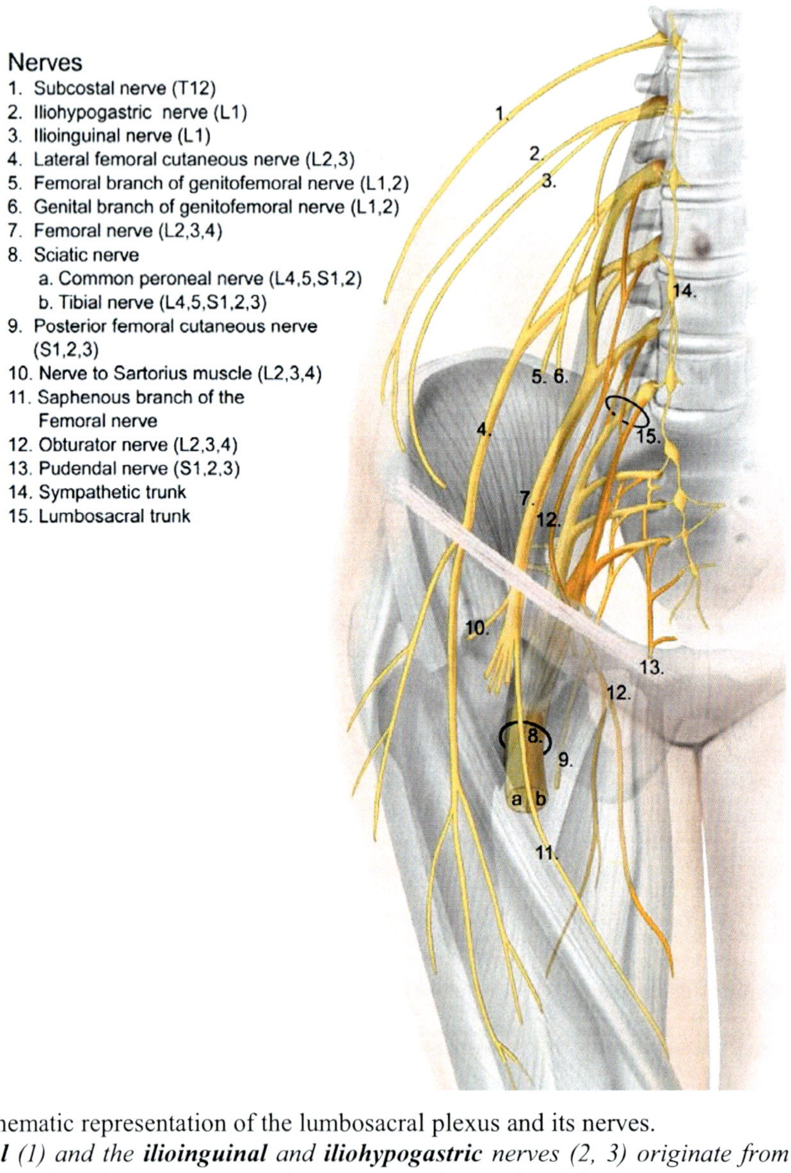

Figure 1: Schematic representation of the lumbosacral plexus and its nerves.
The ***subcostal*** *(1) and the* ***ilioinguinal*** *and* ***iliohypogastric*** *nerves (2, 3) originate from the 12th thoracic (T12) and 1st lumbar (L1) vertebra, respectively. The lateral cutaneous nerve of the thigh (4), and the femoral (5) and genital (6) branches of the genitofemoral nerve originate from the ventral rami of the 2nd and 3rd lumbar vertebrae (L2 and L3), whereas the femoral nerve (7) stems from the dorsal rami of L2, L3, and L4. The 5th lumbar spinal root also gives of a branch to the lumbosacral trunk (15) at the level of L5. The anterior rami of L2 to L4 form the obturator nerve (12), whereas L5 and the first three sacral roots (S1, S2, and S3) form the sciatic nerve. The pudendal nerve also springs from these roots.*

Each lumbar and sacral spinal root of the lumbosacral plexus has its own sensory dermatomal area that it represents (Fig. **2**), as well as its own osteotomal area (Fig. **3**).

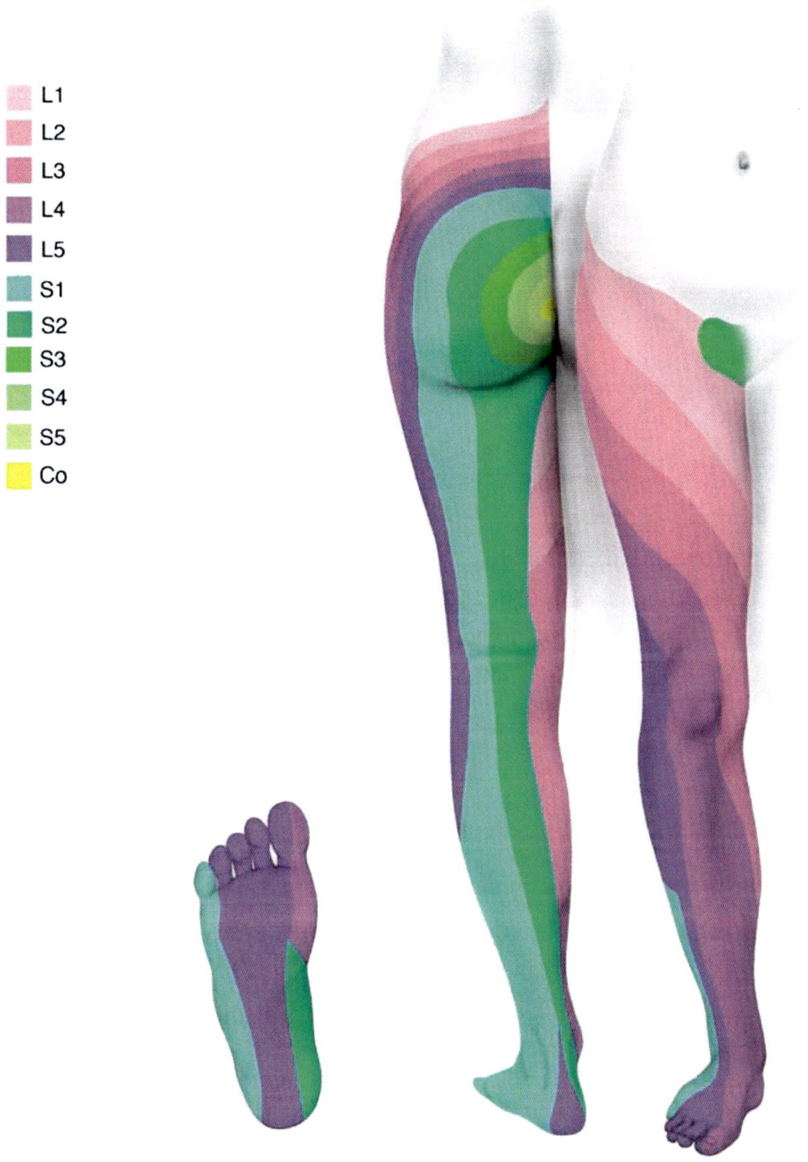

Figure 2: Schematic demarcation of the dermatomes of the lower limb.
These demarcations are not distinct segments as depicted here because there is significant overlap between adjacent dermatomes. L1, L2, L3, L4, and L5 = lumbar roots L2 to L5; S1, S2, S3, S4, and S5 = sacral spinal roots S1 and 2; Co = coccyx.

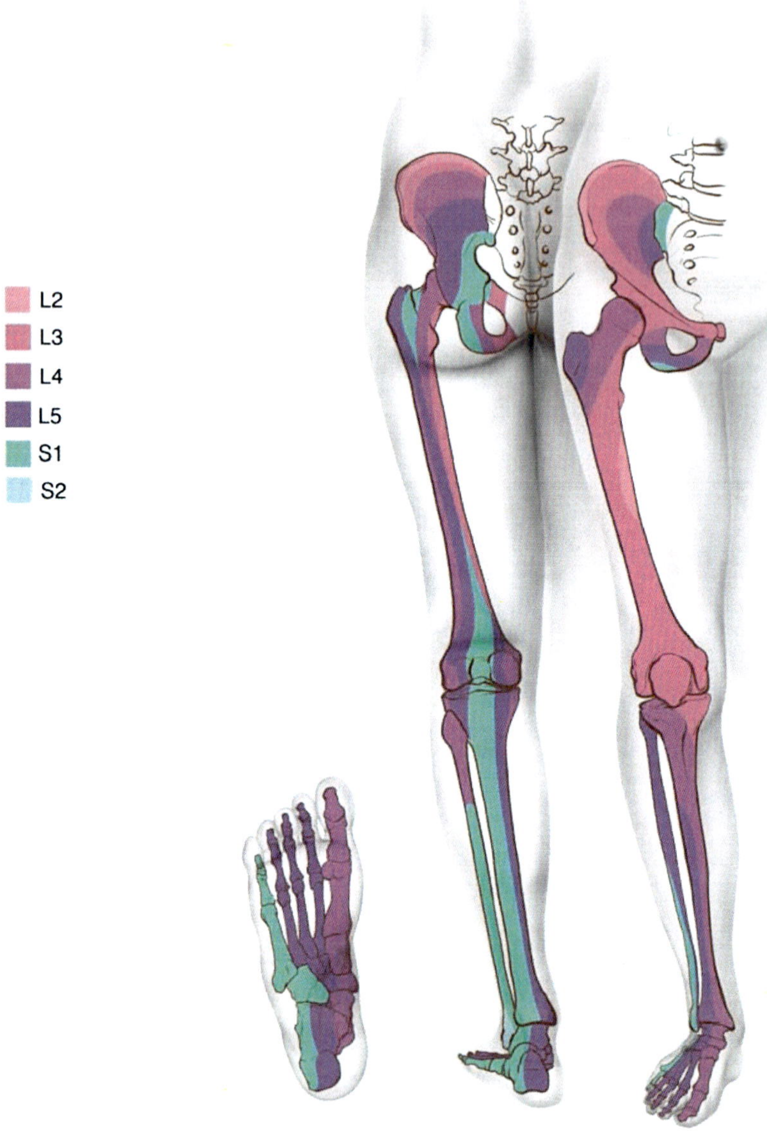

Figure 3: Schematic demarcation of the osteotomes of the lower limb.
These demarcations are not distinct segments as depicted here because there is significant overlap between adjacent osteotomes. L2, L3, L4, and L5 = lumbar roots L2 to L5; S1, S2 = sacral spinal roots S1 and S2.

Although the lumbar and sacral spinal roots represent corresponding sensory dermatomes and osteotomes, the individual peripheral nerves innervate different areas of the lower limb, represented by neurotomes (Fig. **4**).

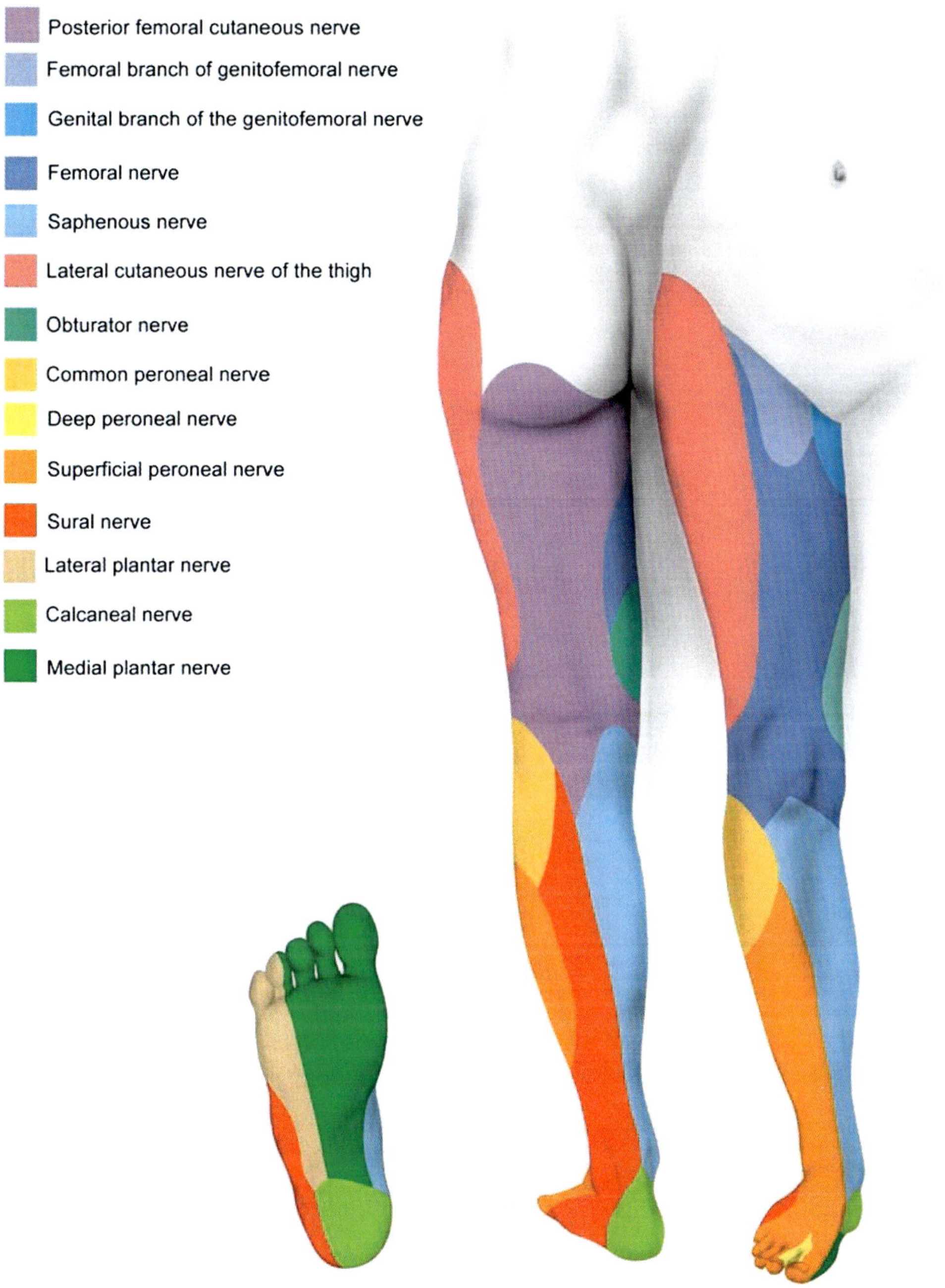

Figure 4: Schematic demarcation of the neurotomes of the upper limb.
These demarcations are not distinct areas as depicted here because there is significant overlap between adjacent neurotomes.

The anatomical dissections depicted in Figs. **5**, **6** and **7** represent the abdominal and pelvic views of the femoral, obturator, and lateral cutaneous nerves of the thigh, while Fig. **8** depicts the trans-sectional view at the level of the inguinal groove.

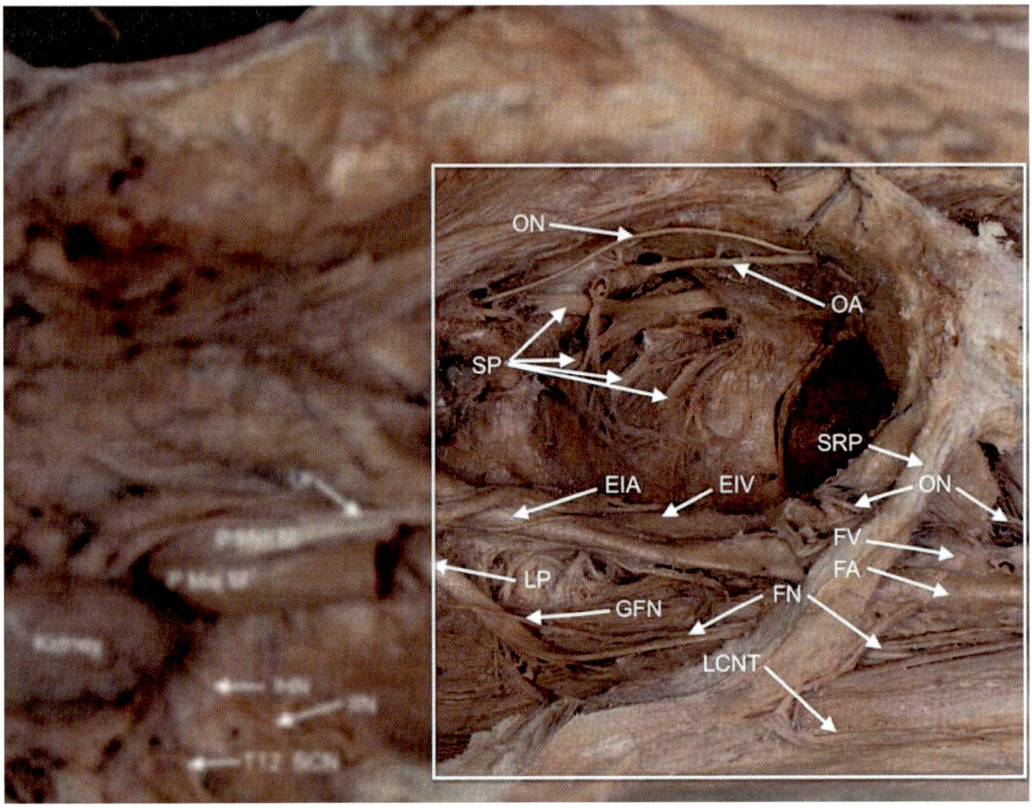

Figure 5: Anatomical dissection of femoral, obturator, and lateral cutaneous nerves of the thigh: abdominal view.
LP = lumbar plexus; SP = sacral plexus; EIA = external iliac artery; EIV = external iliac vein; OA = obturator artery; FA = femoral artery; FV = femoral vein; GFN = genitofemoral nerve; ON = obturator nerve; FN = femoral nerve; LCNT = lateral cutaneous nerve of the thigh; SRP = superior ramus of the pubis.

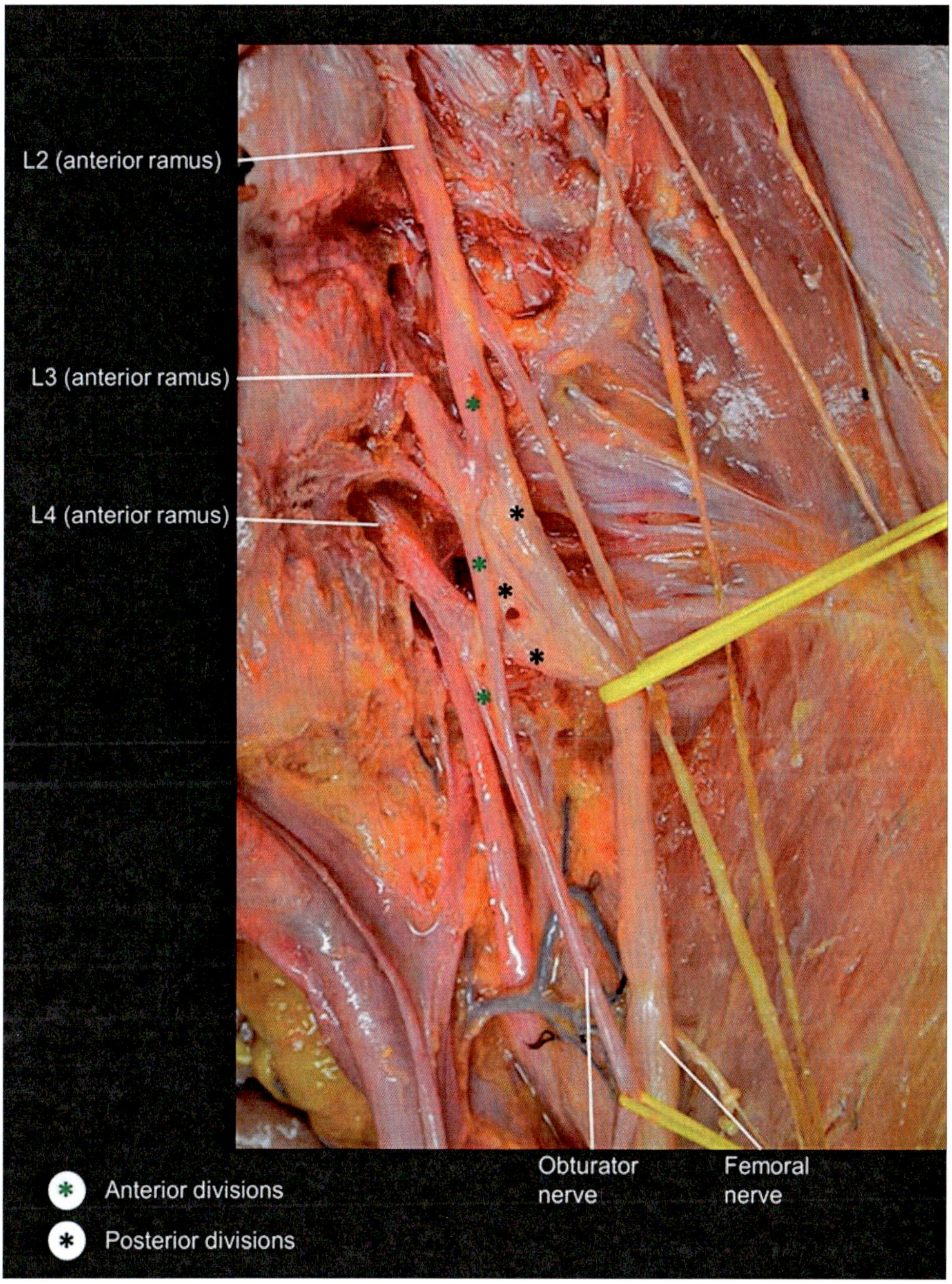

Figure 6: Anatomy of the obturator and femoral nerves: abdominal view.
The anterior and posterior divisions of the lumbar plexus are shown. The anterior divisions merge to form the obturator nerve, whereas the posterior gives rise to the formation of the femoral nerve and lateral cutaneous nerve of the thigh. (Reprinted from Reina, Carrera, Llusé, et al. [4] with permission).

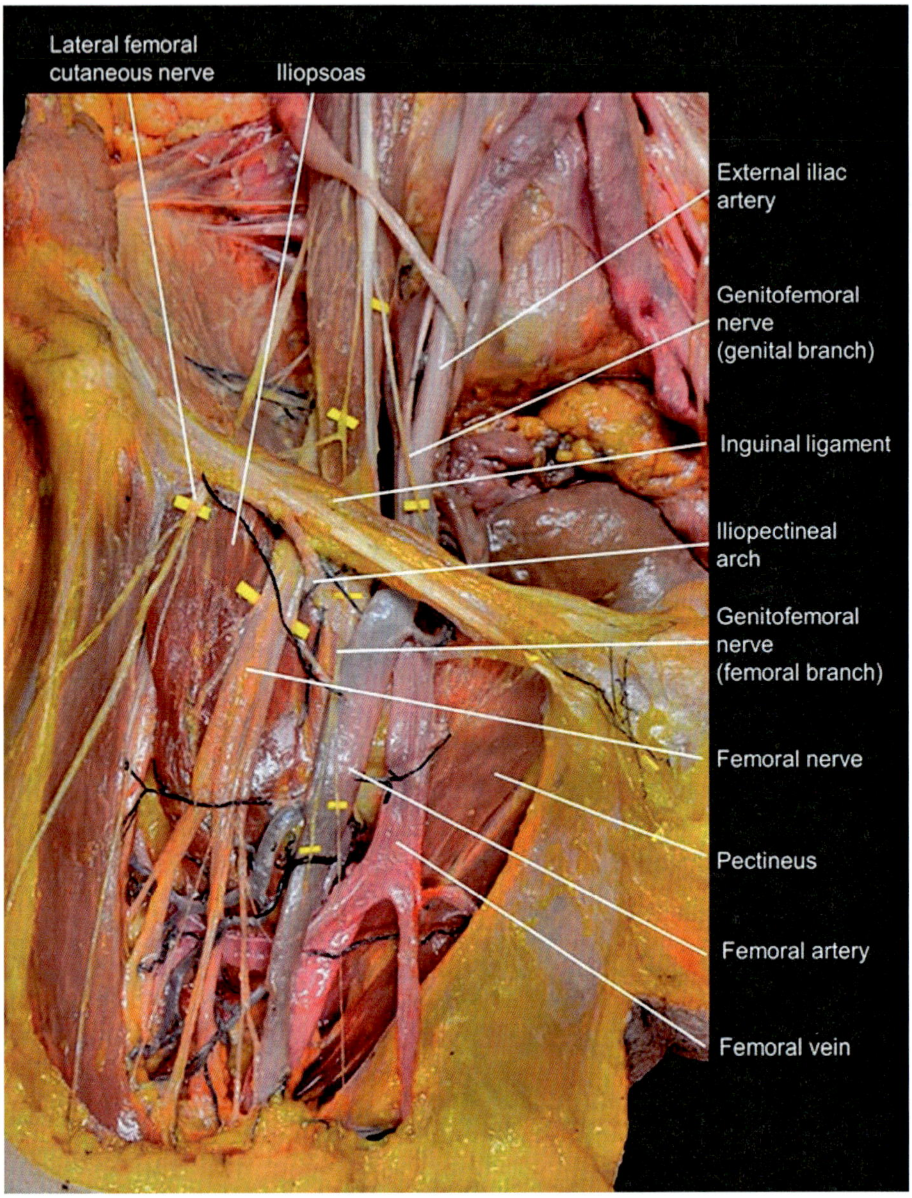

Figure 7: Anatomy of the femoral nerve and lateral cutaneous nerve of the thigh.
This view in the region of the inguinal groove is where a femoral nerve block is usually performed. The femoral nerve gives rise to the branches to the four quadriceps muscles, and the pectinius and sartorius muscles. It also gives off branches that supply sensory innervation to the skin on the medial side of the thigh and leg (saphenous) and the hip joint. In this figure, the lateral cutaneous nerve of the thigh (LCNT), the femoral branch of the genitofemoral nerve, the ilioinguinal nerve, and the genital branch of the genitofemoral nerve can be seen. (Reprinted from Reina, Carrera, Llusá, et al. [4] with permission)

TRANS-SECTIONAL VIEW

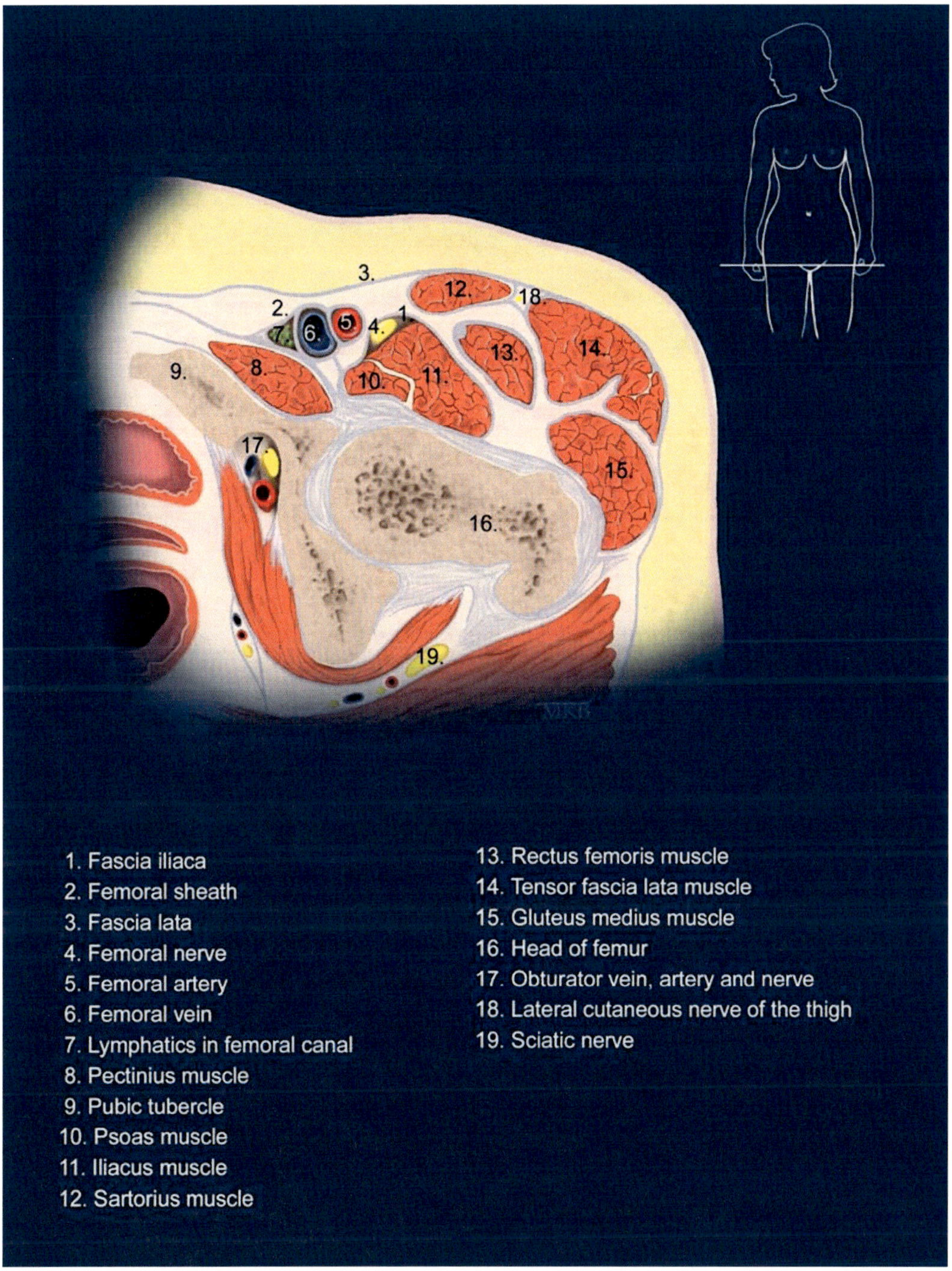

Figure 8: Trans-sectional view at the level of the inguinal groove.

THE FEMORAL NERVE

Surface Anatomy

The surface anatomy of the femoral nerve as is commonly used for femoral nerve block is outlined in Fig. **9**.

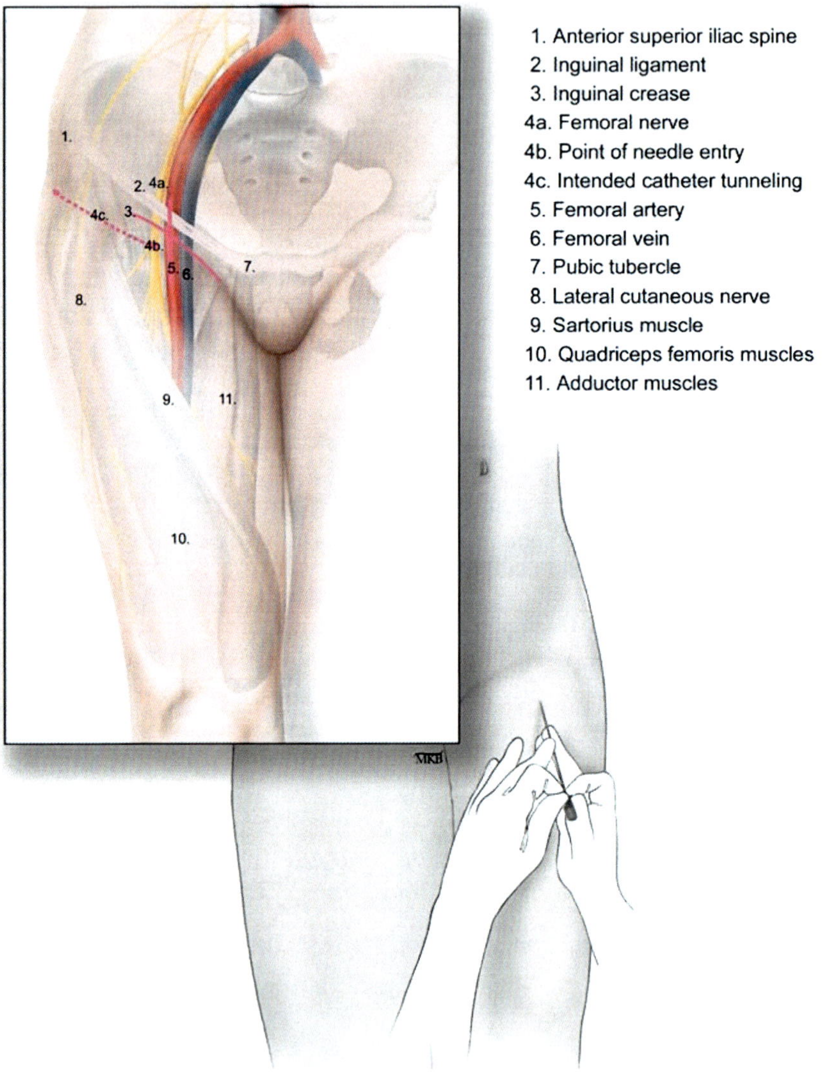

Figure 9: Surface anatomy of the femoral nerve.
The femoral crease (3) and the femoral artery (5) are marked. A point approximately 1 cm caudad and 1 cm lateral of where these lines cross marks to position of the femoral nerve (4a, 4b).

Neurotomes

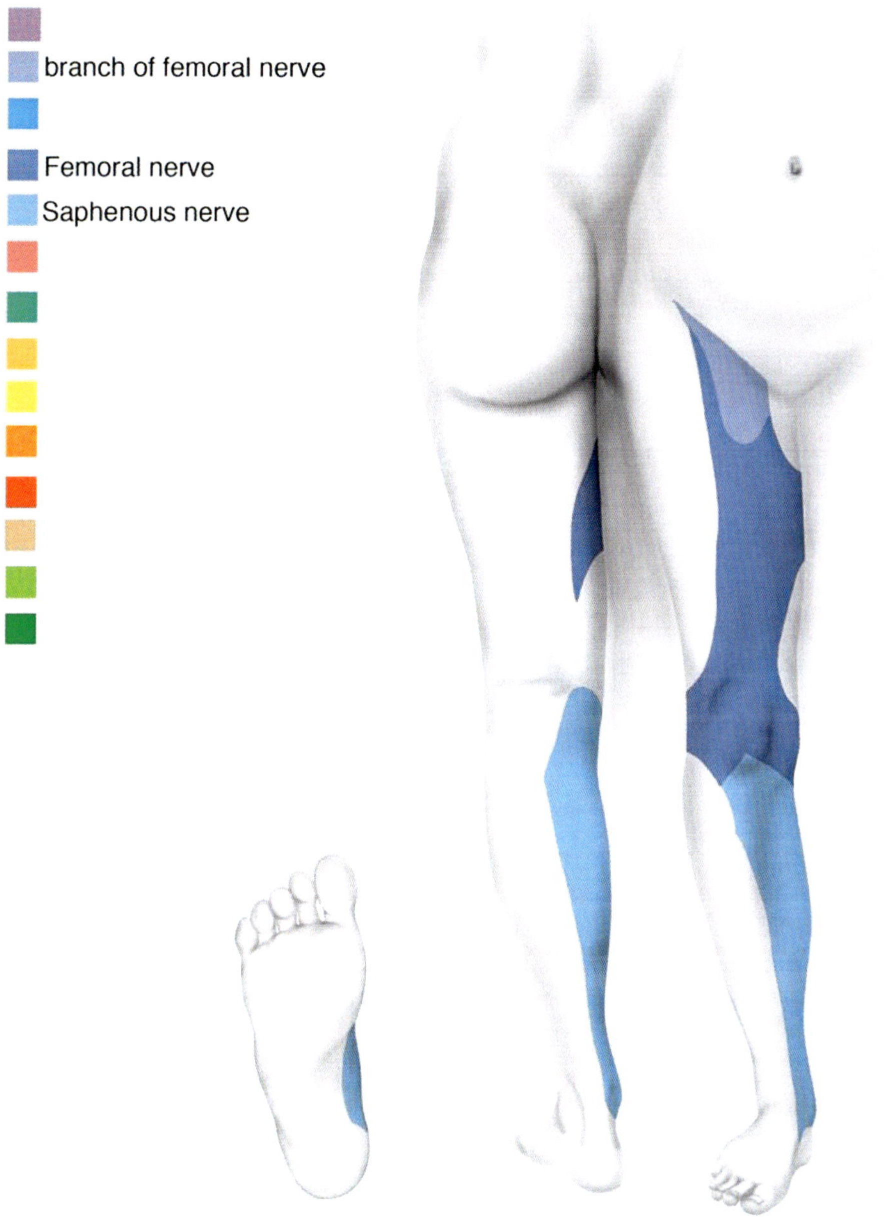

Figure 10: Schematic demarcation of the neurotomes of the lower limb innervated by the femoral nerve and its branches.
*These demarcations as depicted in Fig. **10** are not distinct areas because there is significant overlap between adjacent neurotomes.*

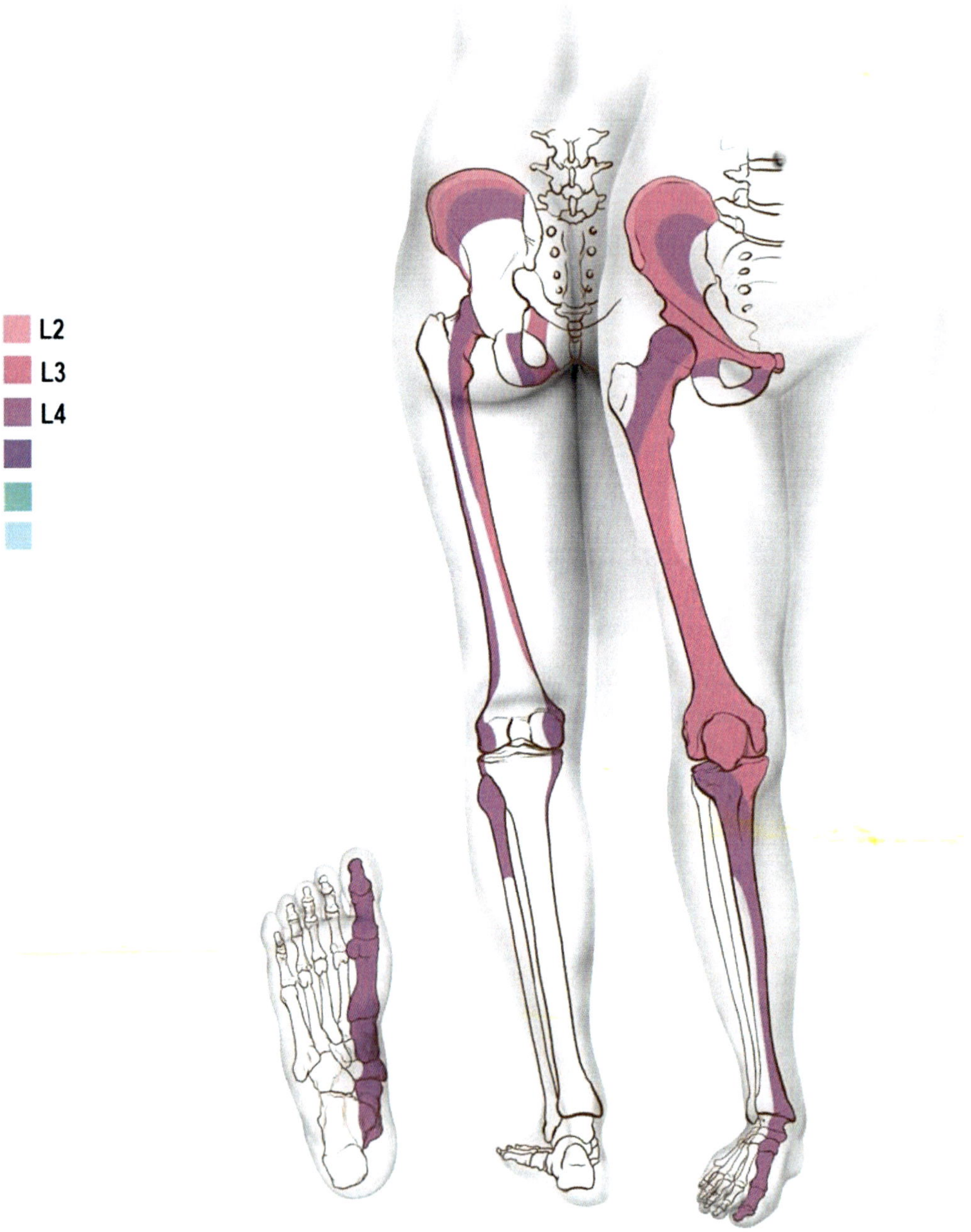

Figure 11: Schematic demarcation of the osteotomes of the lower limb innervated by the femoral nerve and its branches.
These demarcations depicted in Fig. ***11*** *are not distinct areas because there is significant overlap between adjacent osteotomes.*

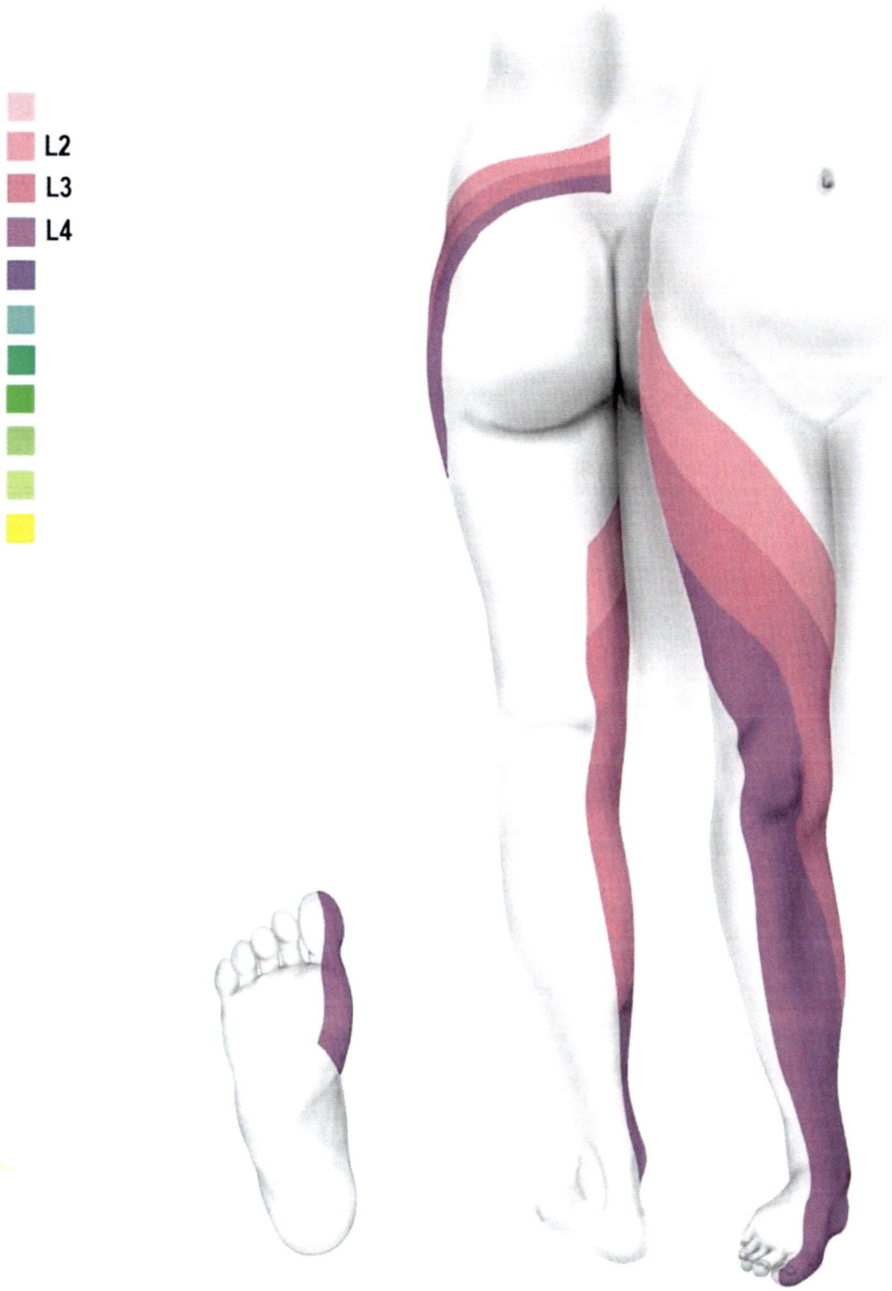

Figure 12: Schematic demarcation of the dermatomes of the lower limb innervated by the femoral nerve and its branches.
These demarcations depicted in Fig. ***12*** *are not distinct areas because there is significant overlap between adjacent dermatomes.*

THE OBTURATOR NERVE

The obturator nerve originates from the anterior rami of the 2nd, 3rd and 4th lumbar spinal roots and leaves the abdomen via the obturator foramen as depicted in the anatomical dissections of Figs. **13a & b**, while the neurotomes of the obturator nerve and lateral cutaneous nerve of the thigh are outlined in Figs. **14** and **15**.

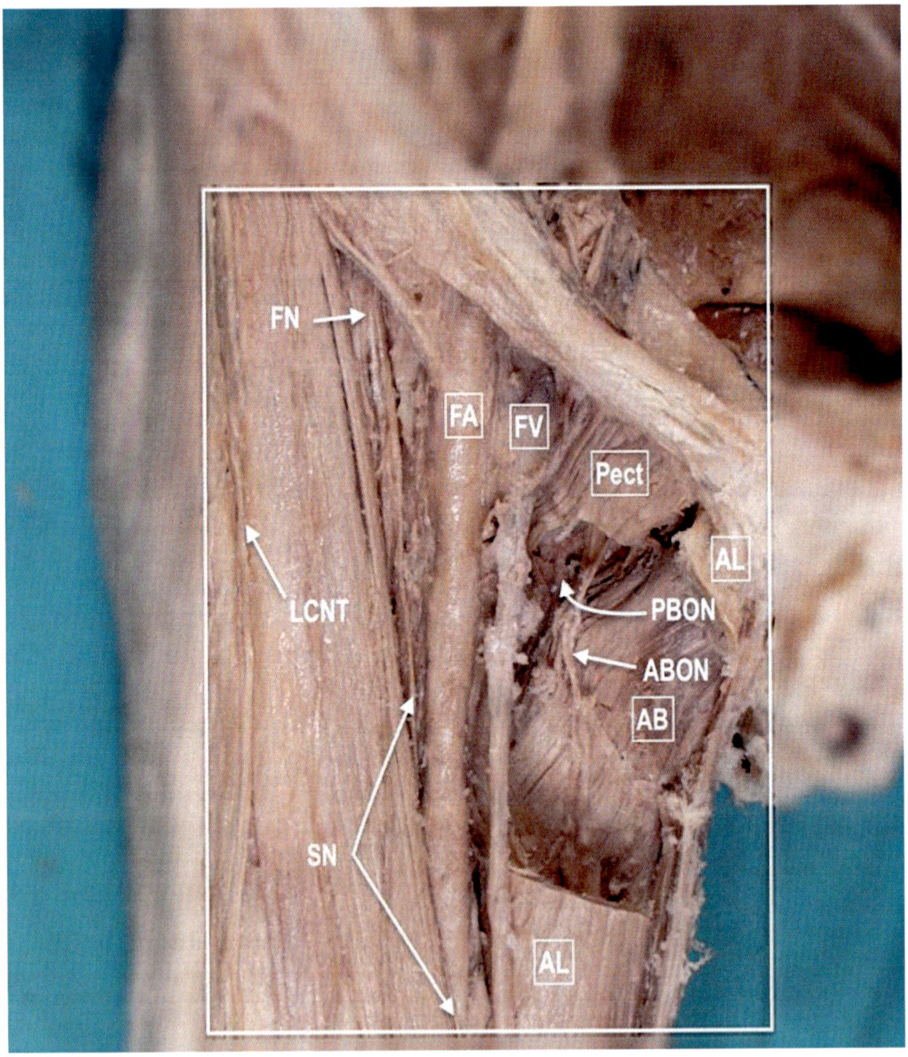

Figure 13a: Dissection of the upper thigh depicting the obturator nerve.
FA = femoral artery; FV = femoral vein; FN = femoral nerve; Pect = pectinius muscle; AL = adductor longus muscle (cut); AB = adductor brevis muscle; LCNT = lateral cutaneous nerve of the thigh; SN = saphenous nerve; ABON = anterior branch of the obturator nerve; PBON = posterior branch of the obturator nerve.

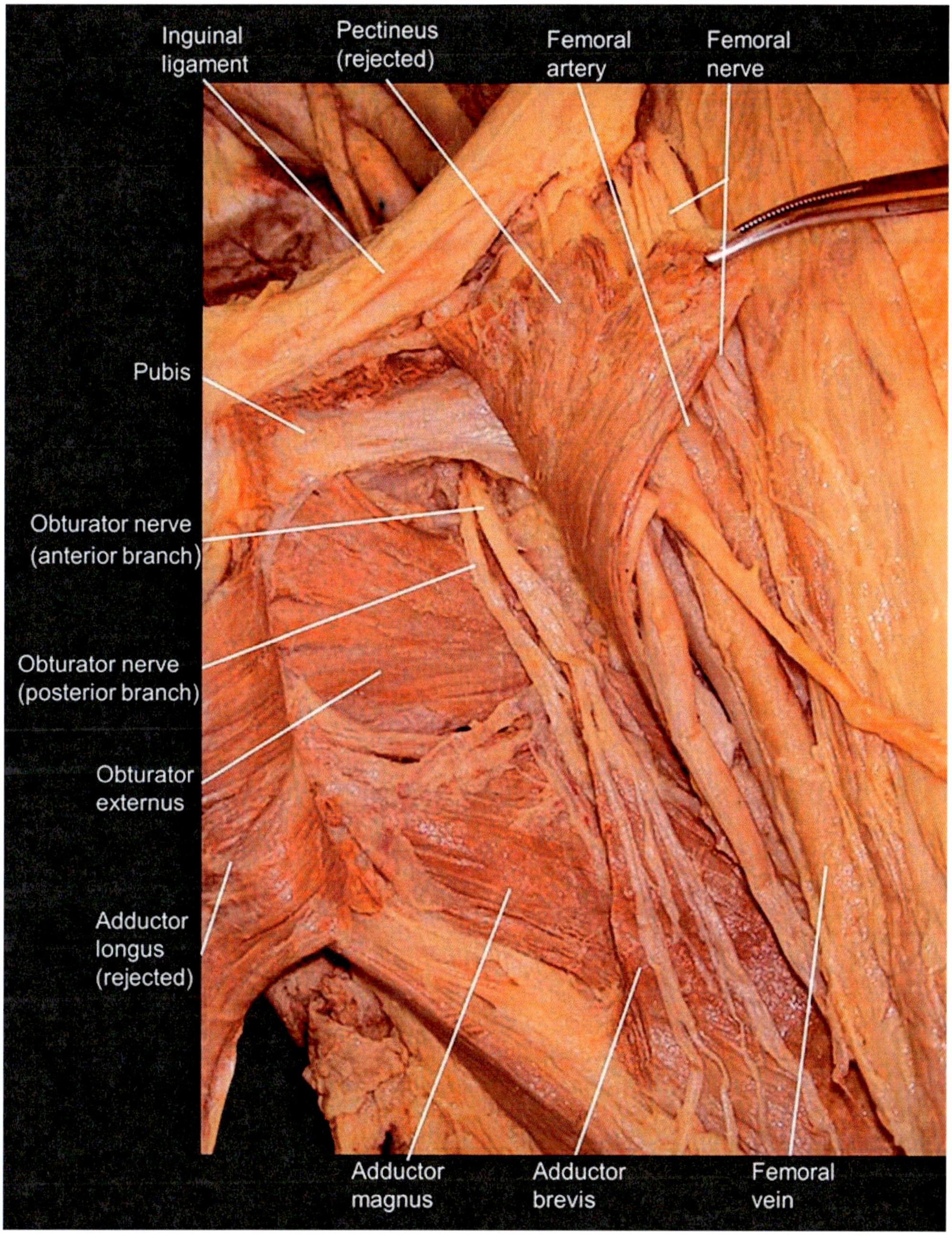

Figure 13b: Macroanatomy of the obturator nerve.
The obturator nerve exits the obturator foramen and then splits into an anterior and posterior branch. The anterior branch descends anterior to the adductor brevis muscle (cut), whereas the posterior branch descends between the adductor brevis and magnus muscles. (Reprinted from Reina, Carrera, Llusá, et al. [4] with permission).

Neurotomes

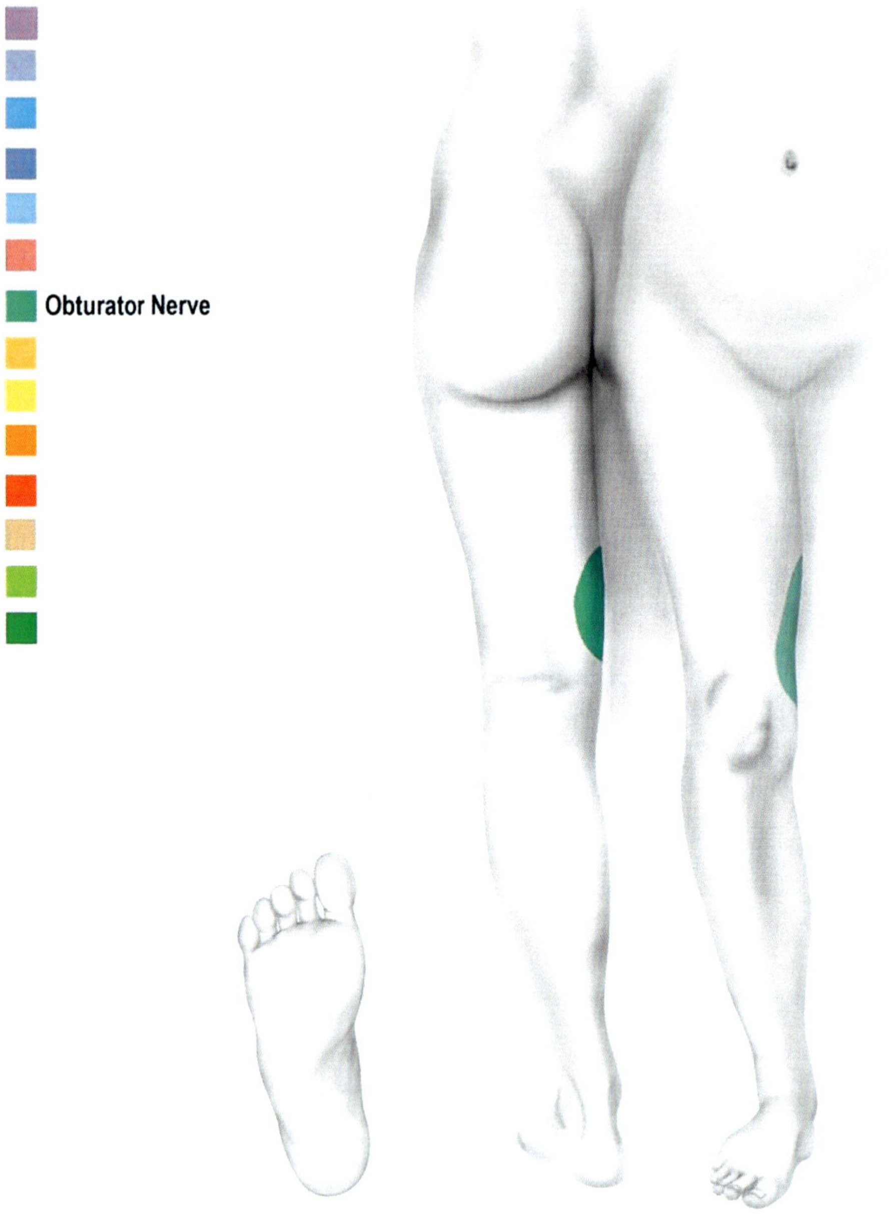

Figure 14: Schematic demarcation of the neurotome of the lower limb innervated by the obturator nerve.
These demarcations are not distinct areas as depicted here because there is significant overlap between adjacent neurotomes.

THE LATERAL CUTANEOUS NERVE OF THE THIGH

Neurotomes

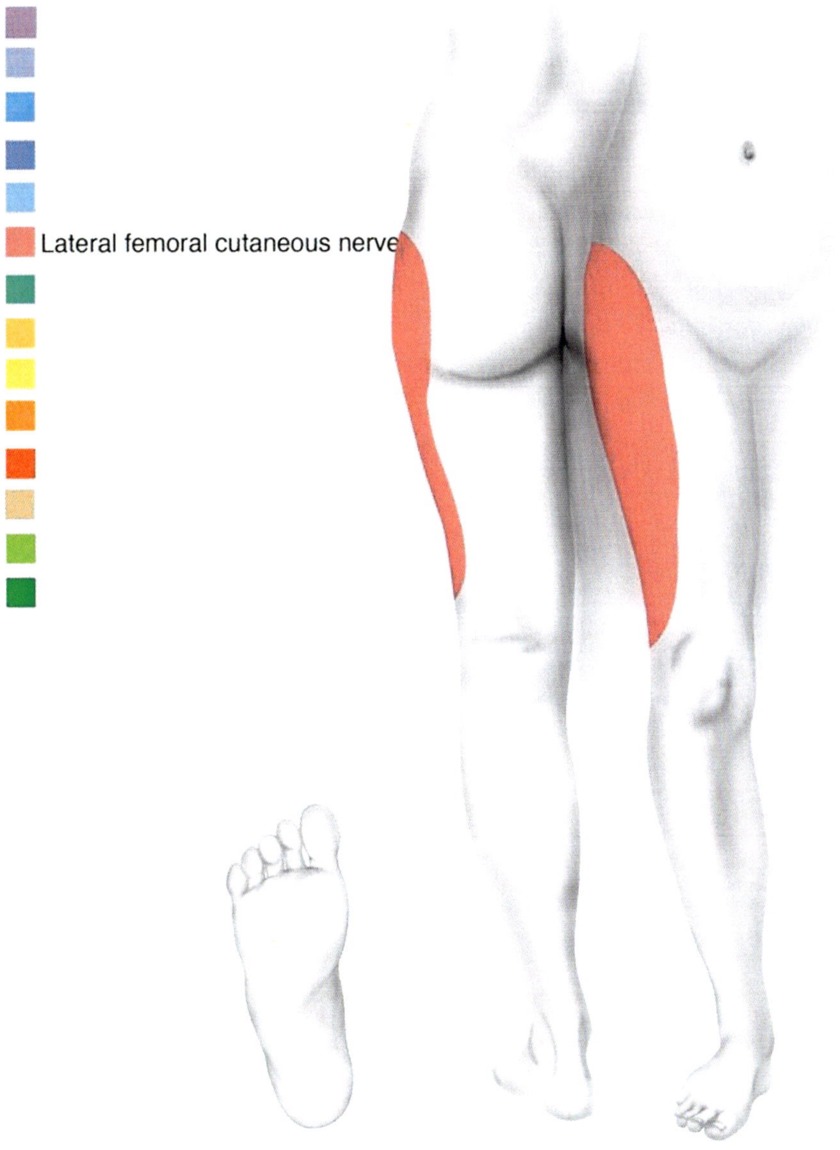

Figure 15: Schematic demarcation of the neurotome of the lower limb innervated by the lateral cutaneous nerve of the thigh.
These demarcations are not distinct areas as depicted here because there is significant overlap between adjacent neurotomes.

THE ADDUCTOR CANAL

This triangular canal in the thigh is also known as Hunter's canal or the subsartorial canal. It is an aponeurotic tunnel in the middle third of the thigh and runs from the apex of the femoral triangle to the opening in the adductor magnus muscle through which the femoral artery and vein reach the popliteal fossa to become the popliteal artery and vein. Anterolaterally, the vastus medialis muscle forms its border. The sartorius muscle is the anterior border, while proximally, the posterior border is formed by the adductor longus muscle and more distally by the aponeurosis that extend between the adductor muscles across the vessels to the vastus medialis. The canal contains not only the femoral artery and vein, but also the descending genicular and muscular branches of the femoral artery and vein, the saphenous nerve, and the nerve to vastus medialis. The subsartorial nerve plexus gets nerve twigs from the medial cutaneous nerve of the thigh and the saphenous and obturator nerves.

SENSORY INNERVATION OF THE KNEE JOINT

The saphenous nerve leaves the adductor canal and gives off an infrapatellar branch that contributes to the peripatellar plexus before it pierces the fascia lata between the sartorius and gracilis muscles to become subcutaneous and supply the prepatellar skin with sensory innervation. It then descends along the medial tibial border to innervate the skin to the medial side of the foot and the ankle joint.

The posterior branch of the obturator nerve usually sends an articular filament to the knee joint, which perforates the adductor magnus muscle distally or joins the femoral artery through the opening in the muscle to enter the popliteal fossa. It joins the popliteal artery to the back of the knee, pierces the oblique posterior ligament and supplies the posterior articular capsule with sensory innervation.

The sciatic nerve contributes to the sensory innervation of the knee joint in that it splits and gives rise to the tibial and common peroneal nerves in the popliteal fossa. The articular branches of the tibial nerve accompany the superior, inferior medial, and middle genicular arteries to the knee joint. They form a plexus with branches of the posterior branch of the obturator nerve that supply the oblique posterior ligament of the knee. The branches that accompany the superior and inferior geniculate arteries also innervate the posterior capsule of the knee joint. The common peroneal nerve has three articular branches, two of which accompany the superior and inferior geniculate arteries; the third ascends with the recurrent tibial artery through the tibialis anterior muscle and supplies the anterolateral part of the knee capsule and the proximal tibiofibular joint.

The principal innervation of the knee is *via* three of the four (deep) muscular branches of the femoral nerve [5]. The branch to the rectus femoris has a branch to the hip joint but not to the knee joint, which interestingly does not violate Hilton's law because this law refers to *groups* of muscles, not individual muscles [1, 2] The largest nerve that innervates the knee goes to the vastus lateralis. The branch to the vastus medialis descends through the upper part of the adductor canal and can usually be traced downward on the surface of the muscle to the knee joint, whereas the branches to the vastus intermedius (two or three of them) descend through the muscle to the knee joint.

SENSORY INNERVATION OF THE HIP JOINT

It is safe to say that virtually all of the nerves of the lumbar and sacral plexus innervate the hip joint because there are no known exceptions to Hilton's Law of Anatomy. Although sensory innervation to the hip joint has been shrouded in mystery for many years and it was thought that the main innervation to the hip capsule came from the obturator nerve, Birnbaum and colleagues [6], after evidently being frustrated by the failure of providing hip analgesia with obturator nerve blocks, comprehensively examined the sensory nerve innervation of the hip joint in formalin-fixed hip joints of cadavers. They found that the innervation of the hip joint was not only complex, but that it also came from a vast number of nerves.

They basically divided the hip joint into segments and the innervation can be summarized as follows:

1. ***Anterior section*** of the hip joint capsule is innervated by:

   a. Articular branches of the ***femoral*** and ***obturator*** nerves.

   b. The ***femoral nerve*** has two articular branches that are responsible for innervation of the anterior and anterolateral region. To some extent, the nerves are accompanied by blood vessels, and in some cases, there is an accessory femoral that is also responsible for sensory innervation to the anterior region of the hip capsule.

   c. The ***obturator nerve*** supplies the anteromedial section of the hip capsule. The articular branches arise from either from the anterior branch, the posterior branch, or the trunk of the obturator nerve. One articular branch passes posterolaterally and over the external obturator muscle, running between the adductor brevis and adductor magnus muscles and originates from the trunk of the obturator nerve.

2. The ***posterior section*** of the hip joint capsule is innervated by:

    a. The articular branches of the ***nerve to the quadratus femoris*** muscle, which passes out of the sciatic nerve immediately after it exits the infrapiriformis foramen. There are usually between one and five articular branches of this nerve.

    b. The articular branches form the ***superior gluteal nerve***, which innervates the posterolateral capsule of the hip joint…

    c. Directly from the ***sciatic nerve***. This nerve passes through the lesser sciatic notch below the sacrotuberous ligament and innervates the internal obturator muscle. It has two articular twigs: one passing posterolaterally and the other posteroinferiorly.

SENSORY INNERVATION OF THE FEMUR

The proximal periosteal innervation for the femur is derived from the nerves that innervate the hip joint, while distally, the femur periostium is innervated by all the nerves that innervate the knee joint. In the areas in between, it gets its sensory innervation form the nerves that innervate the muscles that are attached to the femur.

ACKNOWLEDGEMENTS

The author gratefully acknowledge the following people:

- The Head of the Department of Anesthesiology of the College of Medicine of the University of Florida, Dr. Tim Morey, and his department for their moral support and continuous encouragement.

- The faculty and fellows of the Division of Acute and Perioperative Pain Medicine of the above Department of Anesthesiology for affording the author the time to produce this work by covering his clinical duties.

- Mary K. Bryson for her illustrations of Figs. (**1-4, 8-12, 14** and **15**).
- Corey Astrom of the Department of Anesthesiology of the College of Medicine of the University of Florida for her professional and high quality text editing.
- Raeducation.com LLC for their financial support.

CONFLICT OF INTEREST

The author confirms that this chapter contents have no conflict of Interest

DISCLOSURE

"The summary of the innervation of the hip joint has been adapted from the work of Birnbaum *et al.* [6].

Parts of this work have been previously published in Boezaart A P, Parvataneni HK. Adductor canal block may just be an (unreliable) indirect femoral nerve block. Reg Anesth Pain Med 2014; 39: 556 [7].

ABBREVIATIONS

AB = adductor brevis muscle

ABON = anterior branch of the obturator nerve

AL = adductor longus muscle

EIA = external iliac artery

EIV = external iliac vein

FA = femoral artery

FN = femoral nerve

FV = femoral vein

GFN = genitofemoral nerve

LCNT = lateral cutaneous nerve of the thigh

LP = lumbar plexus

OA = obturator artery

ON = obturator nerve

PBON = posterior branch of the obturator nerve

Pect = pectinius muscle

SN = saphenous nerve

SP = sacral plexus

SRP = superior ramus of the pubis

REFERENCES

[1] Hilton, J. (1863). On Rest and Pain: A Course of Lectures on the Influence of Mechanical and Physiological Rest in the Treatment of Accidents and Surgical Diseases, and the Diagnostic Value of Pain, delivered at the Royal College of Surgeons of England in the years 1860, 1861, and 1862.

[2] Hébert-Blouin M-N, Tubbs RS, Carmichael SW, Spinner RJ. Hilton's Law revisited. Clin Anat 2014; 27: 548-555.

[3] Reina MA, Sala-Blanch X. Cross-sectional microscopic anatomy of the brachial plexus and paraneural sheaths. In: Reina MA, editor. Atlas of functional anatomy for regional anesthesia and pain medicine. New York: Springer Science and Business Media, 2015: 185.

[4] Reina F, Carrera A, Llusá M, Oliva A, Monila JS. Macroscopic view of the lumbar plexus and sacral plexus. In: Reina MA, editor. Atlas of functional anatomy for regional anesthesia and pain medicine. New York: Springer Science and Business Media, 2015: pp. 189-211.

[5] Standring Susan, Ed. Gray's Anatomy: The Anatomical Basis of Clinical Practice. 39th ed. New York: Elsevier/Churchill Livingston, 2005; pp. 1471-1488.

[6] Birnbaum K, Prescher A, Hepler S, Heller KD. The sensory innervation of the hip joint: An anatomical study. Surg Radiol Anat 1998; 19: 371-375.

[7] Boezaart A P, Parvataneni HK. Adductor canal block may just be an (unreliable) indirect femoral nerve block. Reg Anesth Pain Med 2014; 39: 556.

CHAPTER 11

Microanatomy of the Femoral Nerve

André P. Boezaart*

Departments of Anesthesiology and Orthopaedic Surgery and Rehabilitation, Division of Acute and Perioperative Pain Medicine, University of Florida College of Medicine, Gainesville, Florida, USA

Abstract: In this chapter, the author combines the established views of the microstructure of the femoral nerve as an example of a combined peripheral nerve or bundle of nerves with newer concepts that have emerged only recently. The position and importance of the circumneural (paraneural) sheath and subcircumneural (subparaneural) space are discussed, as well as the other membranes and compartments around a peripheral nerve, namely, the endoneurium, perineurium, epineurium, and epimysium. The subepimyseal space is discussed in the context of peripheral nerve block.

Key words: Acute pain medicine, Axon, Circumneural sheath, Combined peripheral nerve, Continuous peripheral nerve block, Endoneurium, Epimysium, Fascia, Fascicles, Femoral nerve, Gliding apparatus, Microanatomy, Nerve axon, Paraneural sheath, Perineurium Epineurium, Peripheral nerve block, Regional anesthesia, Subcircumneural space, Subepimyseal space, Subparaneural space, Ultrastructure.

ULTRASTRUCTURE OF THE FEMORAL NERVE

At the level of the inguinal crease, the femoral nerve is not a single nerve; rather, it is a bundle of nerve branches. The femoral nerve, as an example of a nerve with a number of branches inside a single circumneurium, is considered here. Like other mixed peripheral nerves, the femoral nerve, at this level, comprises numerous nerve branches, all surrounded by a single circumneurium, also known as a paraneurium [1-3].

***Corresponding author André P. Boezaart:** Departments of Anesthesiology and Orthopaedic Surgery, Division of Acute and Peri-operative Pain Medicine, University of Florida College of Medicine, 1600 SW Archer Road, Gainesville, Florida 32610, USA; Tel: 352-846-0913 (Work); Fax: 352-392-7029; E-mail: aboezaart@anest.ufl.edu

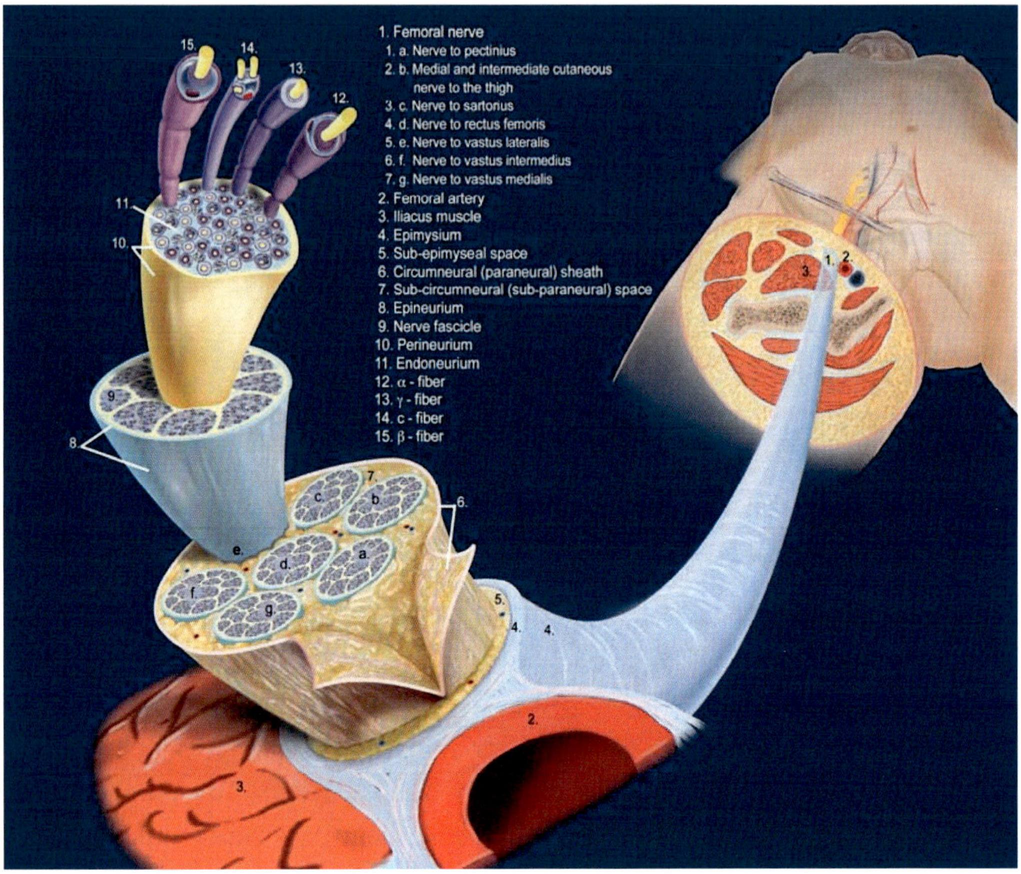

Figure 1: Ultrastructure of the femoral nerve.

1. *The branches of the femoral nerve are enclosed in a common circumneural sheath (6).*
2. *There are eight branches inside the femoral nerve (seven shown here): the nerve to the pectinius, which usually comes off higher up, just above or below the inguinal ligament, the medial and intermediate cutaneous nerves to the thigh, and the nerves to the sartorius, rectus femoris, vastus lateralis, vastus intermedius, and vastus medialis muscles.*
3. *Outside the circumneural sheath is the subepimyseal space (5), which is surrounded by the epimysium (4) - the fascia that surrounds the nerves, muscles, and blood vessels.*
4. *Deep to the circumneural sheath (6) (the paraneural sheath) is the subcircumneural space (7), which is thought to be the ideal space for the needle in catheter placement for a nerve block.*
5. *The next layer, which encloses each individual branch, is the epineurium (8), surrounding the fascicles of each branch.*
6. *In turn, each fascicle is surrounded by its own perineurium (10).*
7. *Inside the perineurium are endoneurium and 12 to 15 nerve axons (Table **1** of Chapter 2).*

The ***endoneurium*** (Fig. **1**, No. 11) is a fine cylindrical lamina that encloses groups of axons with their respective Schwann cells. The axons consist of different axon fiber types, depending of the type of nerve in question (see Table **1** of Chapter 2). Both myelinated and unmyelinated axons are surrounded by the collagen fibers of the endoneurium, but the endoneurium is permeable and thus does not interfere with molecules passage through it. The single-layered endothelial cells of the capillaries in the endoneurium contribute to the blood-nerve barrier [3]. The term endoneurium is sometimes incorrectly used to denote the intrafascicular compartment of the nerve. Its use should be restricted to refer to intrafascicular connective tissue, excluding the perineurial partitions that may subdivide fascicles [1]. Approximately 40% to 50% of the intrafascicular space is occupied by non-neural elements and anywhere from 20% to 30% of this is endoneurial fluid (CSF) and connective matrix - the endoneurium [1, 3].

The ***perineurium*** (Fig. **1**, No. 10) comprises multiple single-cell layers that enclose individual nerve fascicles [3]. They become progressively thinner as the number of fascicles increase. As Key and Retzius [1] describe, the essential structure of the perineurium is a lamellated arrangement of flattened cells separated by layers of collagenous connective tissue that provides an ensheathment for both the somatic and peripheral autonomic nerves and their ganglia. The cellular lamellae are composed of concentric sleeves of flattened polygonal cells that are equipped to function as a metabolically active diffusion barrier, although they do not have the morphologic features of a true epithelium.

The ***epineurium*** (Fig. **1**, No. 8) consists of a condensation of areolar connective tissue that surrounds the perineurial ensheathment of the fascicles of uni- and multifascicular nerves [3, 4]. The attachment of the epineurium to surrounding connective tissue is loose, allowing the nerve to be relatively mobile except where tethered by entering blood vessels or branches [4]. Greater amounts of connective tissue are normally present where nerves cross over joints. In general, the more fascicles there are, the greater the quantity of epineurium.

Variable quantities of adipose tissue are also present in the epineurium, particularly in the larger nerves. After studying the distribution of fat in human nerves and finding predominance in the sciatic nerve, researchers feel that this tissue probably has a protective function in cushioning the fascicles against injury by compression. The susceptibility to compression injury is likely to be less in large multifascicular nerves with considerable quantities of epineurium and fat than in smaller and unifascicular nerves.

The ***vasa nervorum*** enter the epineurium, where they communicate with a longitudinal anastomotic network of arterioles and venules [4]. The epineurium also contains lymphatic vessels, which are not present within the fascicles. These lymphatic channels accompany the arteries of the peripheral nerves and pass into the regional lymph nodes [5].

Anderson and colleagues [6] recently demonstrated the ***circumneural (paraneural) sheath*** [7] in dissections, while Karmakar and his colleagues [8] described the appearance of the circumneural sheath with high-definition ultrasound See Fig. **7** and **8**, Chapter 2). In neurosurgical texts, it has been known as the "gliding apparatus" of the nerve [9]. We now know that injection of a local anesthetic agent or catheter placement in the subcircumneural space (subparaneural space) is ideal for single-injection and continuous nerve block, respectively [9]. Reina and colleagues stained sections through the brachial plexus and peripheral nerves with Masson's trichrome staining to convincingly demonstrate the microscopic ultrastructure of the circumneural (paraneural) sheaths (See Fig. **9**, Chapter 2) [3].

ACKNOWLEDGEMENTS

The author gratefully acknowledge the following people:

- The Head of the Department of Anesthesiology of the College of Medicine of the University of Florida, Dr. Tim Morey, and his department for their moral support and continuous encouragement.
- The faculty and fellows of the Division of Acute and Perioperative Pain Medicine of the above Department of Anesthesiology for affording the author the time to produce this work by covering his clinical duties.
- Mary K. Bryson for her illustrations of Fig **1**.
- Corey Astrom of the Department of Anesthesiology of the College of Medicine of the University of Florida for her professional and high quality text editing.
- Raeducation.com LLC for their financial support.

CONFLICT OF INTEREST

The author invented the "stimulating catheter" and receives royalties from TeleFlex on sales of this product.

DISCLOSURE

Parts of this work have been previously published in Boezaart AP. Microanatomy of the peripheral nervous system revisited, and its implications for paravertebral (para-neuraxial) blocks. Proceedings of the 10th Annual pre-ASA Meeting, Orthopedic Anesthesia Pain Rehabilitation Society (www.OAPRS.org); 2013 October 11; San Francisco, California. United States of America [10].

REFERENCES

[1] Key A, Retzius G. Studies in the anatomy of the nervous system and connective tissue. Stockholm: Samson and Wallin, circa 1876.

[2] Horster H, Whitman L. The method of intraneural injection. [Die Methode der intraneuralen Injektion]. Z Hygiene 1931; 113: 113.

[3] Reina MA, Navarro RA, Mateos EMD. Ultrastructure of myelinated and unmyelinated axons. In: Reina MA, Ed. Atlas of functional anatomy for regional anesthesia and pain medicine. New York: Springer, 2015; pp. 3-126.

[4] French JD, Strain WH, Jones GE. Mode of extension of contrast substances injected into peripheral nerves. J Neuropathol Exp Neurlogy 1948; 7: 47-58.

[5] Moore DC, Hain RF Ward A, Bridenbaugh LD. Importance of the perineural spaces in nerve blocking. JAMA 1954; 156: 1050-5.

[6] Andrerson HL, Anderson SL, Tranun-Jensen J. Injecting inside the paraneural sheath or the sciatic nerve: Direct comparison among ultrasound imaging, macroscopic anatomy and histologic analysis. Reg Anesth Pain Med 2012; 37: 410-4.

[7] Karmakar MK, Shariat AN, Pangthipampai P, Chen J. High-definition ultrasound imaging defines the paraneural sheath and the fascial compartments surrounding the sciatic nerve at the poplitcal fossa. Reg Anesth Pain Med 2013; 38: 447-51.

[8] Millesi H, Zoch G, Rath T. The gliding apparatus of peripheral nerve and its clinical significance. Ann Chir Main Memb Super 1990; 9: 87-97.

[9] Boezaart AP. The sweet spot of the nerve: Is the "paraneural sheath" named correctly, and does it matter? Reg Anesth Pain Med 2014; 39: 557-8.

[10] Boezaart AP. Microanatomy of the peripheral nervous system revisited, and its implications for paravertebral (para-neuraxial) blocks. Proceedings of the 10th Annual pre-ASA Meeting, Orthopedic Anesthesia Pain Rehabilitation Society (www.OAPRS.org); 2013 October 11; San Francisco, California. United States of America.

Chapter 12:
Sonoanatomy of the Nerves in the Anterior Thigh

CHAPTER 12

Sonoanatomy of the Nerves in the Anterior Thigh

Barys V. Ihnatsenka[1], André P. Boezaart[2,*] and Yury Zasimovich[1]

[1]Department of Anesthesiology, Division of Acute and Perioperative Pain Medicine, University of Florida College of Medicine, Gainesville, Florida, USA and [2]Departments of Anesthesiology and Orthopaedic Surgery and Rehabilitation, Division of Acute and Perioperative Pain Medicine, University of Florida College of Medicine, Gainesville, Florida, USA

Abstract: Ultrasound is a dynamic procedure whereby structures can and should be followed to their origins and destinations for optimal identification. Because of this, it is not always satisfactory to study static ultrasound images. When studying sonoanatomy, the authors strongly advise readers to first study the macro- and microanatomy and then to view the accompanying video productions that illustrates the dynamic sonoanatomy (Movies **1-4**). In this chapter, the authors explain the static sonoanatomy of the femoral and obturator nerves and that of the lateral cutaneous nerve of the thigh and the adductor canal, and with the aid of video productions, the dynamic sonoanatomy of these structures and areas.

Keywords: Acute pain medicine, Adductor canal, Adductor canal block, Adductor muscles, Anterior thigh, Dynamic sonoanatomy, Femoral nerve, Genitofemoral nerve., Lateral cutaneous nerve of the thigh, Nerve to sartorius, Obturator nerve, Quadriceps muscles, Rectus femoris, Regional anesthesiologist, Saphenous nerve, Sartorius muscle, Sonoanatomy, Subsartorial plexus, Subsartorial space, Vastus intermedius, Vastus lateralis, Vastus medialis.

SONOANATOMY

Ultrasound is a dynamic process whereby structures can and should be followed to their origins and destinations for optimal identification [1]. Because of this, it is not always satisfactory to study static ultrasound images. When studying sonoanatomy, the authors strongly advise readers to first study the macro- and microanatomy and then to view the accompanying video production (Movie **1**) that illustrate the dynamic sonoanatomy of the structures discussed in this chapter.

***Corresponding author André P. Boezaart:** Departments of Anesthesiology and Orthopaedic Surgery, Division of Acute and Peri-operative Pain Medicine, University of Florida College of Medicine, 1600 SW Archer Road, Gainesville, Florida 32610, USA; Tel: 352-846-0913 (Work); Fax: 352-392-7029;
E-mail: aboezaart@anest.ufl.edu

The ultrasound transducer probe used throughout the scanning for this chapter was a 6 - to 13-MHz linear probe with a 38-mm footprint (HFL - 38, SonoSite Fujifilm, Bothell, WA, USA).

As is the case with almost all sonoanatomy images, the finer and important ultrastructure of the membranes that surround the nerves, similar for that of all major peripheral nerves [2], cannot be readily visualized with regular ultrasound technology. Please refer to Chapter 2 for an explanation of the micro- and ultrastructure of these membranes. For that, high-definition ultrasound technology may be required [3].

FEMORAL NERVE

To obtain the images for this section, we positioned the model ("patient") in the supine position and the leg straight or slightly abducted and externally rotated ("frog-legged" position), as in Fig. (**1**). The femoral artery and tendons of the adductor longus muscle can usually be palpated with ease. We then placed the ultrasound transducer probe axially in the inguinal crease on the artery, which comes into view; medial to it is the femoral vein (Fig. **1**).

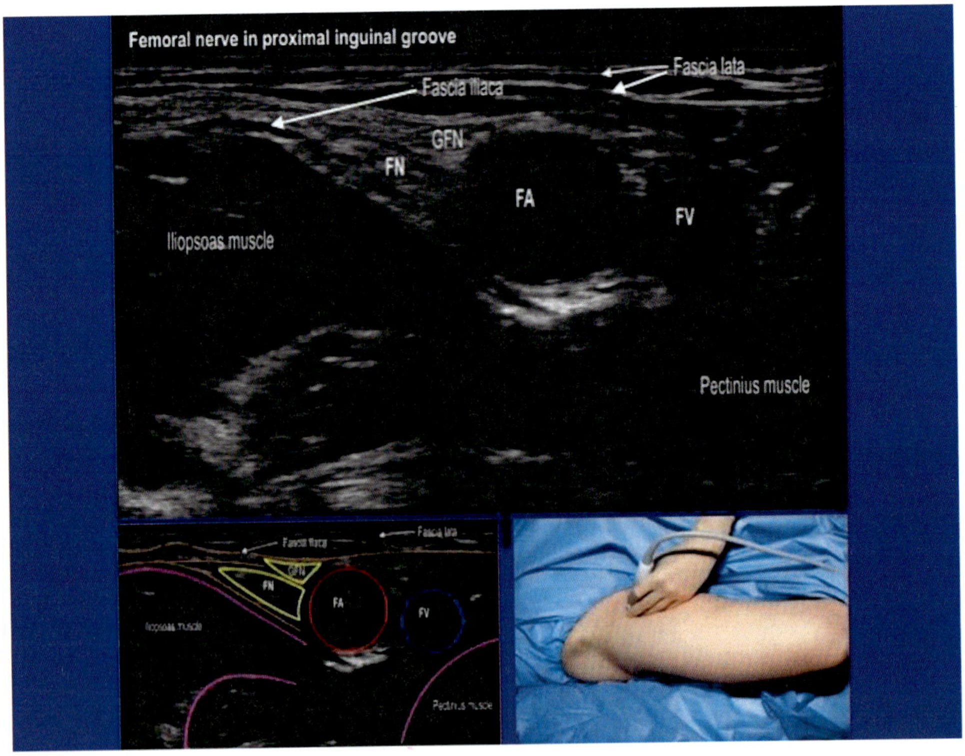

Figure 1: Sonoanatomy of the femoral nerve as viewed in the inguinal crease.
The left side of the image is the lateral side of the model. FA = femoral artery; FV = femoral vein; FN = femoral nerve; GFN =femoral branch of the genitofemoral nerve.

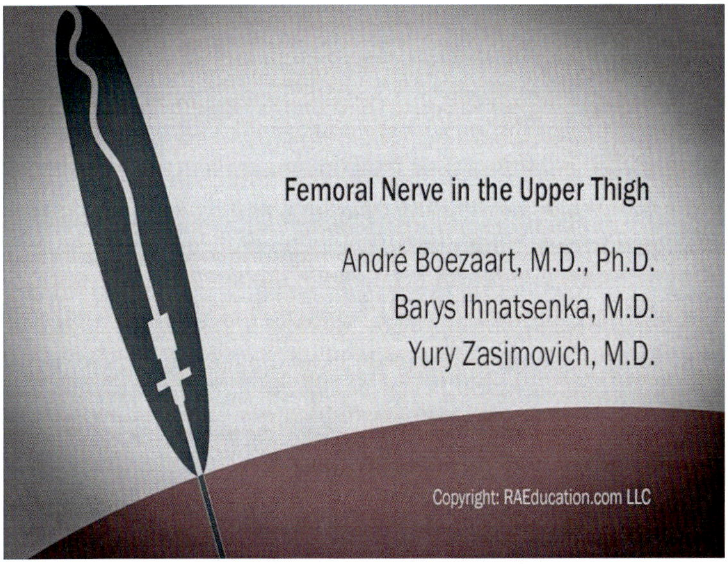

To view this movie click on this link:
https://raeducation.com/ebook

Movie 1: Dynamic sonoanatomy of the femoral nerve.

When ultrasound scanning in this area, it is usually easy to visualize the large, pulsating femoral artery, and just medial to it, the femoral vein. Lateral to the artery is the femoral nerve. This is not one nerve, but a group or bundle of nerves (see Microanatomy section, Chapter 11), with all seven nerves engulfed within one circumneural (paraneural) sheath, and the femoral nerve situated on the iliacus muscle. Anteromedial to it, we can usually find the crural branch of the genitofemoral nerve, which supplies sensory innervation to the upper anterior thigh.

Sliding the probe more distal, the artery and vein split into femoral and deep (profundus) arteries and veins (Fig. **2**). The lateral circumflex femoral artery can also be seen in this area, and which usually courses between the deep and superficial branches or anterior of the femoral nerve. When this comes into view, the probe needs to be moved back more proximally.

The nerve to sartorius is usually more superficial than in this subject, and it can only be positively and accurately identified with transcutaneous nerve stimulation, as is done with nerve stimulator-guided regional anesthesia [4, 5] or percutaneously [6] (see also Functional Anatomy section, Chapter 17). When preparing these images, nerve stimulation confirmation was not sought, but looking at Fig. (**1**), the nerve to sartorius is most likely the nerve structure seen anteromedial between the femoral and genitofemoral nerves. The nerve to sartorius is an exception to Hilton's Law of Anatomy [7] (see Macroanatomy, Chapter 1), and although this muscle moves the knee, its nerve does not supply sensory innervation to the knee joint.

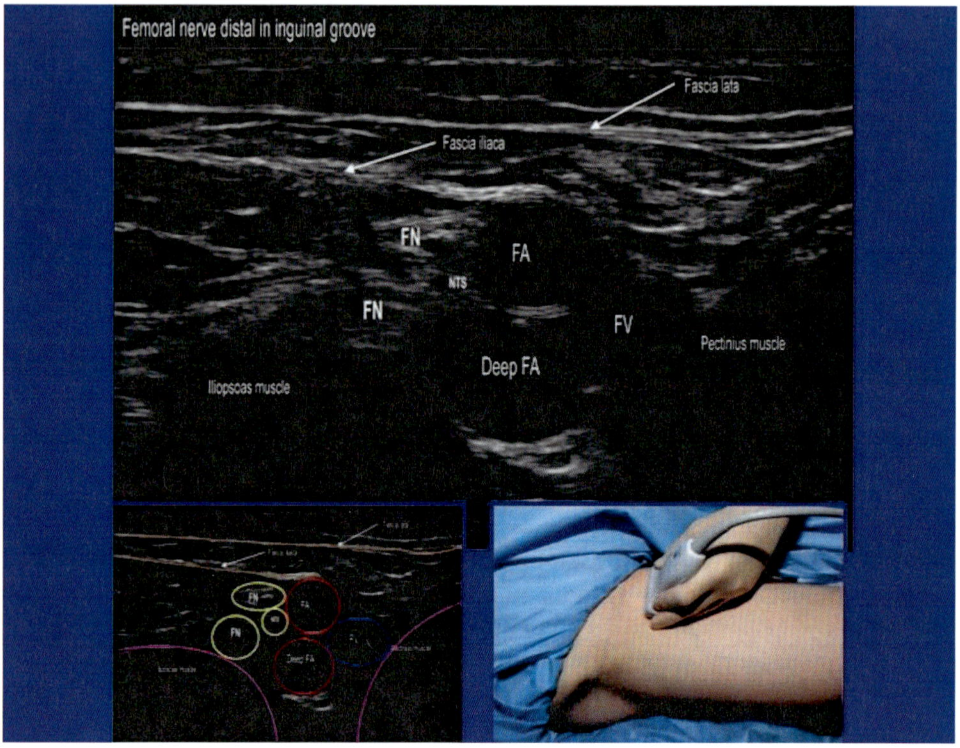

Figure 2: More distal view of the femoral nerve below the inguinal crease.
The left side of the image is the lateral side of the model. FA = femoral artery; FV = femoral vein; FN = femoral nerve; NTS = nerve to sartorius.

The nerve to sartorius may break away from the other nerves in the bundle of nerves in the circumneural (paraneural) sheath of the femoral nerve, higher up, just below the inguinal ligament, thus attempting to block it with a primary block may be successful for knee joint analgesia; the high concentration and volume of drug may diffuse to the other branches of the femoral nerve. A secondary block, however, when a low infusion volume and concentration of drug is infused, will most certainly fail, as the concentration gradient is too small to achieve diffusion through all the tissue layers. If ultrasound guidance is used as the sole technique to place a catheter for continuous nerve block, it is advisable to place it into the posterior deep portion of the nerve, taking care not to penetrate the epineurium or perineurium of individual nerves (see Microanatomy, Chapter 11).

OBTURATOR NERVE

With the patient or model in the supine position and the leg slightly abducted and externally rotated ("frog-legged" position), we move the ultrasound transducer probe medially in the inguinal crease. This brings the femoral vein on the lateral side of the image (Fig. **3**) into view. If there is any doubt about the identity of the vein, slight pressure on the probe will compress the vein, but not the artery. Medial to the femoral vein is the pectinius muscle (Fig. **3**), and if the ultrasound probe is placed over it and the beam of the transducer is tilted cephalad (the handle of the probe moved downward), the bony parts of the superior ramus of the pubis come into view. The obturator nerve, before it splits into its anterior and posterior branches, can now be seen in the corner, formed between the pectinius muscle, the obturator externus and the superior ramus of the pubis (Fig. **3**).

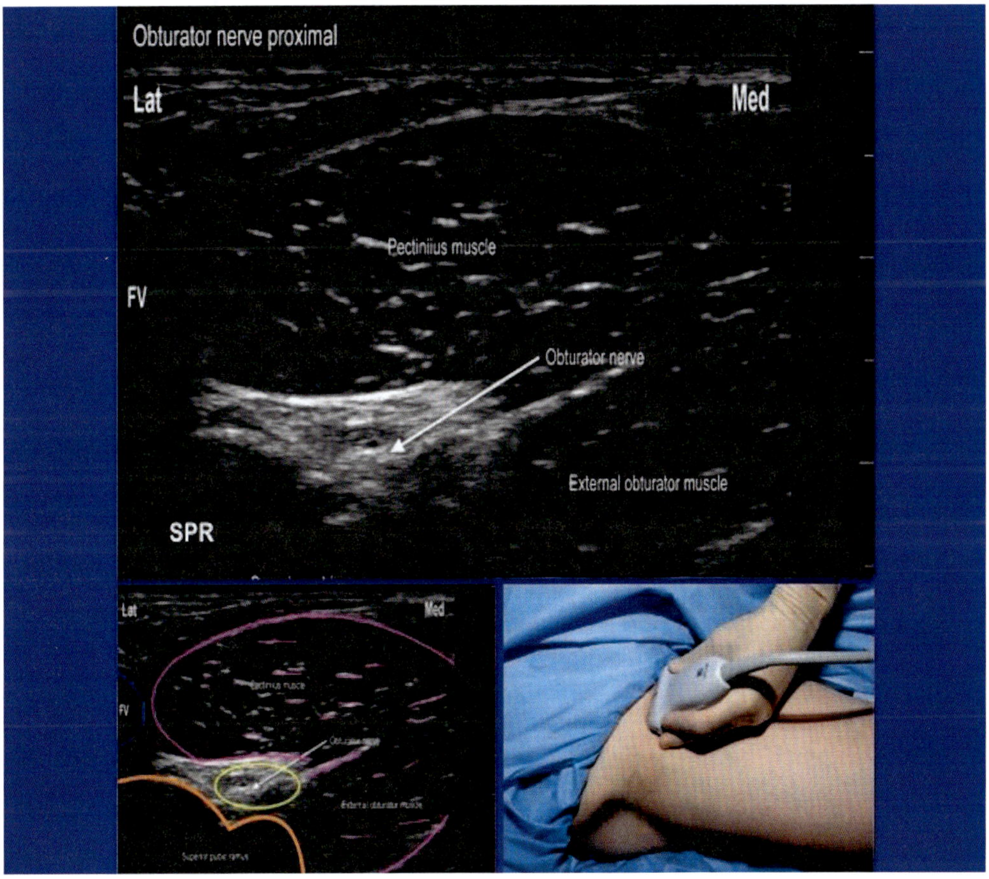

Figure 3: Sonoanatomy of the obturator nerve.
Lat = lateral; Med = medial; FV = femoral vein.

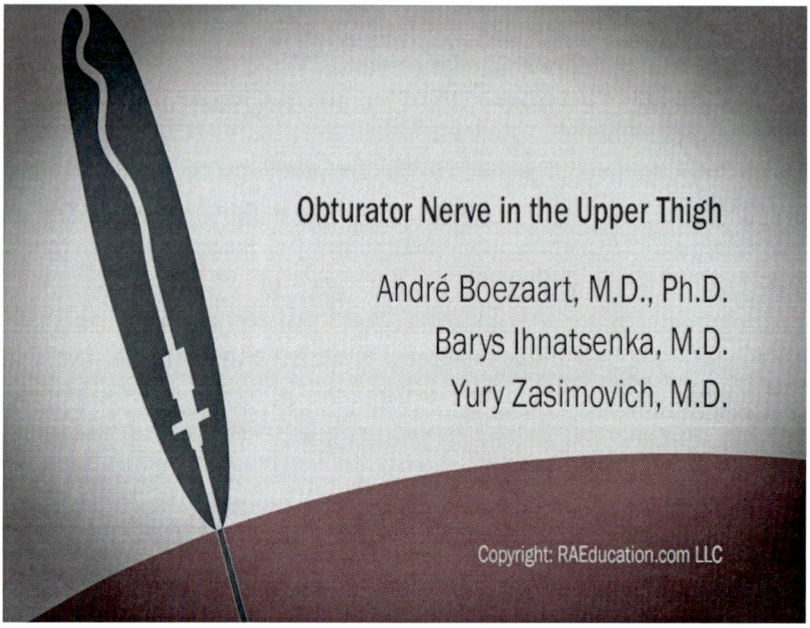

To view this movie click on this link:
https://raeducation.com/ebook

Movie 2: Dynamic sonoanatomy of the obturator nerve.

From this position, we slide the ultrasound transducer probe downward a few centimeters and the three adductor muscles come into view medial to the pectinius muscle (Fig. **4**). The anterior branch of the obturator nerve lies medial to the pectinius muscle between the adductor longus and adductor brevis muscles (Fig. **4**). More posterior, in the fascia layer of the space between the adductor brevis, adductor magnus, and obturator externus muscles, the posterior branch of the obturator nerve can be found. Splitting these fascial layers with local anesthetic agent in these positions will result in reliable obturator nerve blocks. The anterior obturator nerve communicates with the internal cutaneous and internal saphenous nerves to form a subsartorial plexus. Branches of the anterior obturator nerve innervate the hip joint and supply the adductor longus and brevis muscles and pectinius muscles with motor innervation.

The posterior branch of the obturator nerve innervates the obturator externus and adductor brevis and magnus muscles. One of its branches gives off a filament, the articular branch to the posterior capsule of the knee joint (see "innervation of the knee" in Macroanatomy, Chapter 10).

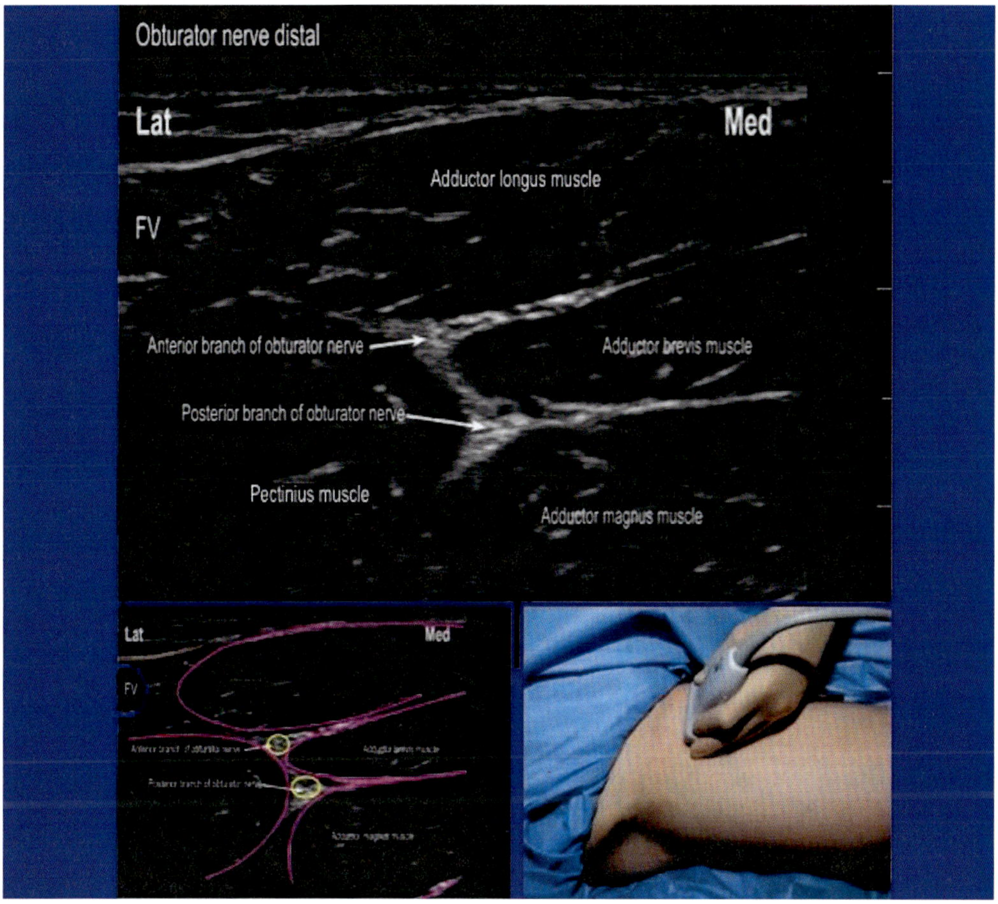

Figure 4: Sonoanatomy of the anterior and posterior branches of the obturator nerve. *Lat = lateral; Med = medial; FV = femoral vein.*

LATERAL CUTANEOUS NERVE OF THE THIGH

The lateral cutaneous nerve of the thigh is relatively easy to find with ultrasound. It lies below the anterior superior iliac spine (ASIS) in the fascial split surrounded by adipose tissue lateral to the sartorius muscle and anterior to where rectus femoris, and tensor fascia lata muscles meet. From here it can be followed up and down, as it lies deep to the sartorius muscle. The subject is positioned in the supine position and the ultrasound transducer probe is placed axially in the inguinal groove over the femoral artery and then moved laterally to over the triangular sartorius muscle. Superficial to where these three muscles come together, we can see a fascial split where the lateral cutaneous nerve of the thigh resides. It is often said to resemble an eye (Fig. **5**).

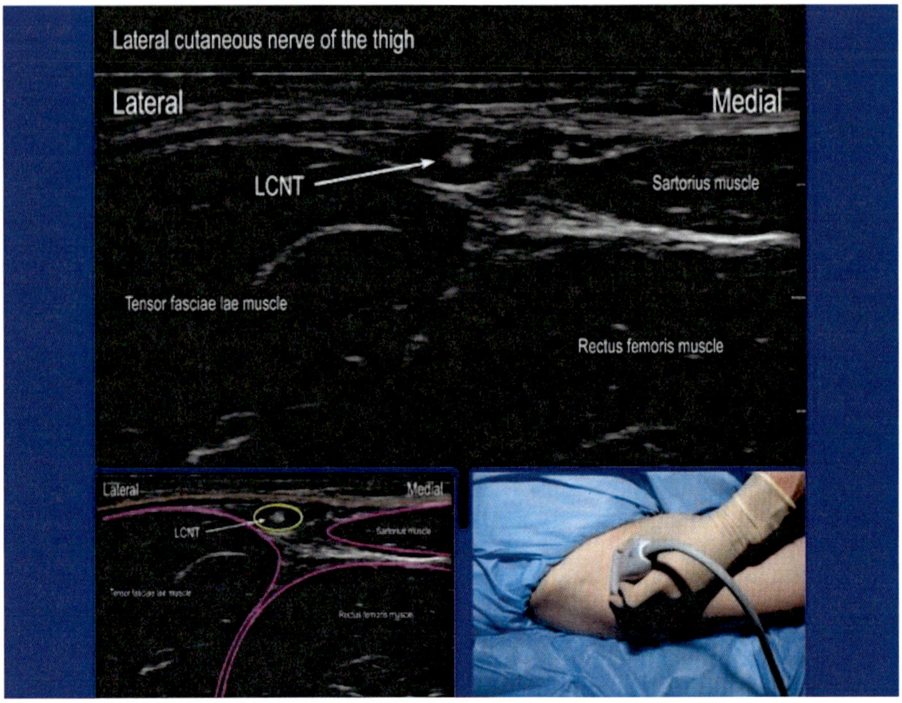

Figure 5: Sonoanatomy of the lateral cutaneous nerve of the thigh.
LCNT = lateral cutaneous nerve of the thigh. Tensor fasciae lae muscle = tensor fascia late muscle.

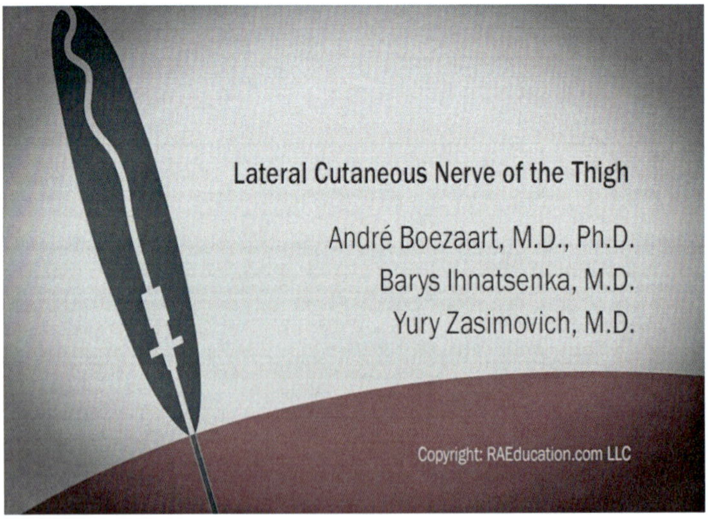

To view this movie click on this link:
https://raeducation.com/ebook

Movie 3: Dynamic sonoanatomy of the lateral cutaneous nerve of the high.

SAPHENOUS NERVE

The saphenous nerve is a branch of the femoral nerve that runs down the anteromedial side of the thigh all the way down to the foot where it supplies sensory innervation to the skin of the inner (medial) side of the lower leg down to the inside of the foot - sometimes to the medial side of the big toe. True to Hilton's Law of Anatomy [7], because it innervates the skin overlying the ankle joint, it also innervates the ankle joint [8].

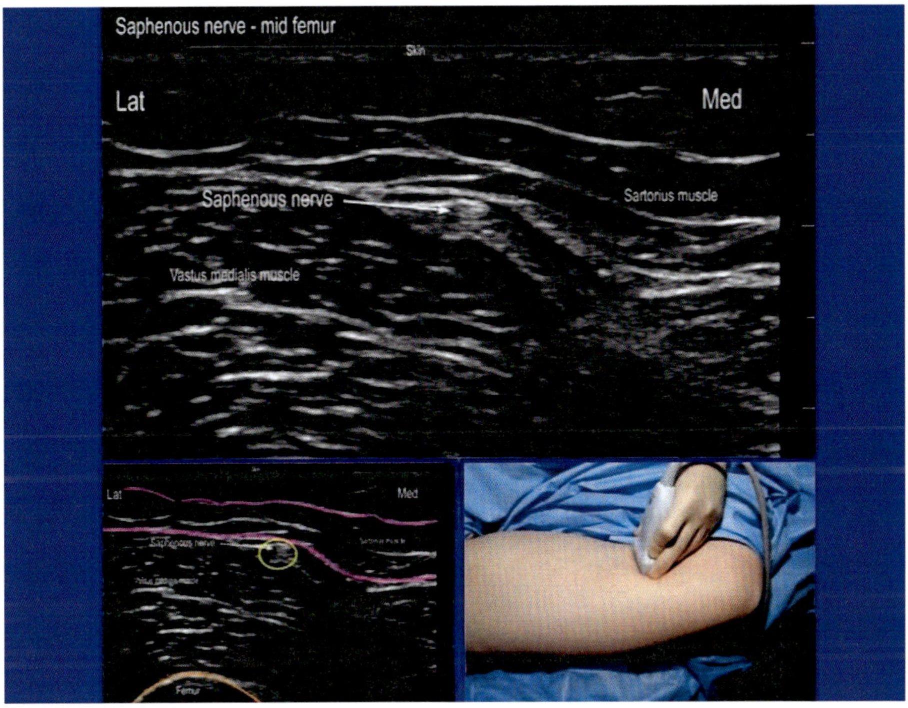

Figure 6: Sonoanatomy of the saphenous nerve in the thigh.
Lat = lateral; Med = medial. ("Saphenous nerve" may well be patellar branch of the saphenous nerve, which usually lies more medial in this same fascial layer).

To obtain the image in Fig. (**6**), we positioned the model in the supine position with the leg slightly abducted and externally rotated in the so-called "frog-legged" position. We then placed the ultrasound transducer probe approximately two-thirds down the thigh in the anteromedial position (Fig. **6**). The triangular sartorius muscle then comes into view and the saphenous nerve can be seen lateral in the fascial plane between the sartorius and vastus medialis muscles, although it is usually on the medial side of the sartorius muscle. The nerve marked here as "saphenous" nerve (Fig. **6**) is most likely the patellar branch of the saphenous nerve, which is at this level in the same fascial layer. Below the knee, it gives off branches that join the plexus patellae, which is always cut during total knee arthroplasty surgery.

ADDUCTOR CANAL

The adductor canal has become topical in recent years [9-13]. Because of this recent attention in the literature, the sonoanatomy of the adductor canal is included in this book.

The subsartorial space (adductor canal) contains the subsartorial plexus (formed by the medial cutaneous nerve of the thigh, the saphenous nerve, and branches of the obturator nerves) and the nerve to the vastus medialis muscle. The saphenous nerve innervates the skin overlying the knee, therefore, according to Hilton's Law of Anatomy [7], it also innervates the knee joint *via* its infrapatellar branch to the plexus patellae. These nerves, however, are irrelevant because the surgeon usually cuts them during surgery [14].

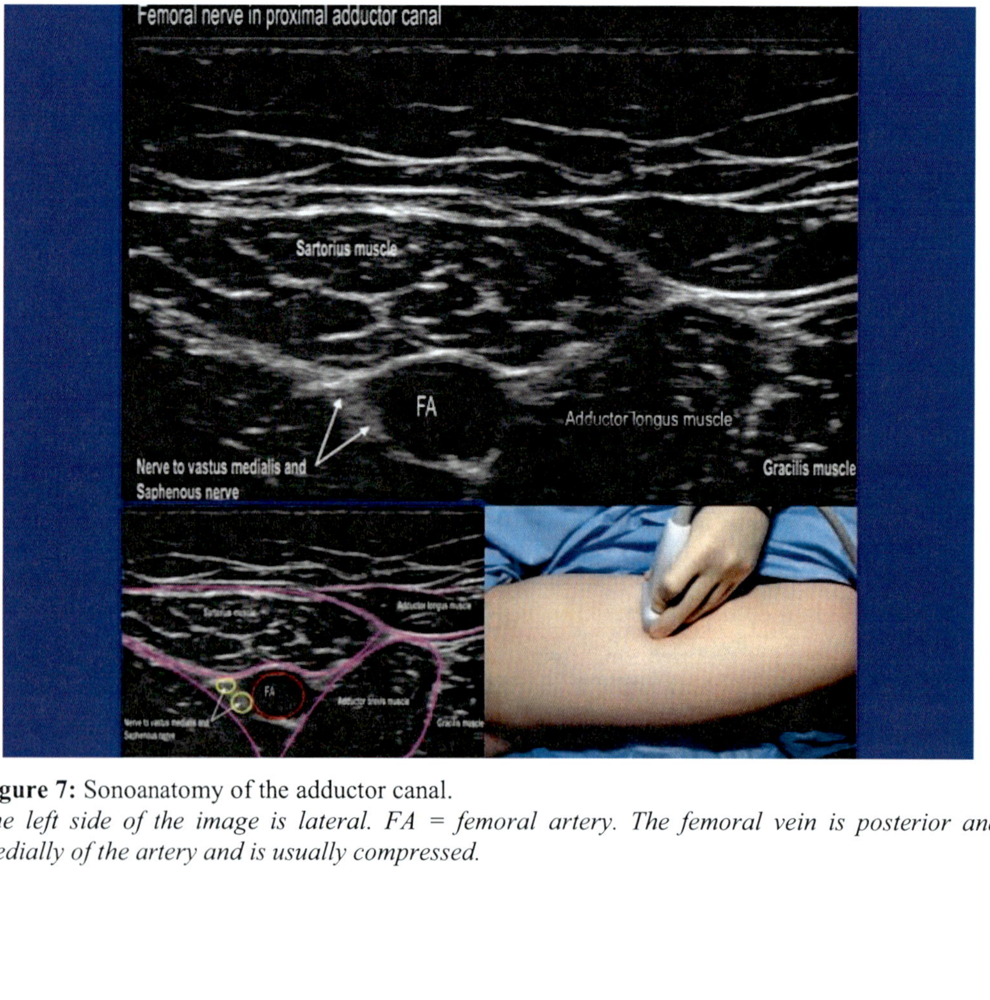

Figure 7: Sonoanatomy of the adductor canal.
The left side of the image is lateral. FA = femoral artery. The femoral vein is posterior and medially of the artery and is usually compressed.

To obtain the image in Fig. (**7**), the model ("patient") was positioned in the supine position with the leg straight or slightly abducted and externally rotated ("frog-legged"), and as in this illustration, the femoral artery and tendons of the adductor longus muscle can usually be palpated. We placed the ultrasound probe in the inguinal crease on the femoral artery, which comes into view.

If we follow the femoral artery distally, we can see the deep or profundus femoral artery splitting off and the femoral artery coursing down the adductor canal. On the lateral side, deep to the sartorius muscle, is the vastus intermedius in the upper thigh, and lower down in the thigh it is replaced by the vastus medialis muscle. On the medial side of the artery (the right side of the image) are the adductor muscles; in the proximal thigh, the adductor longus, and further down, the adductor magnus muscle (Fig. **7**).

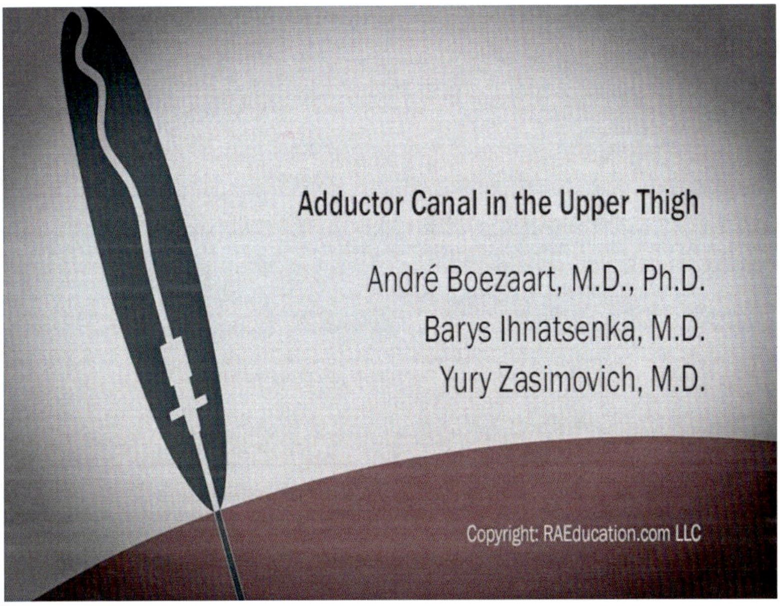

To view this movie click on this link:
https://raeducation.com/ebook

Movie 4: Dynamic sonoanatomy of the adductor canal.

If we follow the artery down, we can see that it runs deeper or posterior as it goes through the adductor hiatus to become the popliteal artery, and the descending genicular artery comes off of the femoral artery in this area. This is one of the positions in which the adductor canal block has been described. Another position is higher up, where the artery is more superficial and the saphenous nerve and the nerve to the vastus medialis can be seen; two of the many nerves that innervate the knee joint (see Macroanatomy, Chapter 10) are lateral to the artery.

ACKNOWLEDGEMENTS

The authors gratefully acknowledge the following people:

- The Head of the Department of Anesthesiology of the College of Medicine of the University of Florida, Dr. Tim Morey, and his department for their moral support and continuous encouragement.
- The faculty and fellows of the Division of Acute and Perioperative Pain Medicine of the above Department of Anesthesiology for affording the authors the time to produce this work by covering their clinical duties.
- Dr. Anastacia Munro for her help with the preparation of the chapter and ultrasound images.
- Corey Astrom of the Department of Anesthesiology of the College of Medicine of the University of Florida for her professional and high quality text editing.
- Nancy Hagen of the Iowa Public Radio for her narration of the movies.
- Raeducation.com LLC for their financial support.

CONFLICT OF INTEREST

The authors confirm that this chapter contents have no conflict of Interest.

REFERENCES

[1] Ihnatsenka BV, Boezaart AP. Ultrasound: Basic understanding and learning the language. Int J Shoulder Surg. 2010;4:55-62.

[2] Reina MA, Sala-Blanch X. Cross-sectional microscopic anatomy of the brachial plexus and paraneural sheaths. In: Reina MA, Ed. Atlas of functional anatomy for regional anesthesia and pain medicine. New York: Springer Science and Business Media; 2015: 237 - 69.

[3] Karmakar MK, Shariat AN, Pangthipampai P, Chen J. High-definition ultrasound imaging defines the paraneural sheath and the fascial compartments surrounding the sciatic nerve at the popliteal fossa. Reg Anesth Pain Med 2013; 38: 447-51.

[4] Salinas FV. Femoral nerve block. In: Boezaart AP, Ed. Anesthesia and orthopaedic surgery. New York, McGraw-Hill 2006; 331-41.

[5] Boezaart AP. Atlas of peripheral nerve blocks and anatomy for orthopaedic anesthesia. Philadelphia: Saunders Elsevier; 2007: pp. 141-59.

[6] Bösenberg AT, Raw R, Boezaart AP. Surface mapping of peripheral nerves in children with a nerve stimulator. Paediatric Anaesthesia 2002; 12: 398-403.

[7] Hébert-Blouin M-N, Tubbs RS, Carmichael SW, Spinner RJ. Hilton's Law revisited. Clin Anat. 2014; 27: 548-55.

[8] Sarrafian SK. Anatomy of the foot and ankle: Descriptive, topographic and functional. Philadelphia, PA; J.B. Lippencott Company 1993; pp. 386 - 7.

[9] Kwofie MK, Shastri UD, Gadsden JC, Sinha SK, Abrams JH, Xu, D, Salviz EA. The effects of ultrasound-guided adductor canal block *versus* femoral nerve block on quadriceps strength and fall risk: A blinded, randomized trial of volunteers. Reg Anesth Pain Med 2013; 68: 321-5.

[10] Boezaart AP, Parvataneni HK. Adductor canal block may just be an (unreliable) indirect femoral nerve block. Reg Anesth Pain Med 2014; 39: 556.

[11] Chen J, Lesse J, Hadzic A, ReissW, Resta-Flarer F. Adductor canal block can result in motor block of the quadriceps muscle. Reg Anesth Pain Med 2014; 39: 170-1.

[12] Davies JJ, Bond TS, Swenson JD. Adductor canal block more than just the saphenous nerve. Reg Anesth Pain Med. 2009;34:618-9.

[13] Veal C, Auyong DB, Hanson NA, Allen CJ, Strodtbeck W. Delayed quadriceps weakness after continuous adductor canal block for total knee arthroplasty: a case report. Acta Anaesth Scan. 2013;58:362-4.

[14] Laffosse J-M, Malo M, Lavigne M, Vendittoli P-A. Hypesthesia after anterolateral *versus* midline skin incision in TKA. Clin Orthop Relat Res. 2011; 469: 3154-63.

Chapter 13:
Applied Macroanatomy of the Sciatic Nerve

CHAPTER 13

Applied Macroanatomy of the Sciatic Nerve

André P. Boezaart*

Departments of Anesthesiology and Orthopaedic Surgery and Rehabilitation, Division of Acute and Perioperative Pain Medicine, University of Florida College of Medicine, Gainesville, Florida, USA

Abstract: There are five areas of interest to the regional anesthesiologist and acute pain physician concerning where the sciatic nerve can be approached. These include the parasacral, the transgluteal, the subgluteal, the mid-femoral, and the popliteal areas. These areas and the relationships of the sciatic nerve to other structures in those specific areas, as well as the areas of sensory distributions of the sciatic nerve and its branches are discussed in this chapter. Other nerves, not part of the sciatic nerve but originating from the sacral plexus, such as the posterior cutaneous nerve of the thigh and the pudendal nerve, are also discussed in this chapter.

Keywords: Acute pain medicine, Common fibular nerve, Common peroneal nerve, Gluteus maximus muscle, Gluteus medius muscle, Gluteus minimus muscle, Mid-femoral approach, Parasacral approach, Popliteal approach, Posterior cutaneous nerve of the thigh, Pudendal nerve, Quadratus femoris muscle, Regional anesthesia, Sacral plexus, Sciatic nerve, Sonoanatomy, Subgluteal approach, Sural nerve, Tibial nerve.

INTRODUCTION

In this chapter, the author will discuss the macroanatomy of the sciatic nerve in the five positions of interest to regional anesthesiologists and acute pain physicians, namely the parasacral, the transgluteal, the subgluteal, the mid-femoral and the popliteal areas. The sensory innervation of the knee, hip and ankle joints will also be discussed.

As a good understanding of anatomy is essential for performing any regional anesthesia technique or invasive procedure for regional anesthesia or acute pain medical condition, it follows that one must understand the most fundamental

***Corresponding author André P. Boezaart:** Departments of Anesthesiology and Orthopaedic Surgery, Division of Acute and Peri-operative Pain Medicine, University of Florida College of Medicine, 1600 SW Archer Road, Gainesville, Florida 32610, USA; Tel: 352-846-0913 (Work); Fax: 352-392-7029;
E-mail: aboezaart@anest.ufl.edu

principle of successful acute or perioperative pain control by regional anesthesia, namely, Hilton's Law of Anatomy [1]. The principles behind Hilton's Law were first espoused in a series of medical lectures given by John Hilton between 1860 and 1862 [1]. John Hilton (1808–1878) was a British surgeon born in Essex (UK) in 1805. He was appointed demonstrator of anatomy in 1828 at Guy's Hospital and assistant surgeon in 1845; he was appointed surgeon four years later. Ten years later, he became Professor of Anatomy and Surgery at the Royal College of Surgeons. From 1859 to 1862, he presented a series of lectures in the form of a course on "Rest and Pain" [1]. The "Law of Anatomy," which has now reached classical status, was revisited and challenged in 2013 using modern technology [2] and was found to be as sound as it was in 1860.

Hilton's Law of Anatomy states: "The same trunks of nerves whose branches supply the groups of muscles moving a joint furnish also a distribution of nerves to the skin over the insertions of the same muscles; and—what at this moment more especially merits our attention—the interior of the joint receives its nerves from the same source" [2].

Upon reflection, we realize that to move any of the joints of the lower limb, all of the muscles around that specific joint are involved. Furthermore, the skin overlying that area receives sensory innervation from branches of the lumbosacral plexus. Because of these two facts, we know that to effectively block painful stimuli from any of the joints of the lower limb, we have to block the entire lumbosacral plexus. In their paper on revisiting Hilton's Law of Anatomy, Marie-Noëlle Hébert-Blouin and colleagues [2] pointed out certain exceptions to this rule, of which the rectus femoris is the most glaring example. While the rectus femoris forms part of the quadriceps group of muscles that move the knee joint, the branch of the femoral nerve that supplies motor innervation to this muscle does not supply sensory innervation to the knee joint, but only to the hip joint, which the rectus femoris muscle also moves. In defense of Hilton's Law, if one reads the law carefully, it does not say "muscle" but "group of muscles." Therefore, the Law remains applicable because the quadriceps group of muscles moves the knee joint, and to provide analgesia to the knee joint, all the nerves to the quadriceps group of muscles must be blocked.

A common misunderstanding that needs our attention is that if, for example, 60% of the nerves that supply sensory innervation to a joint are blocked, the pain generated from that joint would be 60% less. Through the lessons we have learned over the years, especially in obstetric anesthesia where we have seen (and our unfortunate patients have experienced) the unpleasant consequences of unblocked segments or hemi-block with epidurals, and many other scenarios, we now realize that blocking 60% of the nerves that innervate a joint does not reduce pain by 60%. In fact, it only focuses 100% of the pain into the remaining 40% of the joint, therefore, in fact, worsening the pain and suffering of the patient. Although well intended, it is probably not true that we are doing anything positive for the patient by blocking "some" of the nerves and therefore removing "some" of the pain. Disbelief in this misunderstanding, however, is based on clinical experience; it has yet to be challenged by formal research.

Simply put, to provide optimal pain relief due to major surgery or trauma to a joint in the lower extremity, the entire lumbosacral plexus must be blocked. Granted, this is not always possible, especially where the plexus is spread out, as is the case with the lumbosacral plexus. It is especially difficult to achieve during a continuous nerve block, where the catheter is placed on one specific part of the plexus; for example, the lumbar plexus during a continuous lumbar plexus block for pain associated with major hip surgery. When the primary block (high-volume and high-concentration initial block) wears off, the secondary block often fails because the other roots are not close enough or are not in the same circumneural (paraneural) space [3] (see Chapter 2, Fig. **1**) to allow the local anesthetic agent (of too low a volume and concentration) to diffuse to all of the nerve axons of the other more distant roots. Thus, complete coverage of the pain is not achieved (see Microanatomy, Chapters 2, 11, and 14).

It is also not always necessary to block all the nerves that innervate a specific joint. Most of the nerves that innervate a joint reach that joint *via* its joint capsule and during hip replacement surgery or perhaps synovectomy, for example, the joint capsule is destroyed by the surgery, which in effect denervates the joint, making it necessary to block only the nerves that supply sensory innervation to the tissue outside the joint capsule.

MACROANATOMY

Each lumbar and sacral spinal root of the lumbosacral plexus has its own sensory dermatomal area that it represents (Fig. **2**) as well as its own osteotomal area (Fig. **3**), while each nerve has its own neurotomal area of innervation (Fig. **4**).

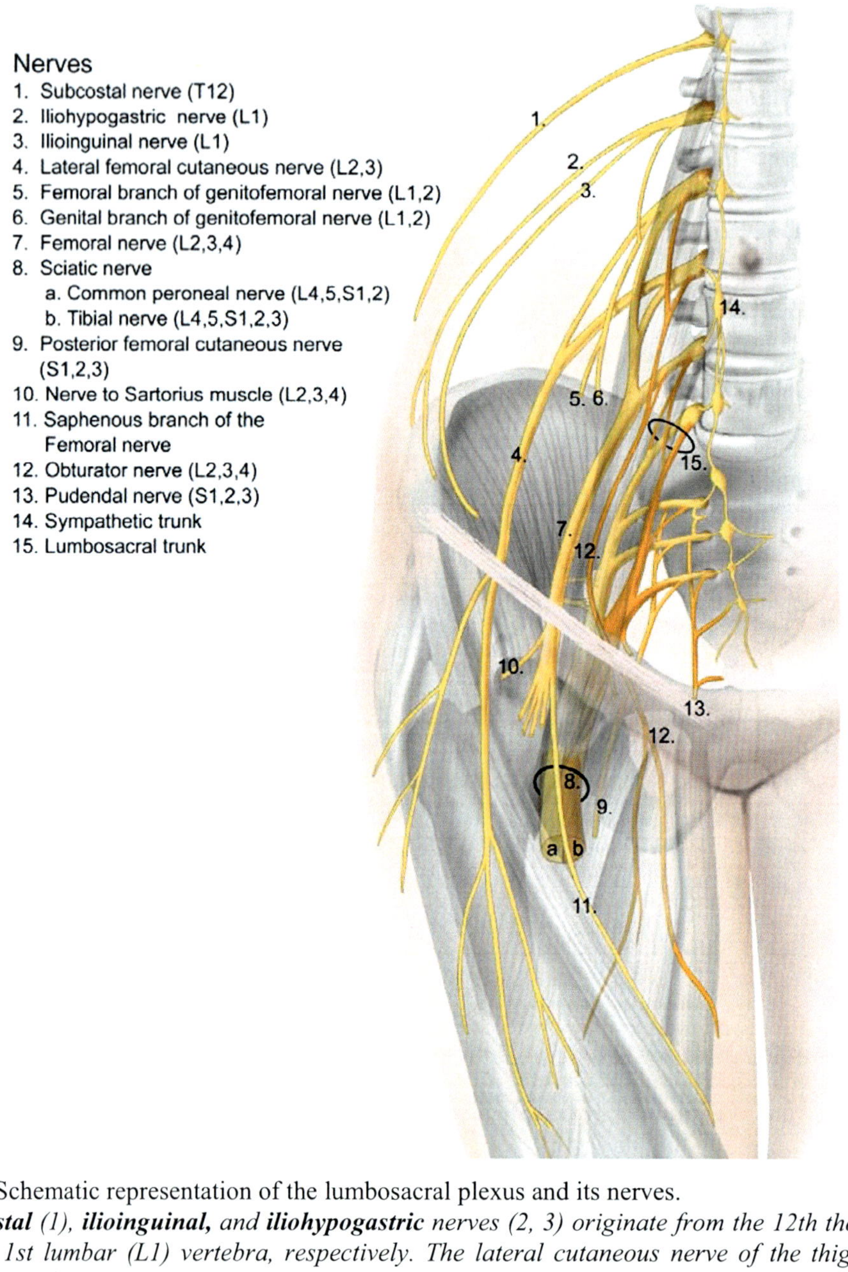

Figure 1: Schematic representation of the lumbosacral plexus and its nerves.
The ***subcostal*** *(1),* ***ilioinguinal,*** *and* ***iliohypogastric*** *nerves (2, 3) originate from the 12th thoracic (T12) and 1st lumbar (L1) vertebra, respectively. The lateral cutaneous nerve of the thigh (4), femoral (5), and genital (6) branches of the genitofemoral nerve originate from the ventral rami of the 2nd and 3rd lumbar vertebrae (L2 and L3), whereas the femoral nerve (7) stems from the dorsal rami of L2, L3, and L4. The 5th lumbar spinal root also gives off a branch to the lumbosacral trunk (15) at the level of L5. The anterior rami of L2 to L4 form the obturator nerve (12), while L5 and the first three sacral roots (S1, S2, and S3) form the sciatic nerve. The pudendal nerve also arises from these roots.*

Dermatomes of the Spinal Roots of the Lower Limb

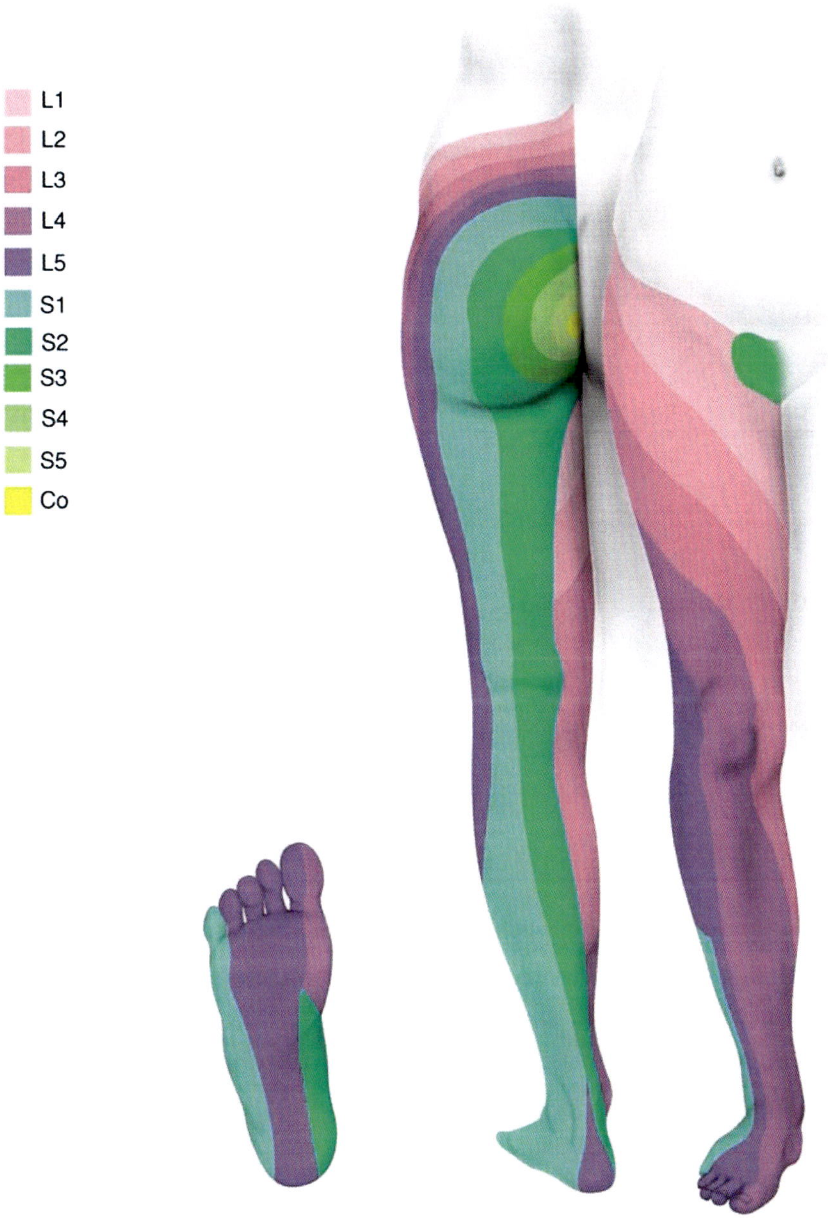

Figure 2: Schematic demarcation of the dermatomes of the lower limb.
These demarcations are not distinct segments as depicted here because there is significant overlap between adjacent dermatomes. L1, L2, L3, L4, and L5 = lumbar roots L2 to 5; S1, S2, S3, S4, and S5 = sacral spinal roots S1 and 2; Co = coccyx.

Osteotomes of the Spinal Roots of the Lower Limb

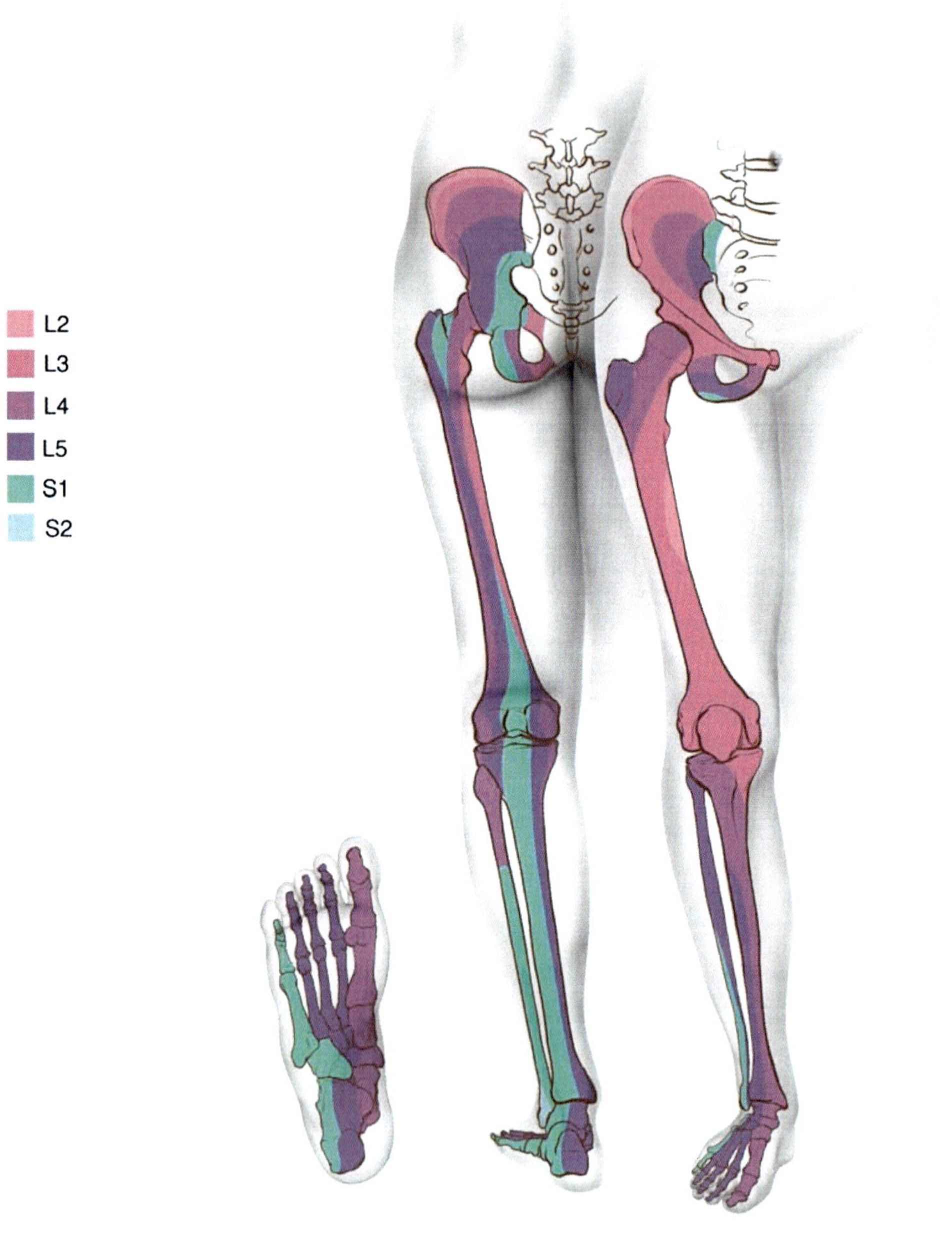

Figure 3: Schematic demarcation of the osteotomes of the lower limb.
These demarcations are not distinct segments as depicted here because there is significant overlap between adjacent osteotomes. L2, L3, L4, and L5 = lumbar roots L2 to 5; S1, S2 = sacral spinal roots S1 and S2.

Neurotomes of the Peripheral Nerves of the Lower Limb

Although the lumbar and sacral spinal roots represent corresponding sensory dermatomes and osteotomes, the individual peripheral nerves innervate different areas of the lower limb represented by neurotomes (Fig. **4** of chapter 10).

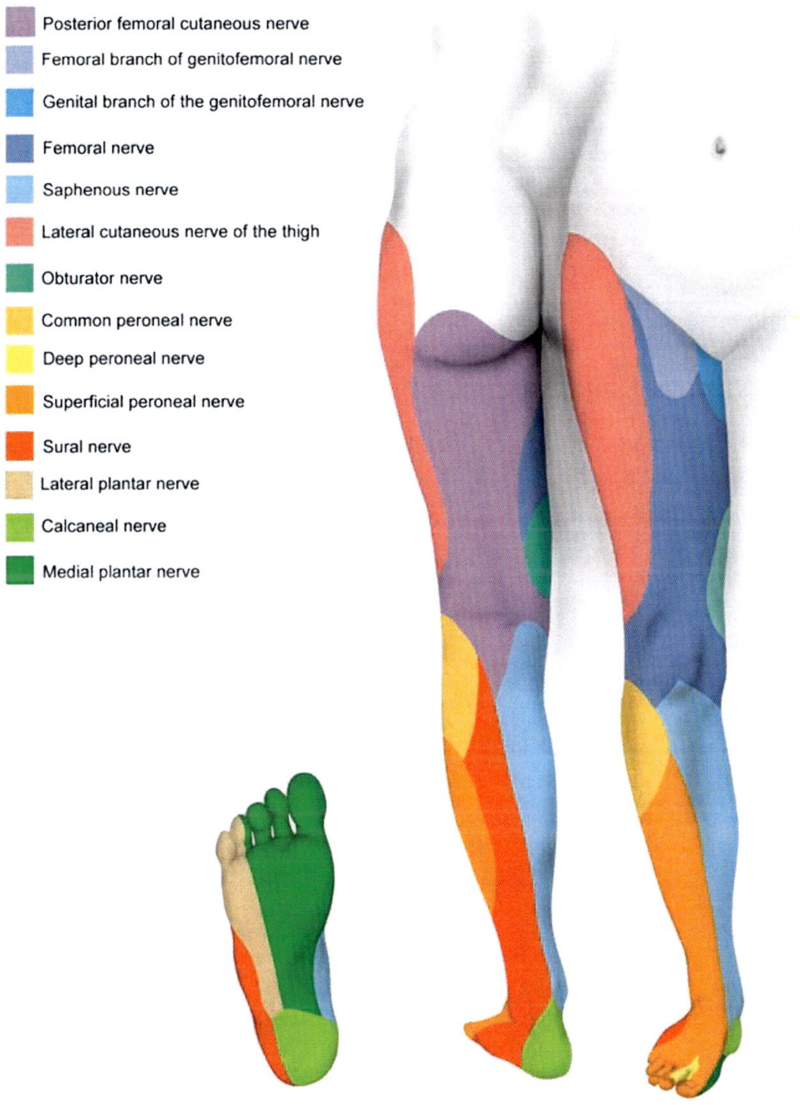

Figure 4: Schematic demarcation of the neurotomes of the upper limb.
These demarcations are not distinct areas as depicted here because there is significant overlap between adjacent neurotomes.

Dissections show that the sciatic nerve originate from the sacral plexus (Figs. **5-8**).

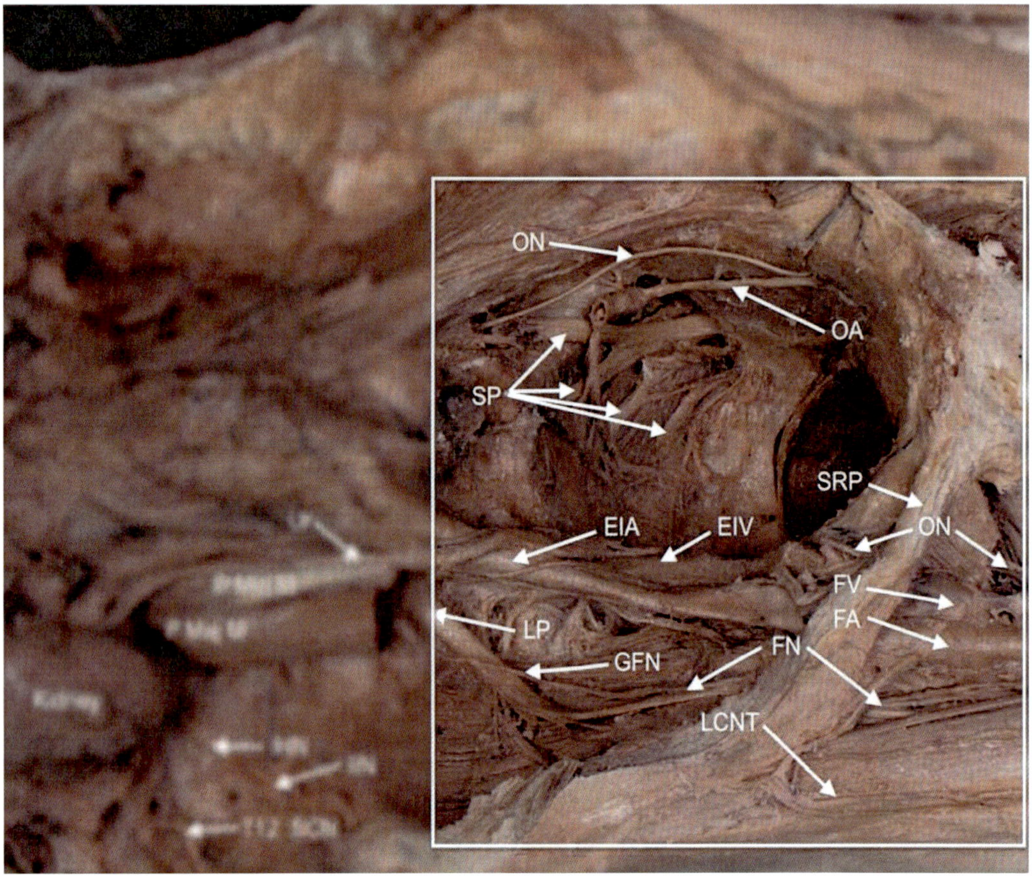

Figure 5: Anatomical dissection of sciatic plexus (SP): abdominal view.
LP = lumbar plexus; SP = sacral plexus; EIA = external iliac artery; EIV = external iliac vein; OA = obturator artery; FA = femoral artery; FV = femoral vein; GFN = genitofemoral nerve; ON = obturator nerve; FN = femoral nerve; LCNT = lateral cutaneous nerve of the thigh; SRP = superior ramus of the pubis.

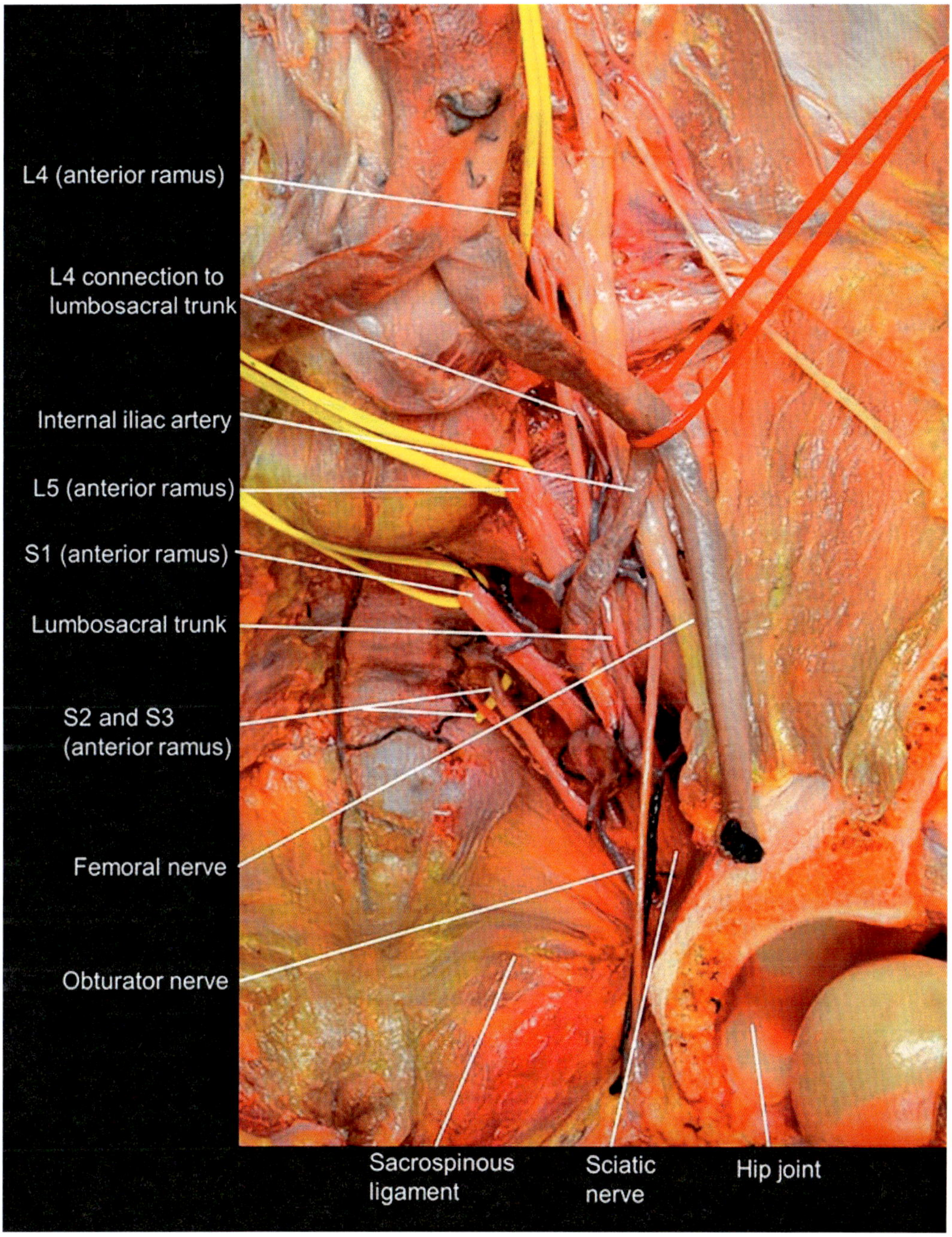

Figure 6: Anatomy of the sacral plexus and sciatic nerve: abdominal view.
The anterior rami of the 4th and 5th lumbar rots and the first three sacral roots (S1–S3) are shown, as well as the lumbosacral trunk. (Reprinted from Reina, Carrera, Llusé, et al. [4] with permission).

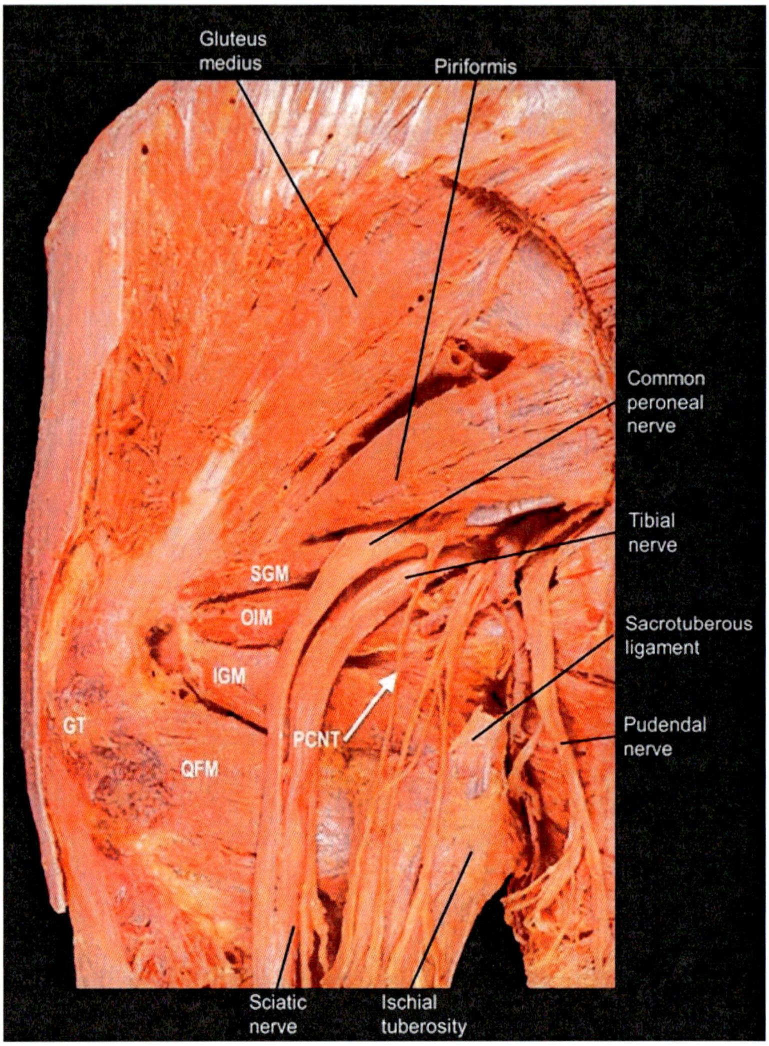

Figure 7: Anatomy of the sciatic nerve.

This view in the region of the subgluteal groove is where a subgluteal sciatic nerve block is usually performed (see surface landmarks in Figs. ***11*** *and* ***12****). The sciatic nerve gives rise to two branches in the popliteal fossa: the tibial nerve and the common peroneal nerve. The lateral sural nerve arises from the common peroneal nerve and the medial sural cutaneous nerve arises from the tibial nerve in the popliteal area, as do the nerves to the soleus and the medial head of the gastrocnemius muscles. Note two parts of the sciatic nerve, the tibial part and the common peroneal part (see Chapter 14). The pudendal nerve is prominent.*
PCNT = posterior cutaneous nerve of the thigh; SGM = superior gemellus muscle; OIM = obturator internus muscle; IGM = inferior gemellus muscle; QFM = quadratus femoris muscle; GT = greater tuberosity of the femur.
(Reprinted from Reina, Carrera, Llusá, et al. [4] with permission).

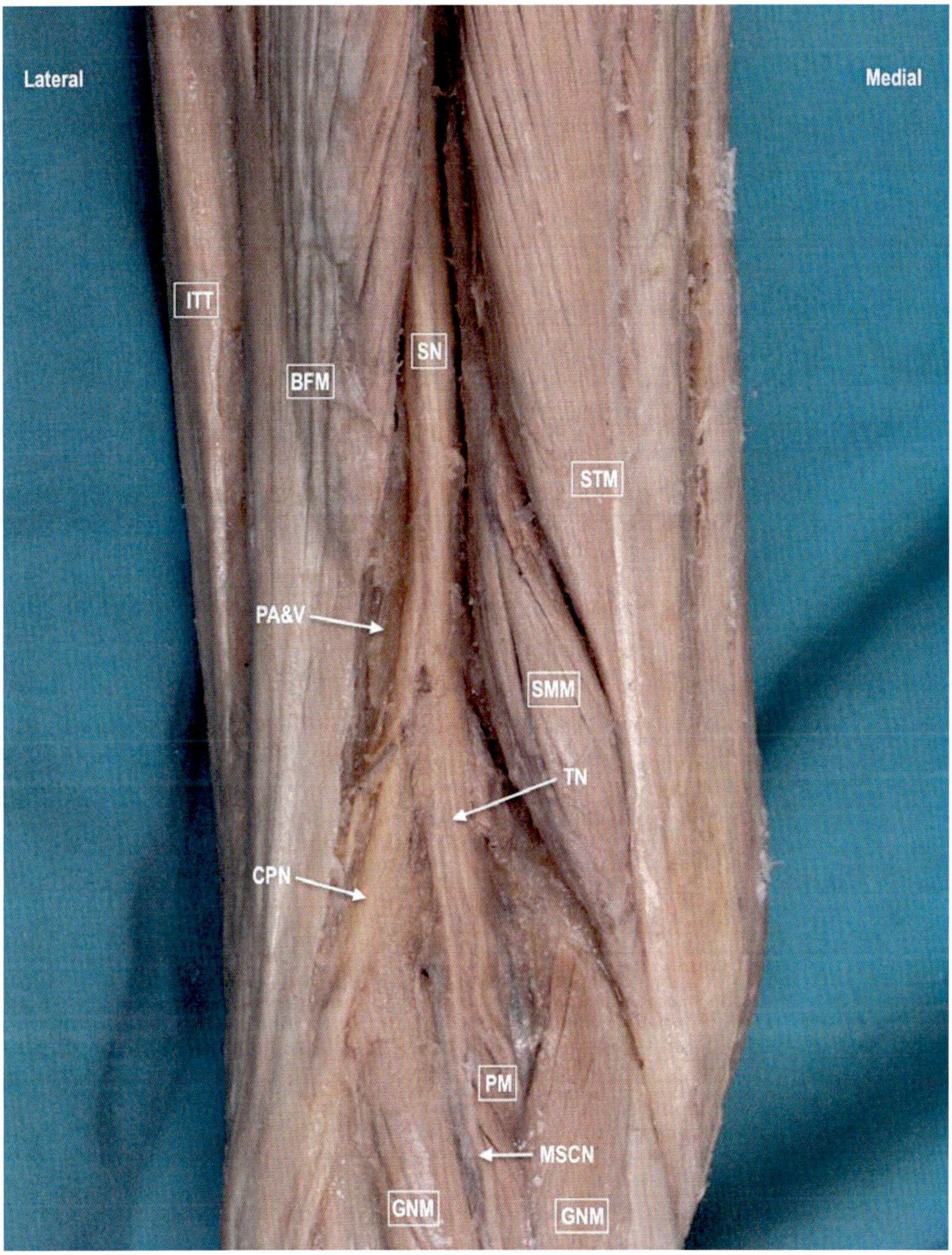

Figure 8: Anatomic dissection of the popliteal fossa.
ITT = iliotibial tract; BFM = biceps femoris muscle; PA&V = popliteal artery and vein; SN = sciatic nerve; STM = semitendinosus muscle; SMM = semimembranosus muscle; TN = tibial nerve; CPN = common peroneal nerve; PM = plantaris muscle; GNM = gastrocnemius muscle; MSCN = medial sural cutaneous nerve.

TRANS-SECTIONAL ANATOMY

The Sciatic Nerve in the Subgluteal Area

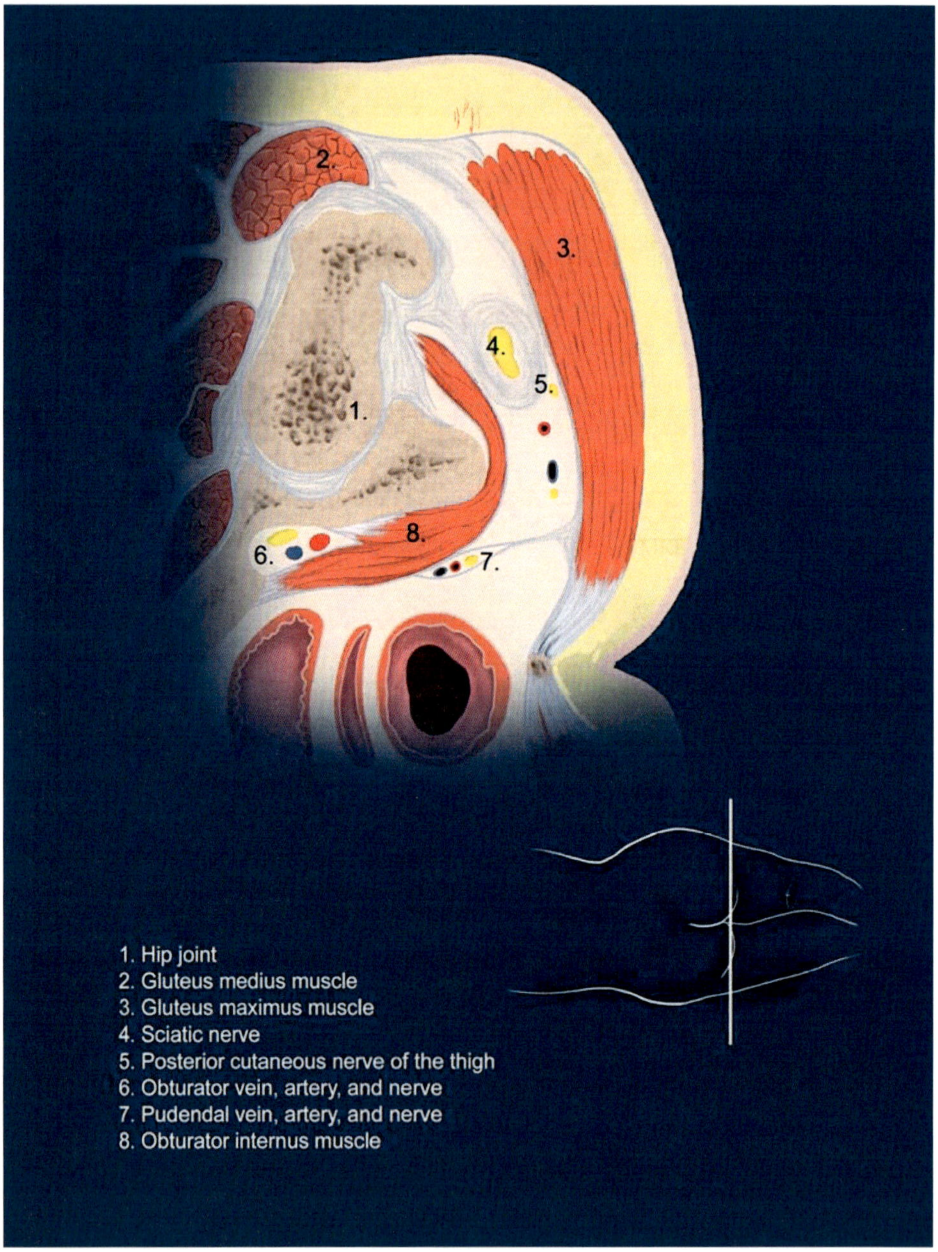

Figure 9: Trans-sectional view of the sciatic nerve in the subgluteal area.
Note that the posterior cutaneous nerve of the thigh is separate from the sciatic nerve (see also Fig. ***1****, Chapter 14)*

The Sciatic Nerve in the Popliteal Area

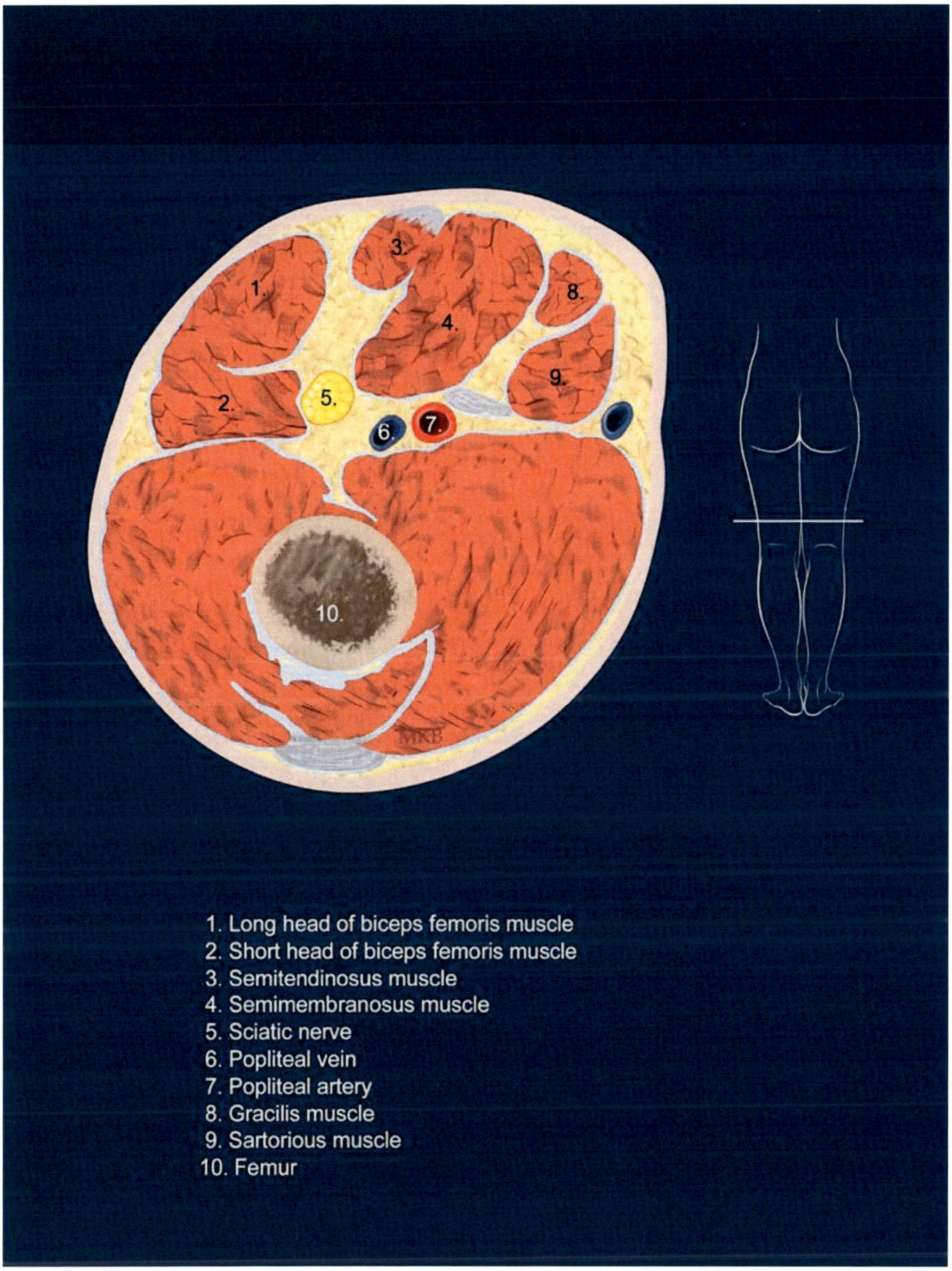

Figure 10: Trans-sectional anatomy of the sciatic nerve in the popliteal fossa.

Surface Anatomy: Subgluteal Sciatic Nerve

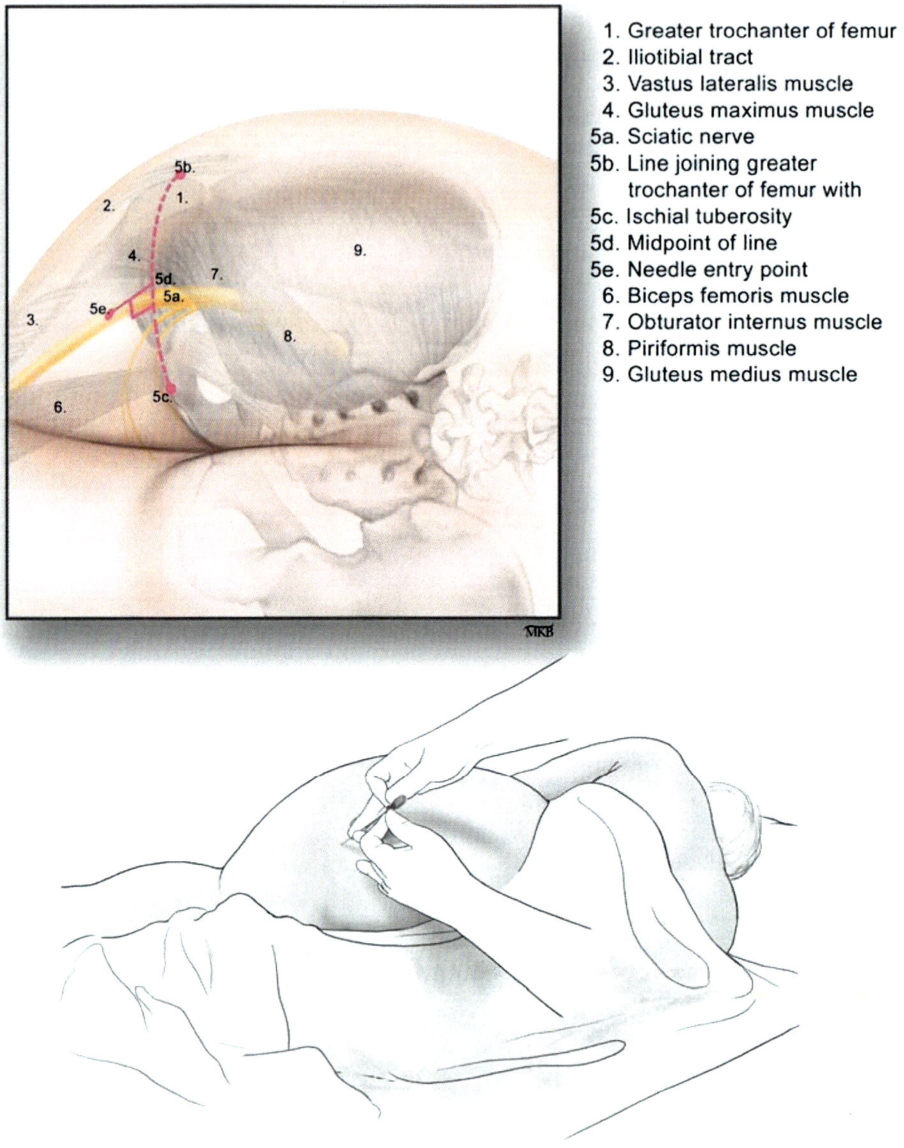

Figure 11: The surface anatomy of the sciatic nerve in the subgluteal area.
A line (5b) is drawn from the greater trochanter (1) that joins it to the ischial tuberosity (5c). A midpoint of this line (5d) and its perpendicular line (5e) outlines the position of the sciatic nerve. The depth of the sciatic nerve from the skin seems to be approximately 43% of the distance between the inguinal to the subgluteal creases from the skin [5]

Surface Anatomy: Parasacral, Transgluteal (Labat), and Subgluteal Sciatic Nerve

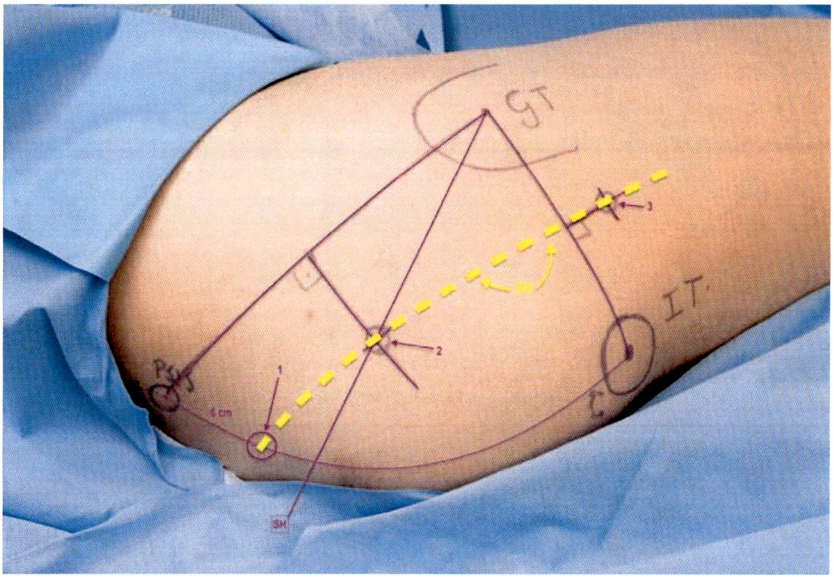

Figure 12: Surface anatomy of the sciatic nerve in the parasacral, transgluteal (Labat, Winnie), and subgluteal areas.
PSIS = posterior superior iliac spine; GT = greater trochanter; IT = ischial tuberosity; SH = sacral hiatus; SN = sciatic nerve. 1, 2, and 3 are the positions where the sciatic nerve can be found:

Position 1: *A line is drawn to join the PSIS with the IT and the sciatic nerve is found 6 cm caudad from the PSIS on this line where it exits the greater sciatic foramen.*

Position 2: *A line is drawn from the GT to the PSIS and a perpendicular line is drawn at the midpoint of this line. In the "Labat" transgluteal approach, the sciatic nerve is found 6 cm down this perpendicular line. In the "Winnie" approach, a further line is drawn from the GT to the SH and the sciatic nerve is found transgluteal where this line crosses the perpendicular line, at Position 2.*

Position 3: *A line is drawn to join the GT with the IT. The sciatic nerve is found in the subgluteal approach on a perpendicular line drawn at the midpoint of this line joining the GR and IT.*

Surface anatomy: popliteal approach to sciatic nerve

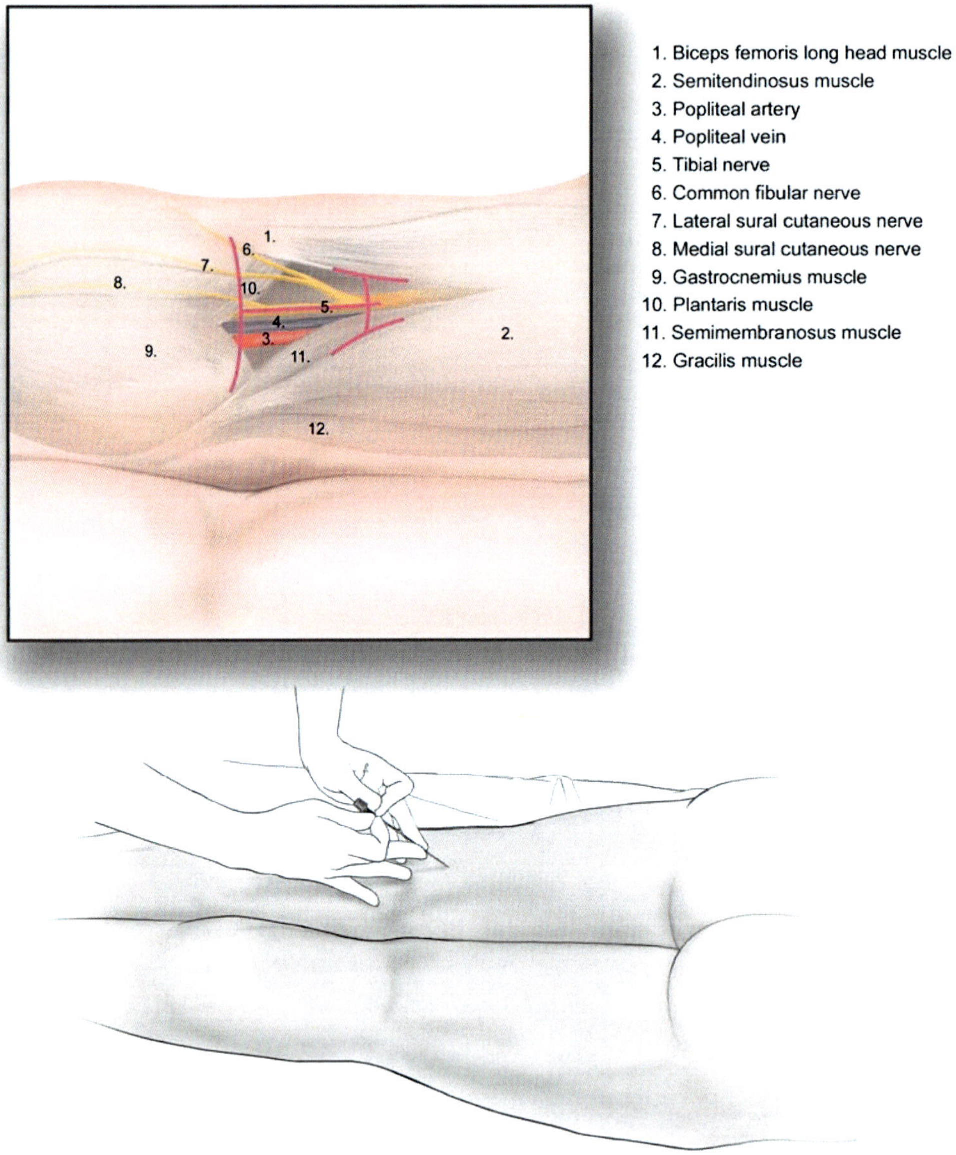

Figure 13: Surface anatomy of the sciatic nerve in the popliteal fossa.
A line (10) is drawn on the popliteal crease line, and two lines are drawn to outline the medial and lateral borders, respectively, of the biceps femoris (1) and semimembranosus and semitendinosus muscles (11). The sciatic nerve is found on a midline (5) that joins the first crease line (10) with a parallel line 7 to 9 cm cephalad that joins the lines outlining the borders of the muscles.

Neurotomes of the Sciatic Nerve

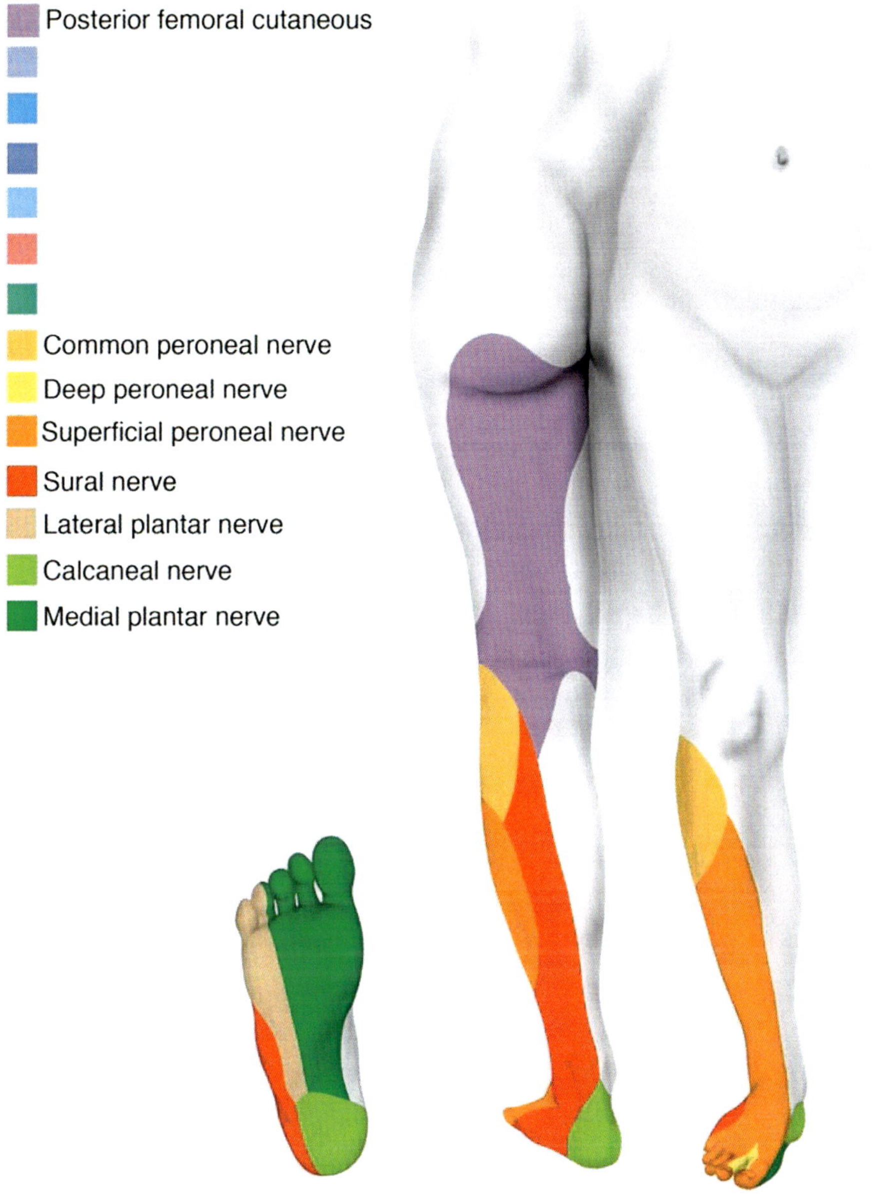

Figure 14: Schematic demarcation of the neurotomes of the lower limb innervated by the sciatic nerve and its branches.
(These demarcations are not distinct areas as depicted here because there is significant overlap between adjacent neurotomes).

Dermatomes of the Sciatic Nerve

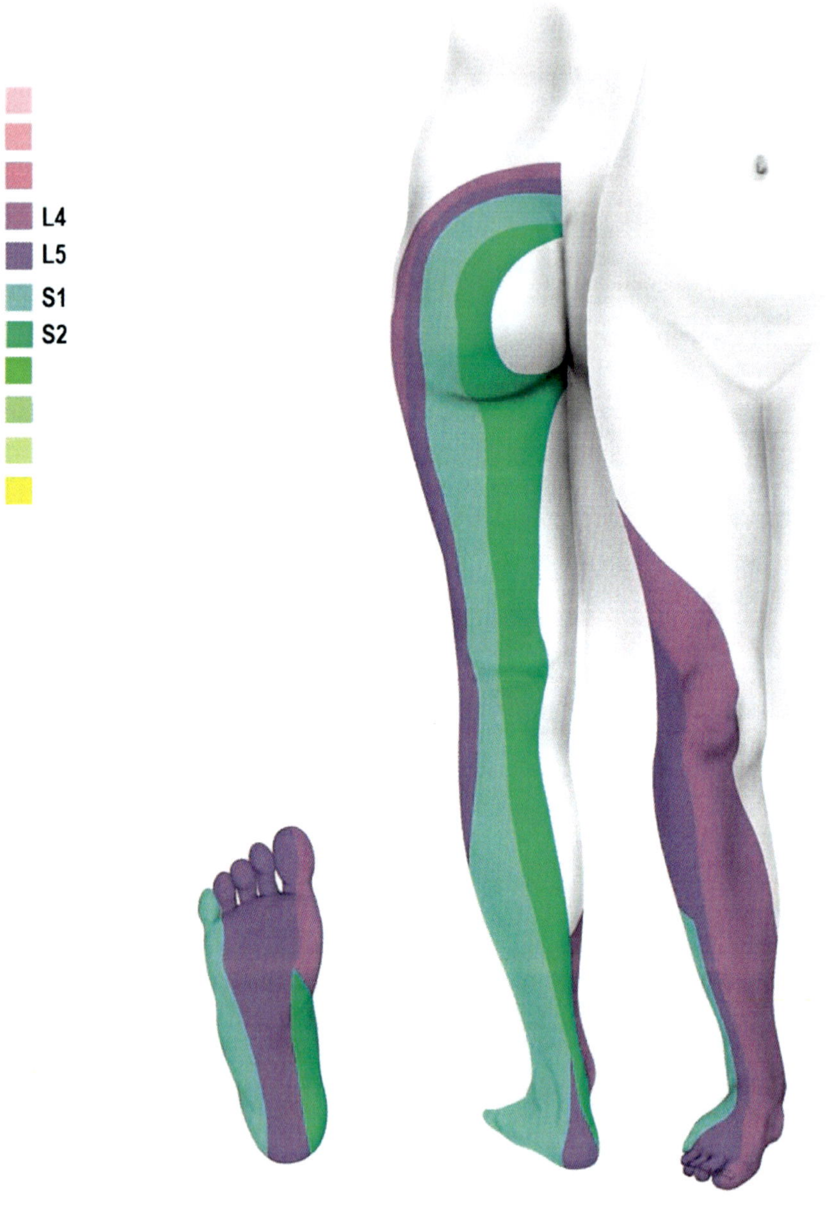

Figure 15: Schematic demarcation of the dermatomes of the lower limb innervated by the sciatic nerve and its branches.
(These demarcations are not distinct areas as depicted here because there is significant overlap between adjacent neurotomes).

Osteotomes of the Sciatic Nerve

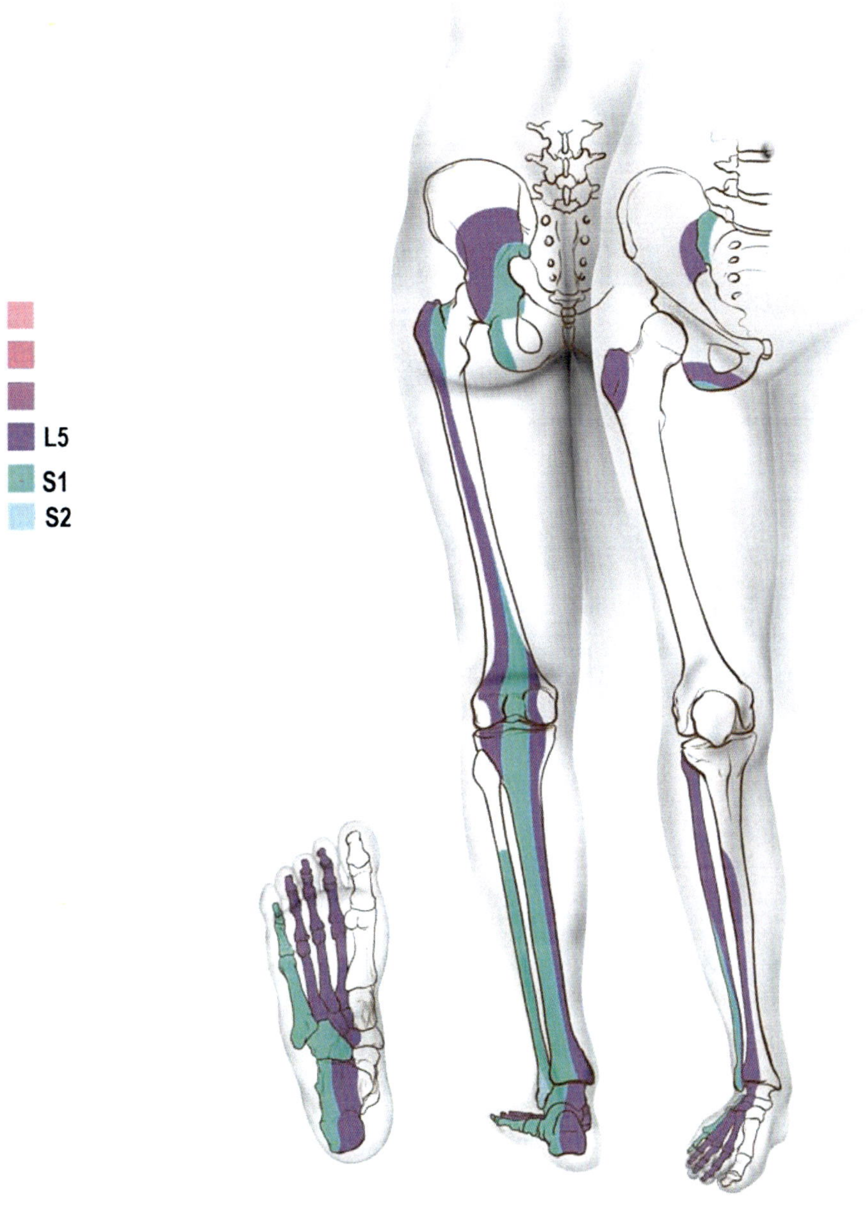

Figure 16: Schematic demarcation of the osteotomes of the lower limb innervated by the sciatic nerve and its branches.
(These demarcations are not distinct areas as depicted here because there is significant overlap between adjacent neurotomes).

INNERVATION OF THE ANKLE JOINT

All the nerves that cross the ankle joint innervate the joint. The more important contributions come from the deep nerves, but the innervation seems to be variable [6]. Three to five articular branches from the ***deep peroneal nerve*** arise at the level of the articular interline. They innervate the anterior aspect of the capsule of the ankle joint, the anterior and inferior tibiofibular ligament, and the anterior talofibular ligament.

The ***posterior tibial nerve*** provides three to five articular branches and innervates the entire medial aspect of the articulation and the posterior and anterior aspect of the medial malleolus. It also innervates the anterior and posterior aspects of the ankle joint.

The ***saphenous nerve***, although being thought of as a pure cutaneous nerve, has a modest but important contribution to the innervation of the ankle joint through its two short articular branches to the anterior medial malleolus and the corresponding capsuloligamentous plane at that level (Fig **15**).

The ***sural nerve*** provides articular branches to the perilateral malleolar capsule and ligament. The superficial peroneal nerve provides inconsistent innervation; it may provide anterolateral and anteromedial branches to the ankle joint.

The talotarsal joint receives nerve supply from the posterior tibial nerve, the ***medial plantar nerve***, and ***accessory deep peroneal nerve*** when present, whereas the cuneonavicular, the intercuneiform, and the cuneometatarsal joints are all innervated on the dorsum by the ***deep peroneal nerve*** and on the plantar side by the medial plantar nerve. The joints of the lateral cuneiform are exceptions in that the ***lateral plantar nerve*** innervates their plantar aspects (see Chapter 16).

SENSORY INNERVATION OF THE KNEE JOINT

The ***saphenous nerve*** leaves the adductor canal and gives off an infrapatellar branch that contributes to the peripatellar plexus before it pierces the fascia lata between the sartorius and gracilis muscles to become subcutaneous and supply the prepatellar skin with sensory innervation. It then descends along the medial tibial border to innervate the skin to the medial side of the foot and the ankle joint.

The ***posterior branch of the obturator nerve*** usually sends an articular filament to the knee joint, which perforates the adductor magnus muscle distally or joins the femoral artery through the opening in the muscle to enter the popliteal fossa. It joins the popliteal artery to the back of the knee, pierces the oblique posterior ligament, and supplies the posterior articular capsule with sensory innervation.

The ***sciatic nerve*** contributes to the sensory innervation of the knee joint in that it splits and gives rise to the ***tibial*** and ***common peroneal nerves*** in the popliteal fossa. The ***articular branches of the tibial nerve*** accompany the superior, inferior medial, and middle genicular arteries to the knee joint. They form a plexus with branches of the ***posterior branch of the obturator nerve*** that supply the oblique posterior ligament of the knee. The branches that accompany the superior and inferior geniculate arteries also innervate the posterior capsule of the knee joint. The ***common peroneal nerve*** has three articular branches, two of which accompany the superior and inferior geniculate arteries; the third ascends with the recurrent tibial artery through the tibialis anterior muscle and supplies the anterolateral part of the knee capsule and the proximal tibiofibular joint.

The principal innervation of the knee is *via* ***three of the four (deep) muscular branches of the femoral nerve*** [7]. The branch to the rectus femoris has a branch to the hip joint but not to the knee joint and therefore, interestingly, does not violate Hilton's law as this law refers to *groups* of muscles, not individual muscles [1, 2]. The largest nerve that innervates the knee is the ***nerve to the vastus lateralis muscle***. The ***branch to the vastus medialis muscle*** descends through the upper part of the adductor canal and can usually be traced downward on the surface of the muscle to the knee joint, whereas the branches of the ***nerve to the vastus intermedius muscle*** (two or three of them) descend through the muscle to the knee joint.

SENSORY INNERVATION OF THE HIP JOINT

It is safe to say that virtually all the nerves of the lumbar and sacral plexus innervate the hip joint because there are no known exceptions to Hilton's Law of Anatomy [7, 8]. Although sensory innervation to the hip joint has been shrouded in mystery for many years and it was thought that the main innervation to the hip capsule came from the obturator nerve, Birnbaum and colleagues [8], after evidently being frustrated by the failure of providing hip analgesia with obturator nerve blocks, comprehensively examined the sensory nerve innervation of the hip joint in formalin-fixed hip joints of cadavers. They found that the innervation of the hip joint was not only complex, but that it also came from a vast number of nerves.

They basically divided the hip joint into segments and the innervation can be summarized as follows:

1. ***Anterior section*** of the hip joint capsule is innervated by:

    a. Articular branches of the ***femoral*** and ***obturator*** nerves.

    b. The ***femoral nerve*** has two articular branches that are responsible for innervation of the anterior and anterolateral region. To some extent, the nerves are accompanied by blood vessels, and in some cases, there is an accessory femoral that is also responsible for sensory innervation to the anterior region of the hip capsule.

    c. The ***obturator nerve*** supplies the anteromedial section of the hip capsule. The articular branches arise from either from the anterior branch, the posterior branch or the trunk of the obturator nerve. One articular branch passes posterolaterally and over the external obturator muscle, running between the adductor brevis and adductor magnus muscles and originates from the trunk of the obturator nerve.

2. The ***posterior section*** of the hip joint capsule is innervated by:

a. The articular branches of the ***nerve to the quadratus femoris*** muscle, which passes out of the sciatic nerve immediately after it exits the infrapiriformis foramen. There are usually between one and five articular branches of this nerve.

b. The articular branches form the ***superior gluteal nerve***, which innervates the posterolateral capsule of the hip joint…

c. Directly from the ***sciatic nerve.*** This nerve passes through the lesser sciatic notch below the sacrotuberous ligament and innervates the internal obturator muscle. It has two articular twigs: one passing posterolaterally and the other posteroinferiorly.

SENSORY INNERVATION OF THE FEMUR

The proximal periosteal innervation for the femur is derived from the nerves that innervate the hip joint, while distally, the femur periostium is innervated by all the nerves that innervate the knee joint [7]. In the areas in between, it gets its sensory innervation form the nerves that innervate the muscles that are attached to the femur (see also Figs. **3** and **16**).

ACKNOWLEDGEMENTS

The author gratefully acknowledge the following people:

- The Head of the Department of Anesthesiology of the College of Medicine of the University of Florida, Dr. Tim Morey, and his department for their moral support and continuous encouragement.
- The faculty and fellows of the Division of Acute and Perioperative Pain Medicine of the above Department of Anesthesiology for affording the author the time to produce this work by covering his clinical duties.
- Mary K. Bryson for her illustrations of Figs. (**1-4** and **9-16**).
- Corey Astrom of the Department of Anesthesiology of the College of Medicine of the University of Florida for her professional and high quality text editing.
- Raeducation.com LLC for their financial support.

CONFLICT OF INTEREST

The author confirms that this chapter contents have no conflict of Interest.

DISCLOSURES

The summary of the innervation of the hip joint has been adapted from the work of Birnbaum, *et al.* [6].

Parts of this work have been previously published in Boezaart A P, Parvataneni HK. Adductor canal block may just be an (unreliable) indirect femoral nerve block. Reg Anesth Pain Med 2014; 39: 556.

ABBREVIATIONS

BFM = biceps femoris muscle

CPN = common peroneal nerve

DP = deep peroneal nerve

EIA = external iliac artery

EIV = external iliac vein

FA = femoral artery

FN = femoral nerve

FV = femoral vein

GFN = genitofemoral nerve

GNM = gastrocnemius muscle

GT = greater trochanter

IGM = inferior gemellus muscle

IT = ischial tuberosity

ITT = iliotibial tract

LCNT = lateral cutaneous nerve of the thigh

LP = lumbar plexus

MSCN = medial sural cutaneous nerve

OA = obturator artery

OIM = obturator internus muscle

ON = obturator nerve

PA&V = popliteal artery and vein

PCNT = posterior cutaneous nerve of the thigh

PM = plantaris muscle

PSIS = posterior superior iliac spine

PT = posterior tibial nerve

QFM = quadratus femoris muscle

SA = saphenous nerve

SGM = superior gemellus muscle

SH = sacral hiatus

SN = sciatic nerve.

SMM = semimembranosus muscle

SN = sciatic nerve

SP = sacral plexus

SRP = superior ramus of the pubis

STM = semitendinosus muscle

SU = sural nerve

TN = tibial nerve

REFERENCES

[1] Hilton, J. On Rest and Pain: A Course of Lectures on the Influence of Mechanical and Physiological Rest in the Treatment of Accidents and Surgical Diseases, and the Diagnostic Value of Pain, delivered at the Royal College of Surgeons of England in the years 1860, 1861, 1862 and 1863.

[2] Hébert-Blouin M-N, Tubbs RS, Carmichael SW, Spinner RJ. Hilton's Law revisited. Clin Anat 2014; 27: 548-55.

[3] Reina MA, Sala-Blanch X. Cross-sectional microscopic anatomy of the brachial plexus and paraneural sheaths. In: Reina MA, Ed. Atlas of functional anatomy for regional anesthesia and pain medicine. New York: Springer Science and Business Media, 2015: 185.

[4] Reina F, Carrera A, Llusá M, Oliva A, Monila JS. Macroscopic view of the lumbar plexus and sacral plexus. In: Reina MA, editor. Atlas of functional anatomy for regional anesthesia and pain medicine. New York: Springer Science and Business Media, 2015: pp. 189-211.

[5] Crabtree EC, Beck M, Lopp BR, Nosovitch M, Edwards JN, Boezaart AP. A Method to estimate the depth of the sciatic nerve during subgluteal block by using thigh diameter as a guide. Reg Anesth Pain Med 2006 31: 358-62.

[6] Sarrafian SK. Anatomy of the foot and ankle: Descriptive, topographic, functional. Philadelphia: J.B. Lippincott Company, 1993; pp. 356-90.

[7] Standring Susan, Ed. Gray's Anatomy: The Anatomical Basis of Clinical Practice. 39th ed. New York: Elsevier/Churchill Livingston, 2005; pp. 1471-88.

[8] K. Birnbaum K, Prescher A, Hepler S, Heller KD. The sensory innervation of the hip joint: An anatomical study. Surg Radiol Anat 1998; 19: 371-5.

CHAPTER 14

Microanatomy of the Sciatic Nerve

André P. Boezaart*

Departments of Anesthesiology and Orthopaedic Surgery and Rehabilitation, Division of Acute and Perioperative Pain Medicine, University of Florida College of Medicine, Gainesville, Florida, USA

Abstract: In this chapter, the author combines the established views of the ultrastructure of the sciatic nerve as an example of a combined peripheral nerve or bundle of nerves with newer concepts that have emerged only recently. The position and importance of the circumneural (paraneural) sheath and subcircumneural or subparaneural space are discussed, as well as the other membranes and compartments around a peripheral nerve, namely, the endoneurium, perineurium, epineurium, and epimysium. The subepimyseal space is discussed in the context of peripheral nerve block.

Keywords: Acute pain medicine, Axon, Circumneural sheath, Combined peripheral nerve, Continuous peripheral nerve block, Endoneurium, Epimysium, Fascia, Fascicles, Gliding apparatus, Microanatomy, Nerve axon, Paraneural sheath, Perineurium Epineurium, Peripheral nerve block, Regional anesthesia, Sciatic nerve, Subcircumneural space, Subepimyseal space, Subparaneural space, Ultrastructure.

ULTRASTRUCTURE OF THE SCIATIC NERVE

At the level of the subgluteal crease, where the subgluteal sciatic nerve block is usually performed, the sciatic nerve is not a single nerve, rather it is a bundle of three nerve branches. The sciatic nerve, as an example of a nerve with a number of branches inside a single circumneurium, is considered here. Like other mixed peripheral nerves, the sciatic nerve, at this level, comprises numerous nerve branches, each surrounded by a single circumneurium, also known as a paraneurium [1-3].

***Corresponding author André P. Boezaart:** Departments of Anesthesiology and Orthopaedic Surgery, Division of Acute and Peri-operative Pain Medicine, University of Florida College of Medicine, 1600 SW Archer Road, Gainesville, Florida 32610, USA; Tel: 352-846-0913 (Work); Fax: 352-392-7029; E-mail: aboezaart@anest.ufl.edu

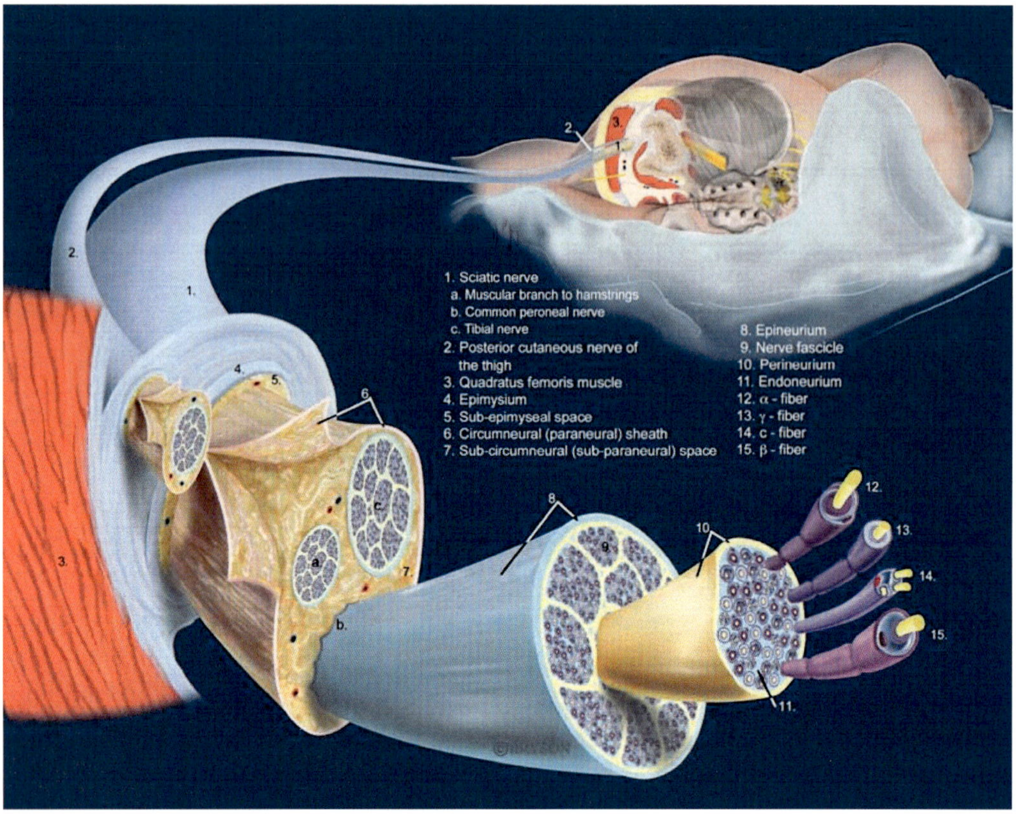

Figure 1: Ultrastructure of the sciatic nerve.

1. *The branches of the sciatic nerve are enclosed in a common circumneural sheath (6).*
2. *There are three branches inside the sciatic nerve: the muscular branch to the hamstring muscles (1a), the common peroneal nerve (1b), and the tibial nerve (1c)*
3. *Outside the circumneural sheath is the subepimyseal space (5), which is surrounded by the epimysium (4) – the fascia that surrounds the nerves, muscles, and blood vessels.*
4. *Deep to the circumneural sheath (6) (also known as the paraneural sheath) is the subcircumneural space (7), which is thought to be the ideal space for the needle in catheter placement for a nerve block.*
5. *The next layer, which encloses each individual branch, is the epineurium (8), surrounding the fascicles of each branch.*
6. *In turn, each fascicle is surrounded by its own perineurium (10).*
7. *Inside the perineurium are the endoneurium and 12 to 15 nerve axons (Table **1** of Chapter 2).*

The ***endoneurium*** (Fig. **1**, No. 11) is a fine cylindrical lamina that encloses groups of axons with their respective Schwann cells. The axons consist of different axon fiber types, depending of the type of nerve in question (see Table **1** of Chapter 2). Both myelinated and unmyelinated axons are surrounded by the collagen fibers of the endoneurium, but the endoneurium is permeable and thus does not interfere with molecules passage through it. The single-layered endothelial cells of the capillaries in the endoneurium contribute to the blood-nerve barrier [3]. The term endoneurium is sometimes incorrectly used to denote the intrafascicular compartment of the nerve. Its use should be restricted to refer to intrafascicular connective tissue, excluding the perineurial partitions that may subdivide fascicles [1]. Approximately 40% to 50% of the intrafascicular space is occupied by non-neural elements and anywhere from 20% to 30% of this is endoneurial fluid (CSF) and connective matrix – the endoneurium [1, 3].

The ***perineurium*** (Fig. **1**, No. 10) comprises multiple single-cell layers that enclose individual nerve fascicles [3]. They become progressively thinner as the number of fascicles increase. As Key and Retzius [1] describe, the essential structure of the perineurium is a lamellated arrangement of flattened cells separated by layers of collagenous connective tissue that provides an ensheathment for both the somatic and peripheral autonomic nerves and their ganglia. The cellular lamellae are composed of concentric sleeves of flattened polygonal cells that are equipped to function as a metabolically active diffusion barrier, although they do not have the morphologic features of a true epithelium.

The ***epineurium*** (Fig. **1**, No. 8) consists of a condensation of areolar connective tissue that surrounds the perineurial ensheathment of the fascicles of uni- and multifascicular nerves [3, 4]. The attachment of the epineurium to surrounding connective tissue is loose, allowing the nerve to be relatively mobile except where tethered by entering blood vessels or branches [4]. Greater amounts of connective tissue are normally present where nerves cross over joints. In general, the more fascicles there are, the greater the quantity of epineurium.

Variable quantities of adipose tissue are also present in the epineurium, particularly in the larger nerves. After studying the distribution of fat in human nerves and finding predominance in the sciatic nerve, researchers feel that this tissue probably has a protective function in cushioning the fascicles against injury by compression. The susceptibility to compression injury is likely to be less in large multifascicular nerves with considerable quantities of epineurium and fat than in smaller and unifascicular nerves.

The ***vasa nervorum*** enter the epineurium, where they communicate with a longitudinal anastomotic network of arterioles and venules [4]. The epineurium also contains lymphatic vessels, which are not present within the fascicles. These lymphatic channels accompany the arteries of the peripheral nerves and pass into the regional lymph nodes [4].

Anderson and colleagues [5] recently demonstrated the ***circumneural (paraneural) sheath*** [3] in dissections, while Karmakar and his colleagues [6] described the appearance of the circumneural sheath with high-definition ultrasound (see Figs. **7** & **8** of Chapter 2). In neurosurgical texts, it has been known as the "gliding apparatus" of the nerve [7]. We now know that injection of a local anesthetic agent or catheter placement in the subcircumneural space (subparaneural space) is ideal for single-injection and continuous nerve block, respectively [8]. Reina and colleagues stained sections through the brachial plexus and peripheral nerves with Masson's trichrome staining to convincingly demonstrate the microscopic ultrastructure of the circumneural (paraneural) sheaths (See Fig. **9**, Chapter 2) [3].

ACKNOWLEDGEMENTS

The author gratefully acknowledge the following people:

- The Head of the Department of Anesthesiology of the College of Medicine of the University of Florida, Dr. Tim Morey, and his department for their moral support and continuous encouragement.
- The faculty and fellows of the Division of Acute and Perioperative Pain Medicine of the above Department of Anesthesiology for affording the author the time to produce this work by covering his clinical duties.
- Mary K. Bryson for her illustrations of Fig. (**1**).
- Corey Astrom of the Department of Anesthesiology of the College of Medicine of the University of Florida for her professional and high quality text editing.
- Raeducation.com LLC for their financial support.

CONFLICT OF INTEREST

The author confirms that this chapter contents have no conflict of Interest.

DISCLOSURE

Parts of this work have been previously published in Boezaart AP. Microanatomy of the peripheral nervous system revisited, and its implications for paravertebral (para-neuraxial) blocks. Proceedings of the 10th Annual pre-ASA Meeting, Orthopedic Anesthesia Pain Rehabilitation Society (www.OAPRS.org); 2013 October 11; San Francisco, California. United States of America [9].

REFERENCES

[1] Key A, Retzius G. Studies in the anatomy of the nervous system and connective tissue. Stockholm: Samson and Wallin, circa 1876.

[2] Horster H, Whitman L. The method of intraneural injection. [Die Methode der intraneuralen Injektion]. Z Hygiene 1931; 113: 113.

[3] Reina MA, Navarro RA, Mateos EMD. Ultrastructure of myelinated and unmyelinated axons. In: Reina MA, Ed. Atlas of functional anatomy for regional anesthesia and pain medicine. New York: Springer, 2015; pp. 3-126.

[4] French JD, Strain WH, Jones GE. Mode of extension of contrast substances injected into peripheral nerves. J Neuropathol Exp Neurlogy 1948; 7: 47-58.

[5] Andrerson HL, Anderson SL, Tranun-Jensen J. Injecting inside the paraneural sheath or the sciatic nerve: Direct comparison among ultrasound imaging, macroscopic anatomy and histologic analysis. Reg Anesth Pain Med 2012; 37: 410-4.

[6] Karmakar MK, Shariat AN, Pangthipampai P, Chen J. High-definition ultrasound imaging defines the paraneural sheath and the fascial compartments surrounding the sciatic nerve at the popliteal fossa. Reg Anesth Pain Med 2013; 38: 447-51.

[7] Millesi H, Zoch G, Rath T. The gliding apparatus of peripheral nerve and its clinical significance. Ann Chir Main Memb Super 1990; 9: 87-97.

[8] Boezaart AP. The sweet spot of the nerve: Is the "paraneural sheath" named correctly, and does it matter? Reg Anesth Pain Med 2014; 39: 557-8.

[9] Boezaart AP. Microanatomy of the peripheral nervous system revisited, and its implications for paravertebral (para-neuraxial) blocks. Proceedings of the 10th Annual pre-ASA Meeting, Orthopedic Anesthesia Pain Rehabilitation Society (www.OAPRS.org); 2013 October 11; San Francisco, California. United States of America.

Chapter 15:
Sonoanatomy of the Sciatic Nerve

CHAPTER 15

Sonoanatomy of the Sciatic Nerve

Barys V. Ihnatsenka[1], André P. Boezaart[2,*] and Yury Zasimovich[1]

[1]Department of Anesthesiology, Division of Acute and Perioperative Pain Medicine, University of Florida College of Medicine, Gainesville, Florida, USA and [2]Departments of Anesthesiology and Orthopaedic Surgery and Rehabilitation, Division of Acute and Perioperative Pain Medicine, University of Florida College of Medicine, Gainesville, Florida, USA

Abstract: Ultrasound is a dynamic process whereby structures can and should be followed to their origins and destinations for optimal identification. Because of this, it is not always satisfactory to study static ultrasound images. When studying sonoanatomy, the authors strongly advise readers to first study the macro- and microanatomy and then to view the accompanying video productions that illustrates the dynamic sonoanatomy (Movies **1-3**). In this chapter, the authors explain the static sonoanatomy of the sciatic nerve at the parasacral, the subgluteal, mid-femoral and the popliteal areas, and with the aid of a video production, the dynamic sonoanatomy of these structures and areas.

Keywords: Acute pain medicine, Common fibular nerve, Common peroneal nerve, Dynamic ultrasound, Gluteus maximus muscle, Gluteus medius muscle, Gluteus minimus muscle, Mid-femoral approach, Parasacral approach, Popliteal approach, Posterior cutaneous nerve of the thigh, Pudendal nerve, Quadratus femoris muscle, Regional anesthesia, Sacral plexus, Sciatic nerve, Sonoanatomy, Subgluteal approach, Sural nerve, Tibial nerve, Ultrasound.

INTRODUCTION

Ultrasound is dynamic whereby structures can and should be followed to their origins and destinations for optimal identification [1]. Because of this, it is not always satisfactory to study static ultrasound images alone. When studying sonoanatomy, the authors strongly advise readers to first study the macro- and microanatomy and then to view the accompanying video productions (Movies **1-3**) that illustrate the dynamic sonoanatomy of the structures discussed in this chapter. After studying this text, it is advisable to recruit a model, sometimes yourself, and reproduce the images in this chapter with an ultrasound machine.

***Corresponding author André P. Boezaart:** Departments of Anesthesiology and Orthopaedic Surgery, Division of Acute and Peri-operative Pain Medicine, University of Florida College of Medicine, 1600 SW Archer Road, Gainesville, Florida 32610, USA; Tel: 352-846-0913 (Work); Fax: 352-392-7029;
E-mail: aboezaart@anest.ufl.edu

The ultrasound transducer probe used throughout the scanning for this chapter was a 2 - to 5 -MHz curvi-linear probe with a 60 mm footprint (C-60, SonoSite Fujifilm, Bothell, WA, USA).

As is the case with almost all the sonoanatomy images, the finer and important ultrastructure of the membranes that surround the nerves, similar for that of all major peripheral nerves [2], cannot readily be visualized with regular ultrasound technology. Please refer to Chapter 2 (Microanatomy) for an explanation of the ultrastructure of these membranes. For that, high-definition ultrasound technology may be required [3].

PARASACRAL SCIATIC NERVE

There may be some clinical situations in which it is necessary to approach the sciatic nerve at this level to place continuous or single-injection nerve blocks. As with every nerve block, the decision to use this approach should be made after careful consideration of the indications and risks. The risks of using this approach are based on the anatomical fact that we approach the sciatic nerve as exits the sciatic notch. With it are other nerves that perhaps do not need to be blocked or we do not particularly want to block, such as the pudendal nerve, which is situated medially. Furthermore, entering the sciatic notch places the needle inside the pelvis, and there are structures nearby that should be avoided such as major blood vessels, the rectum and colon, and ureters, to name a few. The posterior cutaneous nerve of the thigh exits with the sciatic nerve, and if it must be blocked, this, with the transgluteal approach ("Labat approach" [4], presents a reasonable area to approach both the sciatic nerve and the posterior cutaneous nerve of the thigh. Further caudad in the sciatic notch is the nerve to the levator ani and coccygeus muscles; blocking these may lead to fecal incontinence.

To create the images in this section, we positioned the model ("patient") in the lateral or Simms position, as in Fig. (**1**), with the buttock area exposed. We placed the ultrasound transducer probe axially on the ala or wing of the ilium (Fig. **1**), which brings the gluteus maximus, medius and minimus muscles into view as well as the hard line of the wing of the ilium.

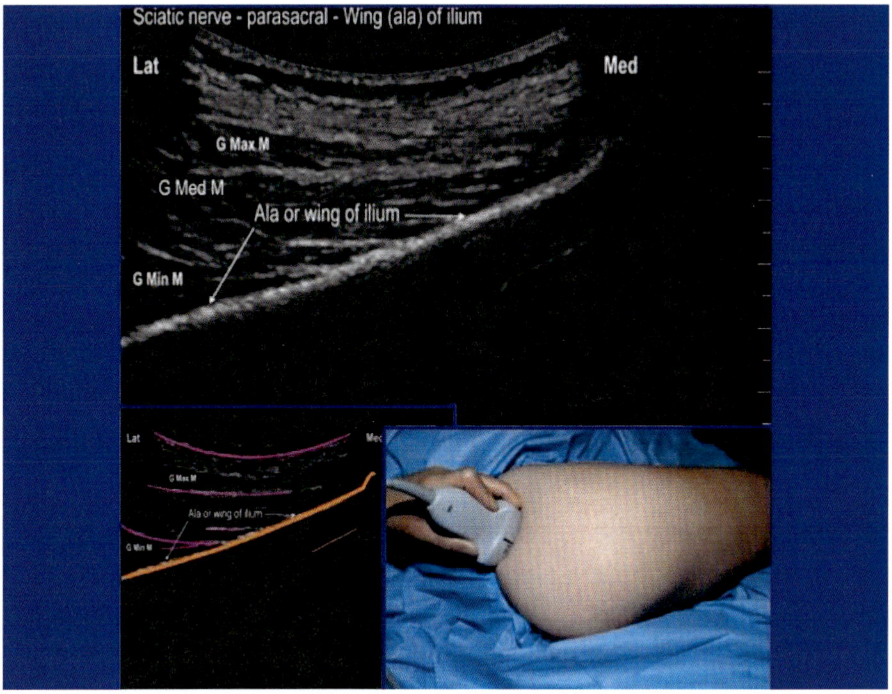

Figure 1: Sonoanatomy of the parasacral approach to the sciatic nerve.
Lat = lateral; Med = medial; G Max M = gluteus maximus muscle; G Min M = gluteus minimus muscle; G Med M = gluteus medius muscle.

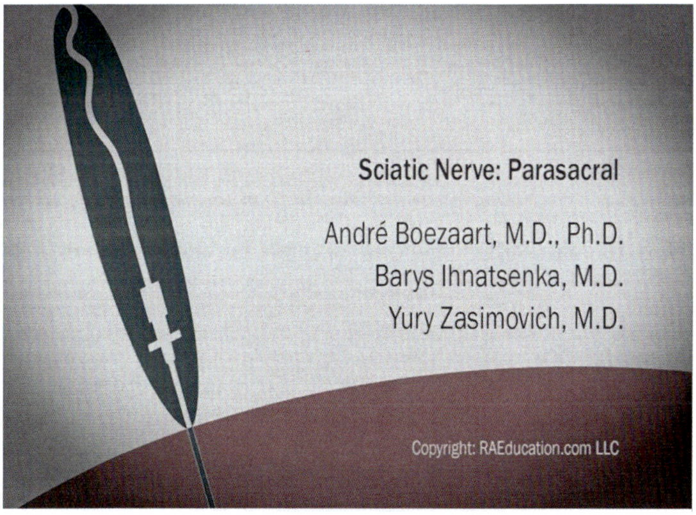

To view this movie click on this link:
https://raeducation.com/ebook

Movie 1: Dynamic sonoanatomy of the parasacral sciatic nerve.

We now slide the ultrasound transducer probe caudally and the sciatic notch comes into view with the body of the ischium bone inferolaterally and the sacrum medially. If we slide the probe more caudad the body of the ilium bone becomes the ischial spine, posteromedially and eventually the ischial tuberosity. In addition to the gluteus muscles, the piriformis muscle can also be seen here (Fig. **2**). The sciatic nerve starts here at the confluence of the 4th and 5th lumbar roots and first three sacral roots. At times, we see spinal roots and other times, the sciatic nerve, which renders a high sciatic nerve block in this area a paravertebral block with all the attributes (good and bad) that accompany a paravertebral block [5]. Chief of these is that the spinal roots may, similar to all spinal roots, be surrounded by dura, which essentially creates a sacral paravertebral and extradural block (see Microanatomy, Chapter 2).

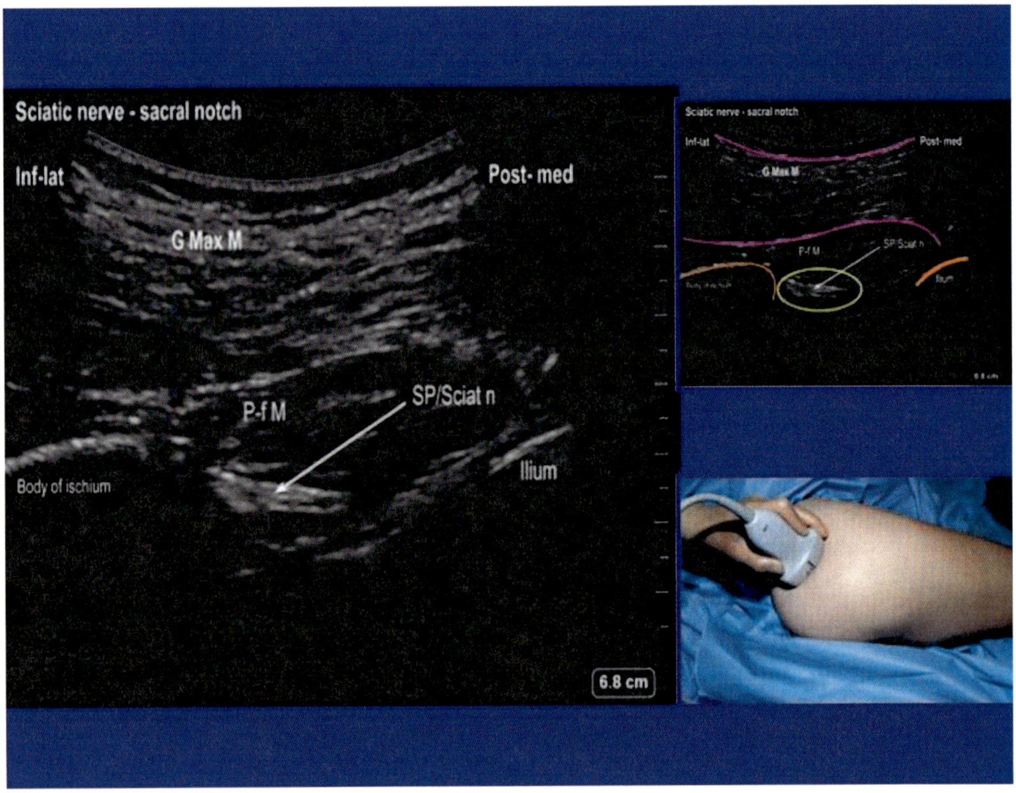

Figure 2: Sonoanatomy of the sciatic nerve or sacral plexus in the sciatic notch or sacral paravertebral space.
Inf-lat = inferolateral; Post-med = posteromedially; G Max M = gluteus maximus muscle; P-f M = piriformis muscle; SP/Sciat nerve = sacral plexus or sciatic nerve. 6.8 cm is the distance from the skin in centimeters in this particular model.

The depth in centimeters obviously varies from one patient to another, depending on the size of the gluteal muscles and the amount of subcutaneous adipose tissue, which was very minimal in this particular model. Having such a minimal amount of adipose tissue, however, is seldom the situation and the deeper (further anterior) the structures are situated, the worse the ultrasound image becomes.

We can now slide the ultrasound transducer probe further distally and follow the sciatic nerve down to the area of the body of the ischium where the "Labat block" or transgluteal sciatic block is performed [4], and even more distally to the subgluteal area, where the nerve is no longer in a confined space. In the mid-buttock or Labat area, the nerve is still in a relatively tight space between the piriformis muscle and the ischial bone and there are a large number of blood vessels in the same area as the nerve, making this an unfavorable area to place continuous or single-injection blocks of the sciatic nerve, but in this position, the posterior cutaneous nerve is still in close proximity to the sciatic nerve. Some important nerves to the hip joint are also located here. As we move the ultrasound probe further distally, we reach the subgluteal area where the sciatic nerve is no longer under the piriformis muscle, the blood vessels are fewer, and the posterior cutaneous nerve of the thigh has course away from the nerve. This makes this an ideal and safe position to place single-injection and continuous blocks of the sciatic nerve if posterior cutaneous nerve or hip capsule blocks are not also sought (Fig. **3**). The posterior cutaneous nerve of the thigh gives off inferior cluneal nerves and perineal branches that one may or may not want to avoid blocking. The depth at which the nerve is situated is again very variable and depends mainly on the amount of subcutaneous adipose tissue in this area -very minimal in this model. The deeper (or more anterior) the nerve is situated, the more difficult it becomes to visualize it with ultrasound. As a rule of thumb, the nerve will consistently be approximately 45% to 50% of the distance from the anterior inguinal crease to the posterior subgluteal crease from the skin [6].

SUBGLUTEAL SCIATIC NERVE

The hamstring muscles implant on the ischial tuberosity and it is not possible to distinguish, nor is it necessary to distinguish, whether this is the biceps femoris or semitendinosus muscle, although the biceps femoris is the most likely because it implants more lateral on the ischial tuberosity than the latter.

The position of the nerve has often been described as in a "hammock" of fascia spanning the femur and the ischial tuberosity [7-9]. We do not need much

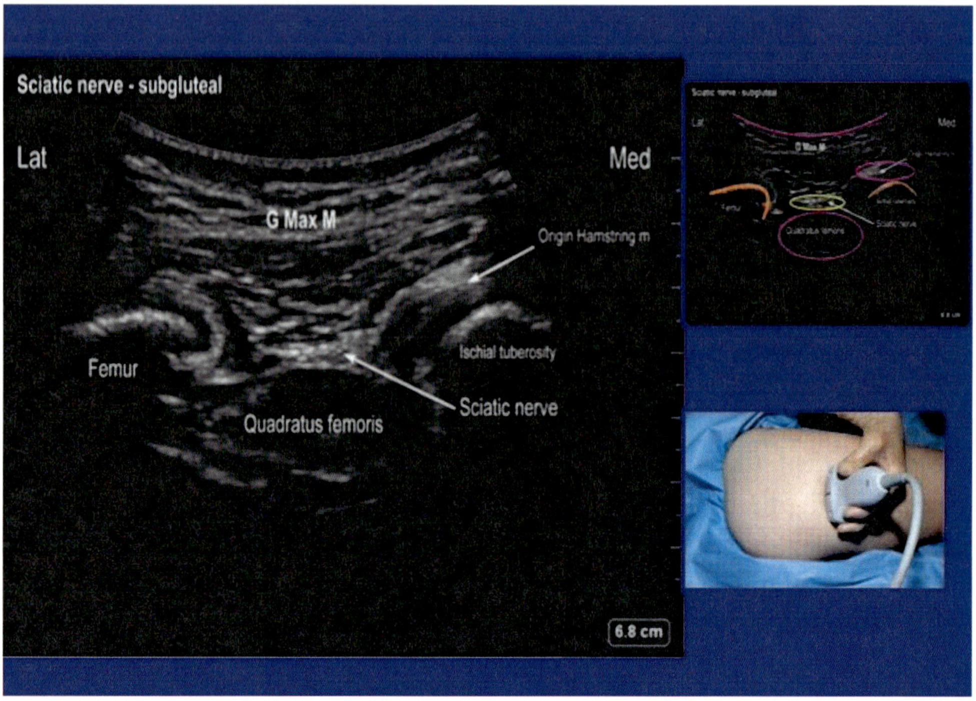

Figure 3: Sonoanatomy of the sciatic nerve in the subgluteal area.
Lat = lateral; Med = medial; G Max M = gluteus maximus muscle (inferior edge); Origin of hamstring m = origin of hamstring muscle. 6.8 cm = distance from the skin in centimeters.

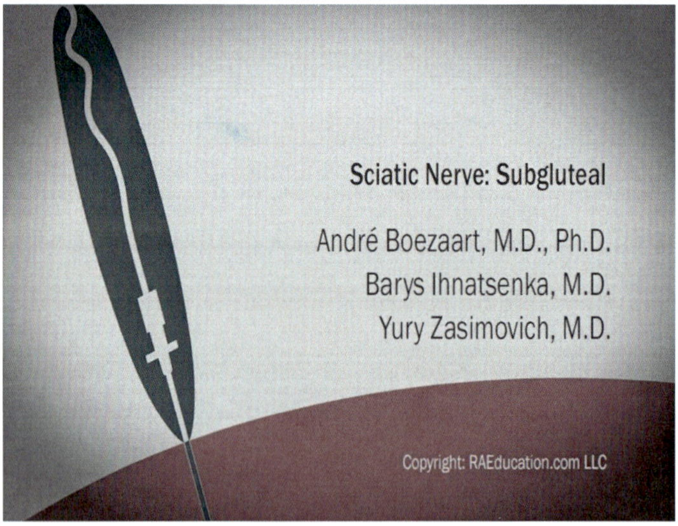

To view this movie click on this link:
https://raeducation.com/ebook

Movie 2: Dynamic sonoanatomy of the subgluteal sciatic nerve.

imagination to see this in this image (Fig. **3**). The nerve courses distally on the quadratus femoris muscle and further down on the adductor minimus, part of the adductor magnus, and further down on the adductor magnus itself. If we follow the nerve down from underneath the piriformis muscle, it lies from superior to inferior, first on the superior gemellus muscle, and then on the obturator internus, and finally on the inferior gemellus muscle before it lies on the quadratus femoris muscle.

We can now follow the sciatic nerve further down to the mid-femoral area. This is an especially valuable exercise if the clinical situation, patient habitus, or positioning dictates a more distal approach. Furthermore, if it is essential to preserve hamstring function in a patient for some reason (mobilization, for example), a more distal approach may be indicated because the nerves to the hamstring muscles branch off of the sciatic nerve just distal to the subgluteal area - usually just distal to its position on the quadratus femoris muscle. When using nerve stimulation to identify the sciatic nerve, it may be of value to know that the muscular branches of the sciatic nerve branch off medially [10]. Thus, if one encounters a hamstring motor response, the stimulating needle needs to be repositioned slightly more laterally.

To prepare the images of Fig. (**4**), the model was positioned in the Sim's position, and the HFL-38 ultrasound probe was used. We can also obtain the same results with the patient lateral or even supine, as in the next section (popliteal).

MID-THIGH SCIATIC NERVE

We now follow the nerve further down with the patient still in the Sim's position. This view of the sciatic nerve in the popliteal area can be obtained from this Sim's position or from a number of other positions, depending on the clinical situation. The images for this section were obtained from the model in the supine position and her lower leg on a specially designed pillow that allows for the ultrasound transducer probe to be placed on the posterior aspect of the leg in the popliteal fossa (Fig. **5**).

The sciatic nerve enters the popliteal fossa and is situated posterior to the femoral artery after it penetrates the adductor hiatus and becomes the popliteal artery. It varies from one patient to another, but the sciatic nerve is usually a solitary nerve high up in the popliteal fossa and splits into the tibial nerve and common peroneal (sometimes referred to as the common fibular) nerve at around 7 to 9 cm above the popliteal crease [11]. This may be an overestimation of the distance. The nerve probably splits closer to 3 - 5 cm abo the crease. The medial and lateral sural nerves also originate from the tibial and common peroneal nerves, respectively, in the popliteal fossa [10], but these are seldom seen with routine ultrasound scanning.

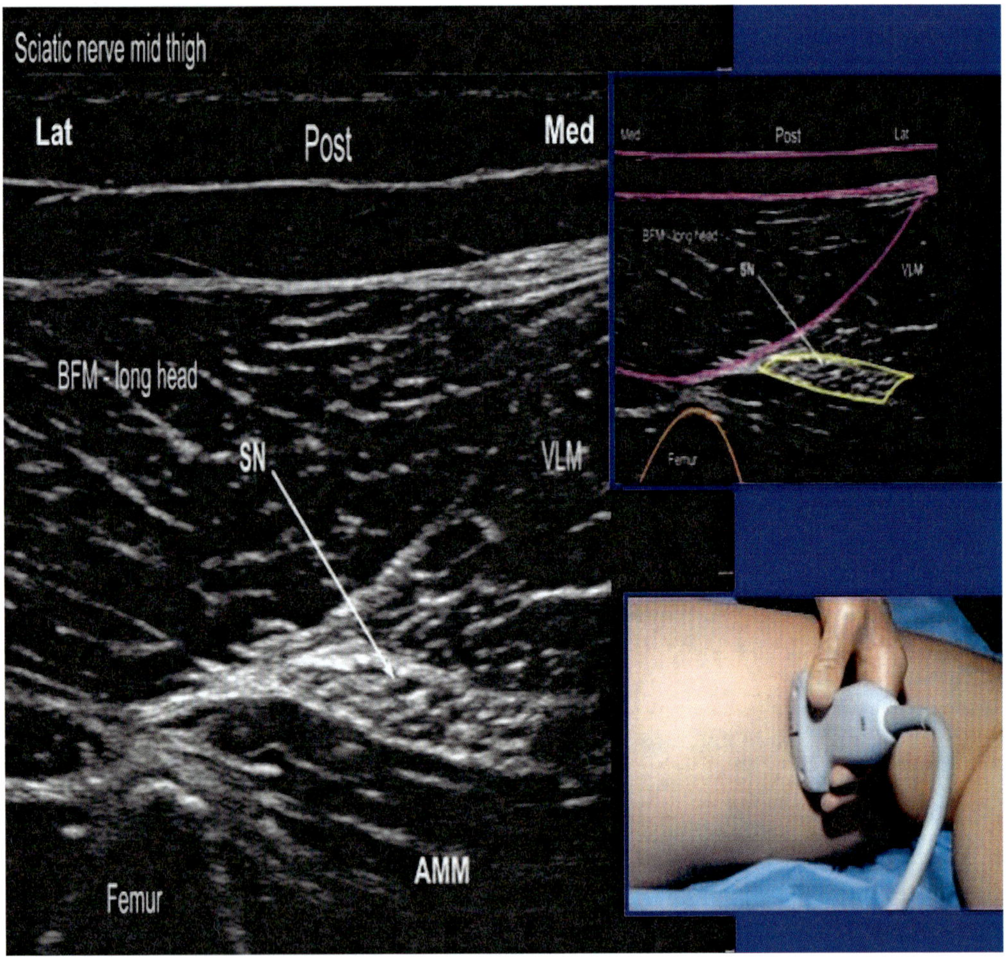

Figure 4: Sonoanatomy of the sciatic nerve in the mid-femoral area.
Med = medial; Post = posterior; Lat = lateral; BFM - long head = long head of the biceps femoris muscle; VLM = vastus lateralis muscle; AMM = adductor magnus muscle; SN = sciatic nerve.

POPLITEAL SCIATIC NERVE

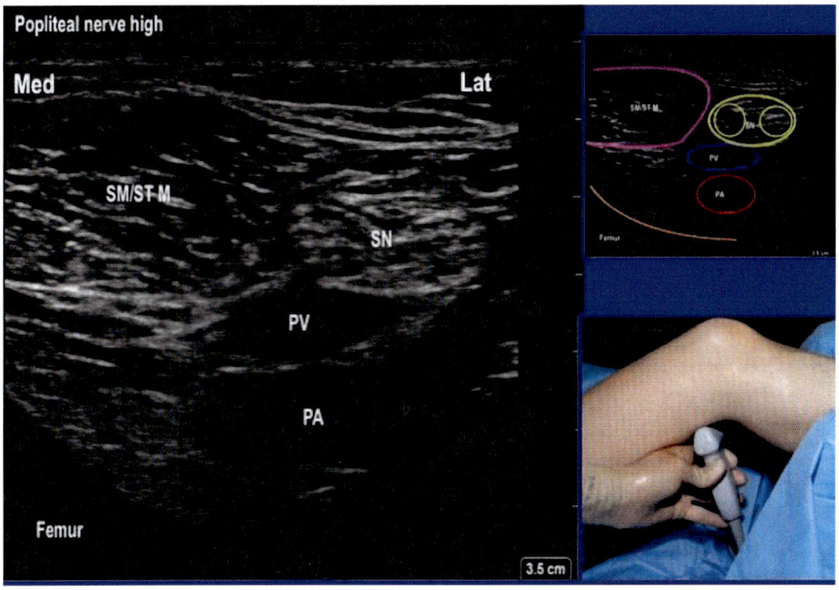

Figure 5: Sonoanatomy of the sciatic nerve (popliteal nerve) in the popliteal fossa behind the knee.
Med = medial; Lat = lateral; SM/ST M = semimembranosus and semitendinosus muscles; PV = popliteal vein; PA = popliteal artery; SN = sciatic nerve (popliteal part of...). 3.5 cm refers to the distance in centimeters from the skin.

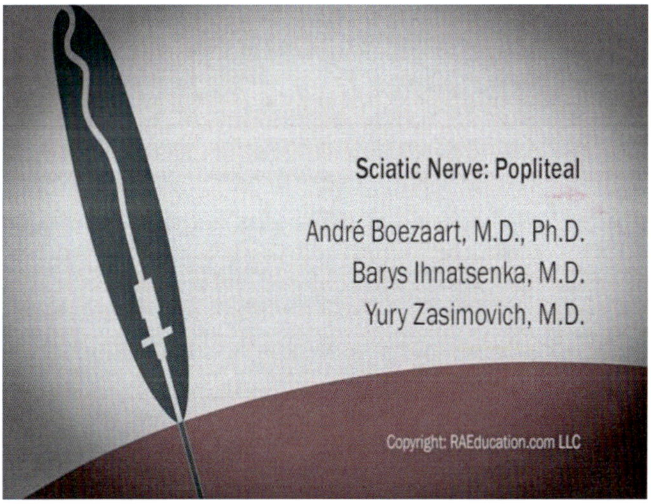

To view this movie click on this link:
https://raeducation.com/ebook

Movie 3: Dynamic sonoanatomy of the popliteal sciatic nerve.

If the nerve can now be followed further distally, it can be seen to split into its common peroneal branch laterally and tibial branch medially.

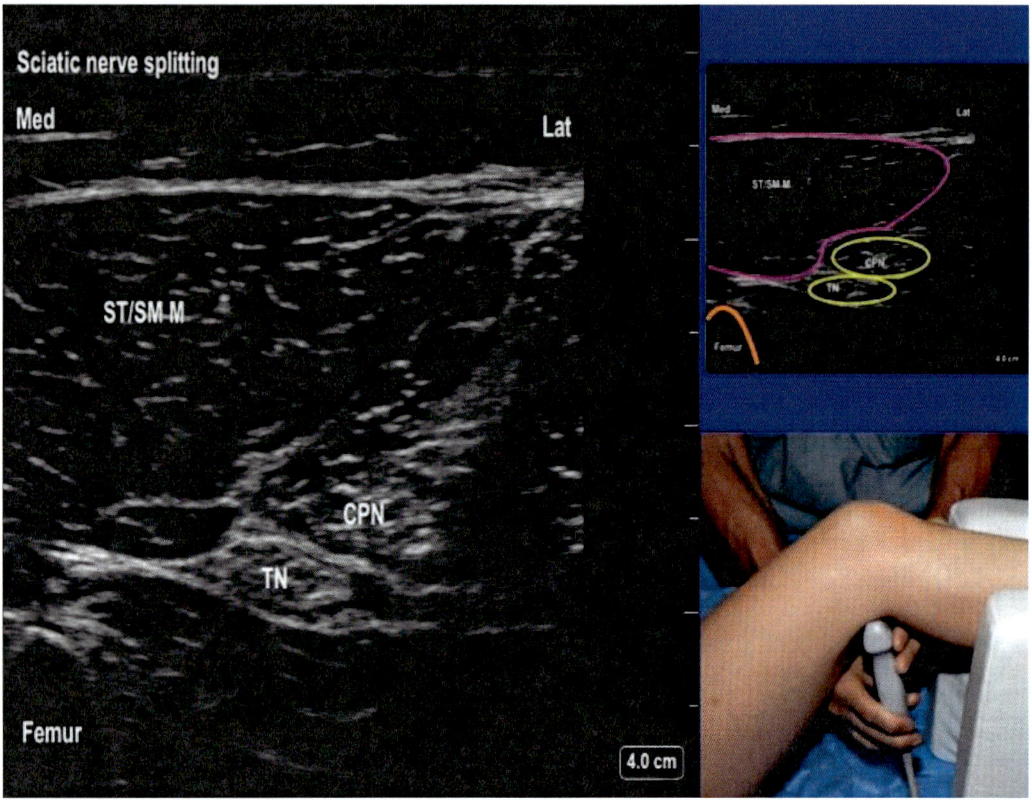

Figure 6: Sonoanatomy of the sciatic (popliteal) nerve in the popliteal fossa showing the early splitting of the nerve.
Med = medial; Lat =lateral; ST/SM M = semimembranosus and semitendinosus muscles; CPN = common peroneal nerve (also called common fibular nerve); TN = tibial nerve. 4.0 cm is the depth in centimeters from the skin.

Following these nerves further distally will show them splitting away totally, as depicted in Fig. (**7**) (from another model), and the lateral common peroneal nerve courses laterally around the femur and later fibular head, while the tibial nerve runs further distally with the popliteal artery and vein.

Lateral to the common peroneal nerve is the long head of the biceps femoris muscle. Medial to the tibial nerve are the semimembranosus and semitendinosus muscles. The pulsating artery and compressible vein can almost always be seen ventral and medial to the nerves.

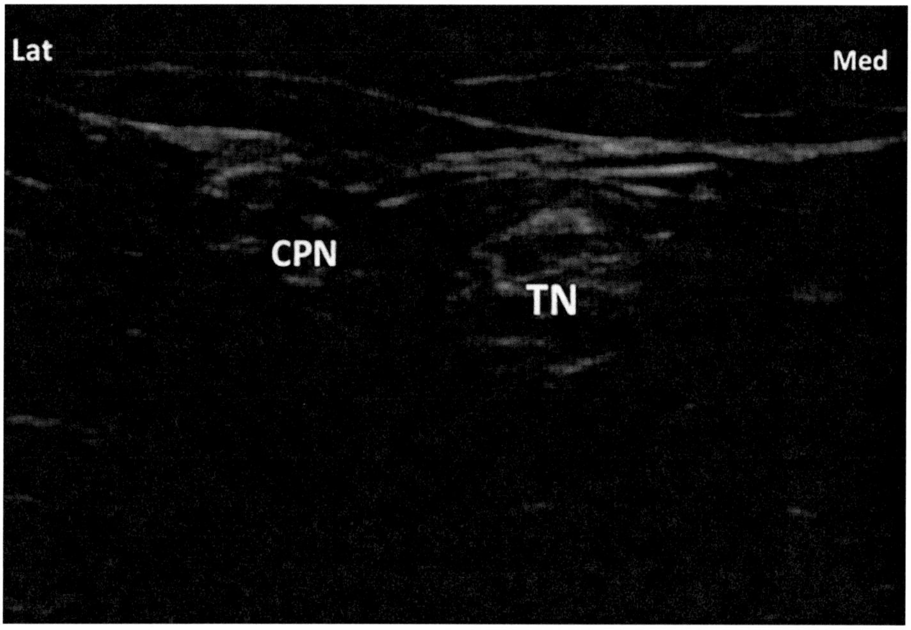

Figure 7: Sonoanatomy of the sciatic nerve (popliteal nerve) in the popliteal fossa after the sciatic nerve has split.
Lat = lateral; Med = medial; CPN = common peroneal nerve; TN = tibial nerve.

ACKNOWLEDGEMENTS

The authors gratefully acknowledge the following people:

- The Head of the Department of Anesthesiology of the College of Medicine of the University of Florida, Dr. Tim Morey, and his department for their moral support and continuous encouragement.
- The faculty and fellows of the Division of Acute and Perioperative Pain Medicine of the above Department of Anesthesiology for affording the authors the time to produce this work by covering their clinical duties.
- Dr. Anastacia Munro for her help with the preparation of the chapter and ultrasound images.
- Corey Astrom of the Department of Anesthesiology of the College of Medicine of the University of Florida for her professional and high quality text editing.

- Nancy Hagen of the Iowa Public Radio for her narration of the movies.

- Raeducation.com LLC for their financial support.

CONFLICT OF INTEREST

The authors confirm that this chapter contents have no conflict of Interest.

ABBREVIATIONS

AMM	=	adductor magnus muscle
BFM	=	biceps femoris muscle
CPN	=	common peroneal nerve
G Max M	=	gluteus maximus muscle
G Med M	=	gluteus medius muscle
G Min M	=	gluteus minimus muscle
Inf-lat	=	inferolateral
Lat	=	lateral
long head	=	long head of the biceps femoris muscle
Med	=	medial
Origin of hamstring m	=	origin of hamstring muscle
P-f M	=	piriformis muscle
PA	=	popliteal artery
Post	=	posterior
Post-med	=	posteromedially
PV	=	popliteal vein

SM/ST M = semimembranosus and semitendinosus muscles

SN = sciatic nerve

SP/Sciat nerve = sacral plexus or sciatic nerve

ST/SM M = semimembranosus and semitendinosus muscles

TN = tibial nerve

VLM = vastus lateralis muscle

REFERENCES

[1] Ihnatsenka BV, Boezaart AP. Ultrasound: Basic understanding and learning the language. Int J Shoulder Surg. 2010;4:55-62.
[2] Reina MA, Sala-Blanch X, Fernández P. Cross-sectional microscopic anatomy of the brachial plexus and paraneural sheaths. In: Reina MA, Ed. Atlas of functional anatomy for regional anesthesia and pain medicine. New York, Springer Science and Business Media; 2015: pp. 237-69.
[3] Karmakar MK, Shariat AN, Pangthipampai P, Chen J. High-definition ultrasound imaging defines the paraneural sheath and the fascial compartments surrounding the sciatic nerve at the popliteal fossa. Reg Anesth Pain Med 2013; 38: 447-51.
[4] Labat G. Regional Anesthesia: Its technic and clinical application (first edition). Philadelphia, PA: W.B. Saunders Company 1923; pp. 289-91.
[5] Boezaart AP, Lucas SD, Elliott CE. Paravertebral block: cervical, thoracic, lumbar and sacral. Curr Opin Anaesthesiol 2009; 22: 637-43.
[6] Crabtree EC, Beck M, Lopp BR, Nosovitch M, Edwards JN, Boezaart AP. A Method to estimate the depth of the sciatic nerve during subgluteal block by using thigh diameter as a guide. Reg Anesth Pain Med 2006 31:358-62.
[7] Karmakar MK, Kwok WH, Ho AM, Tsang K, Chui PT, Gin T. Ultrasound-guided sciatic nerve block: description of a new approach at the subgluteal space. Br J Anaesth 2007; 98: 390-5.
[8] Chan VWS. The use of ultrasound for peripheral nerve block. In: Boezaart AP, Ed. Anesthesia and orthopaedic surgery. New York: McGraw-Hill 2006; pp. 283-90.
[9] Boezaart AP. Atlas of peripheral nerve block and anatomy for orthopaedic anesthesia. Philadelphia, PA: Saunders Elsevier; pp. 171-89.
[10] Netter F H. Atlas of human anatomy, Second Edition. East Hanover, NJ: Novartis 1997; plate 468.
[11] Vloka JD, Hadzic A, April E, Thys DM. The Division of the Sciatic Nerve in the Popliteal Fossa: Anatomical Implications for Popliteal Nerve Blockade. Anesth Analg 2001; 92: 215-7.

Chapter 16:
Applied Macro- and Sonoanatomy of the Nerves Around the Ankle

CHAPTER 16

Applied Macro- and Sonoanatomy of the Nerves Around the Ankle

André P. Boezaart[1,*] and Barys V. Ihnatsenka[2]

[1]Departments of Anesthesiology and Orthopaedic Surgery and Rehabilitation, Division of Acute and Perioperative Pain Medicine, University of Florida College of Medicine, Gainesville, Florida, USA and [2]Department of Anesthesiology, Division of Acute and Perioperative Pain Medicine, University of Florida College of Medicine, Gainesville, Florida, USA

Abstract: To ensure a successful ankle block, it is important to realize that there are two nerves that are deep to the fascia layer and three nerves that are superficial to it. An electrical current can readily cross fascia layers, but local anesthetics cannot, therefore, it is important to deposit the local anesthetic on the correct side of the fascia. The deep nerves are the posterior tibial and deep peroneal nerves. The superficial nerves are the sural, saphenous, and superficial peroneal nerves. If the name of the nerve starts with an "s," it lies superficial to the fascia. The macroanatomy, which includes the trans-sectional anatomy and surface anatomy, and the sonoanatomy of all the nerves around the ankle are discussed in this chapter, as well as the sensory areas that these nerve innervate and the innervation of the ankle joint.

Keywords: Ankle block, Ankle joint, Deep peroneal nerves, Electrical current, Electrical nerve stimulation, Fascia layer, Macroanatomy, Posterior tibial nerve, Saphenous nerve, Sonoanatomy, Superficial peroneal nerve, Sural nerve, Surface anatomy, Trans-sectional anatomy.

MACROANATOMY

The posterior tibial nerve is the terminal branch of the tibial nerve that innervates most of the sole of the foot and is also the only motor nerve at the ankle and can thus be identified with a nerve stimulator. Fig. (**2**) illustrates the sensory innervation of the foot.

***Corresponding author André P. Boezaart:** Departments of Anesthesiology and Orthopaedic Surgery, Division of Acute and Peri-operative Pain Medicine, University of Florida College of Medicine, 1600 SW Archer Road, Gainesville, Florida 32610, USA; Tel: 352-846-0913 (Work); Fax: 352-392-7029; E-mail: aboezaart@anest.ufl.edu

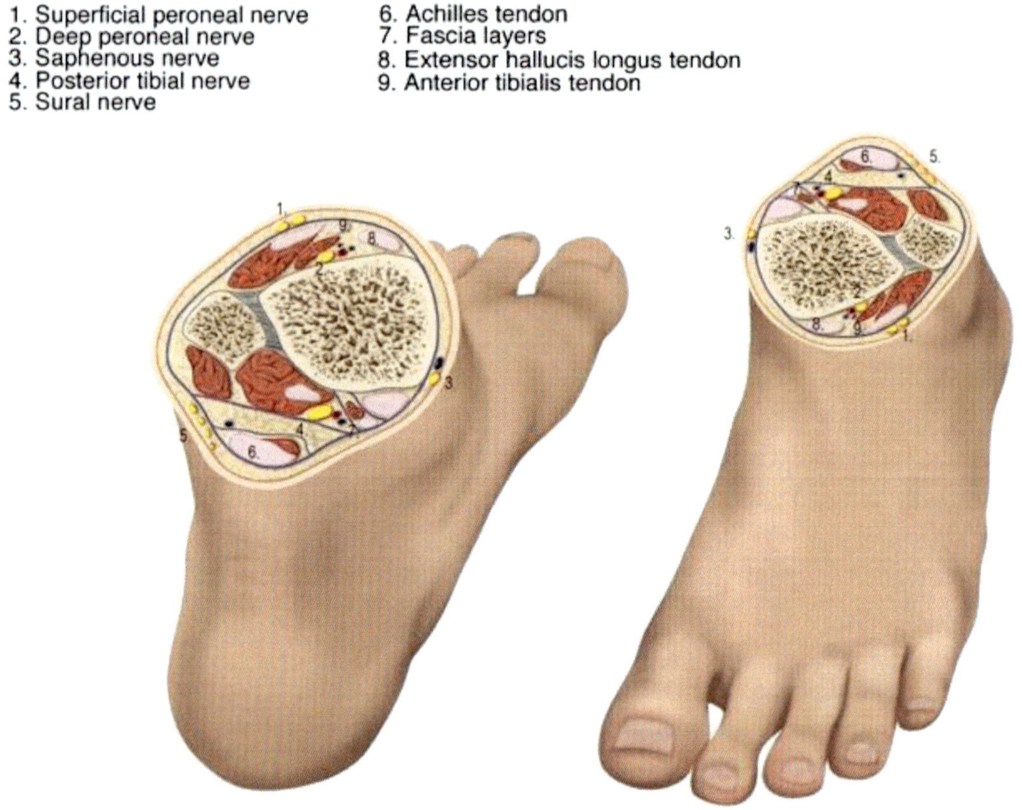

Figure 1: Macroanatomy of the nerves at the ankle: transection through ankle.
This illustration identifies the five nerves of the foot in the context of the fascial layers in which they lie. There are 5 nerves around the ankle; two deep to the fascia layer and three superficial to it. The two deep nerves are the posterior tibial nerve and the deep peroneal nerve, whereas the three superficial nerves are the superficial peroneal, saphenous and sural nerves. Note that the names of all the superficial nerves start with "s".

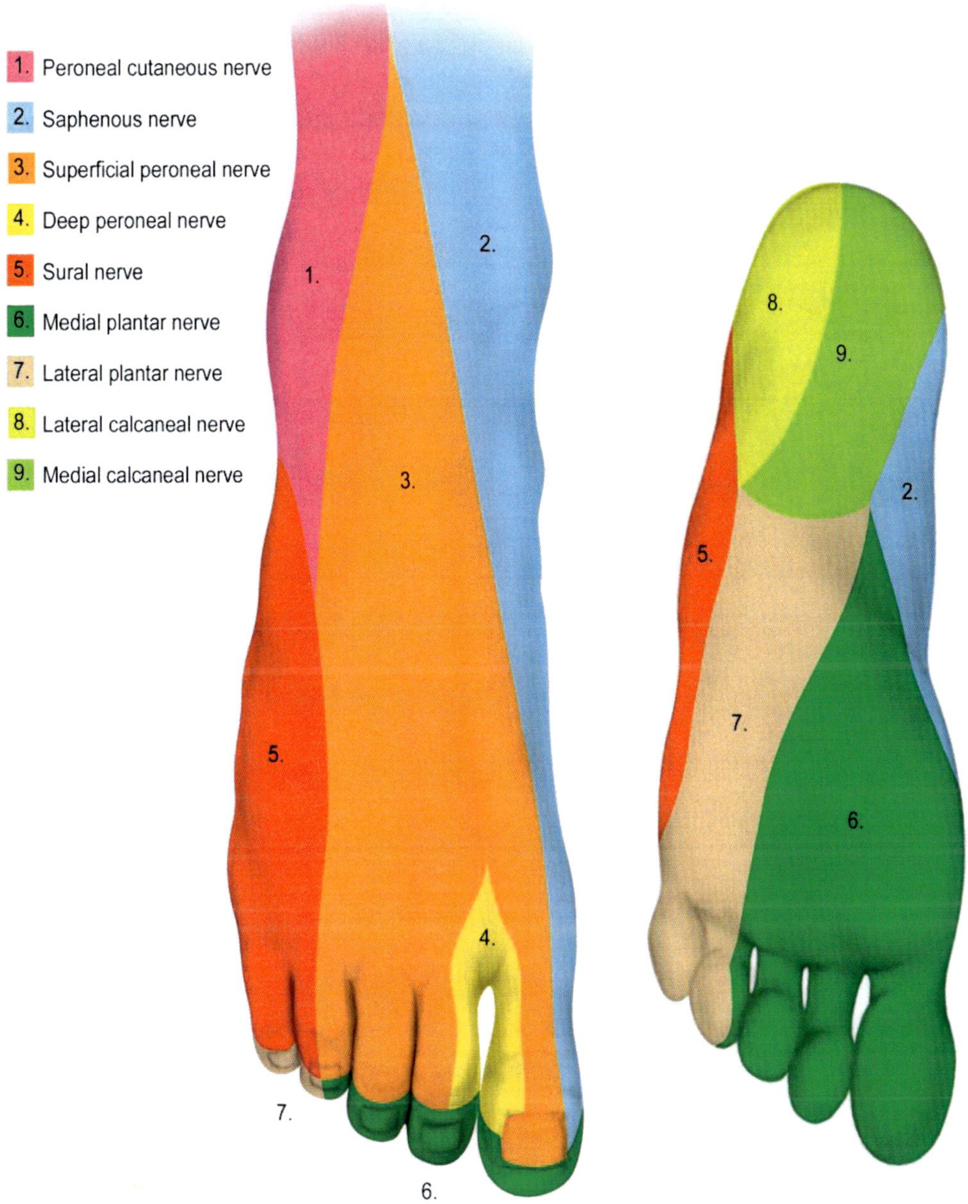

Figure 2: Sensory distribution of the nerves of the foot and ankle.

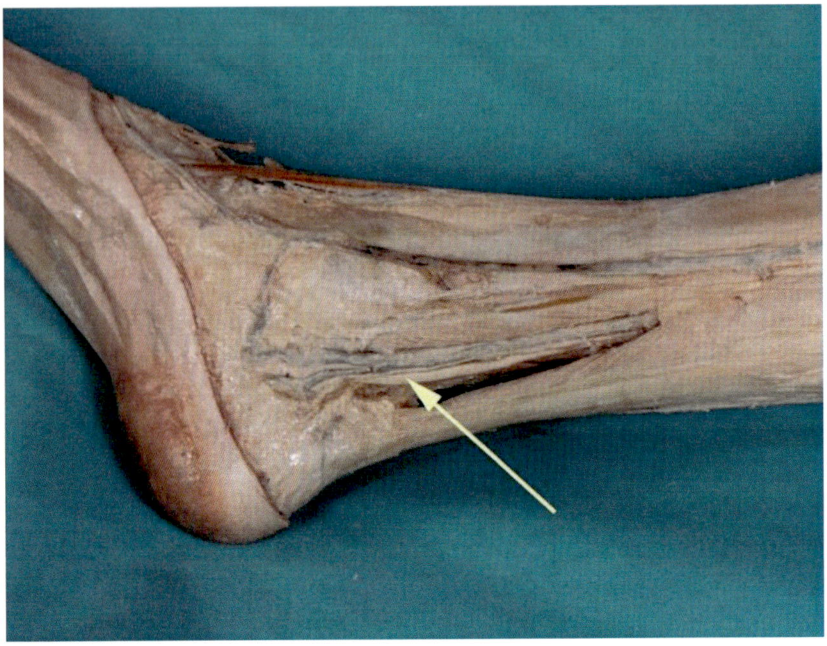

Figure 3: Macroanatomy of the posterior tibial nerve.
Posterior tibial, indicated with the arrow, is usually posterior to the tibial artery.

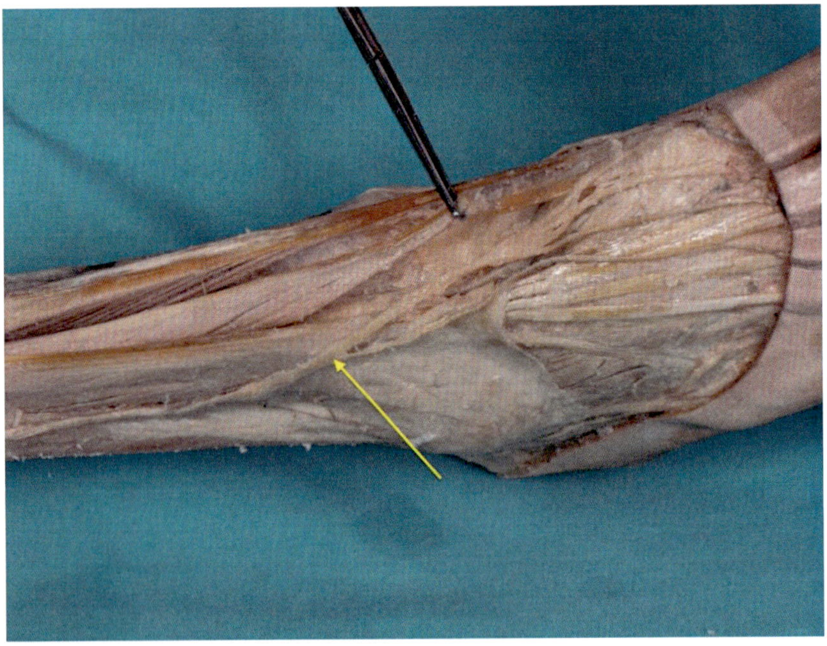

Figure 4: Macroanatomy of the superficial peroneal nerve.
Superficial peroneal nerve is indicated with the arrow.

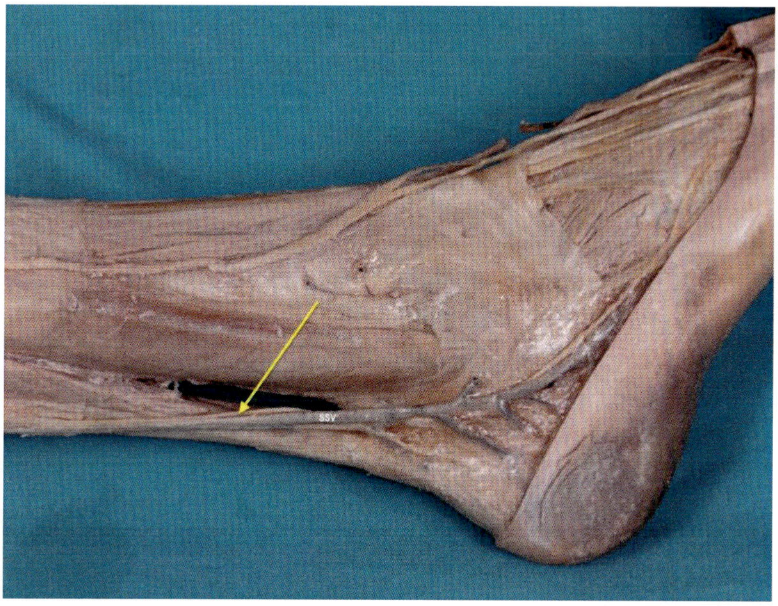

Figure 5: Macroanatomy of the sural nerve.
Sural nerve is indicated with the arrow. SSV = small saphenous vein.

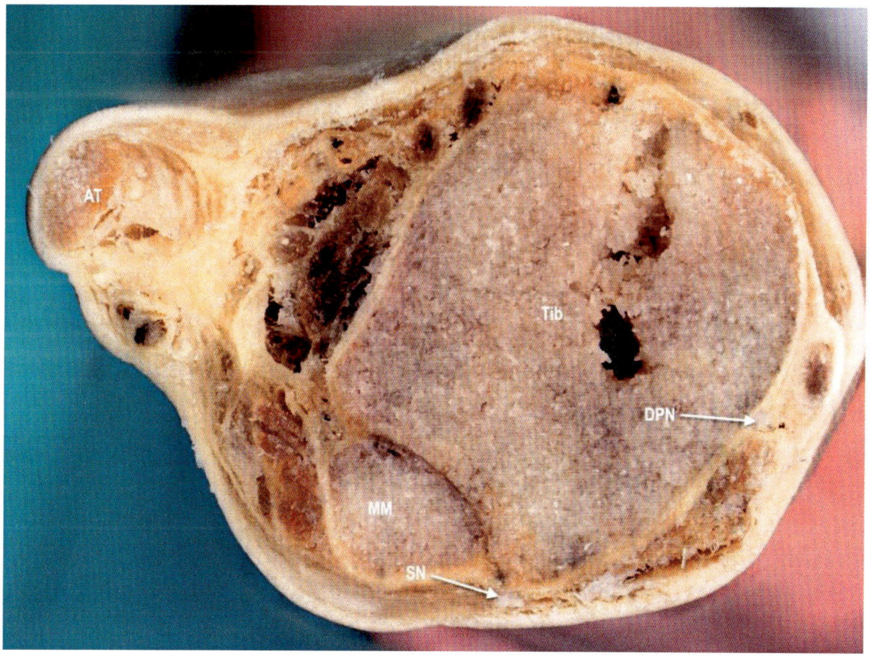

Figure 6: Macroanatomy of the deep peroneal and saphenous nerves.
DPN = deep peroneal nerve; SN = saphenous nerve, Tib = tibia; MM = medial malleolus; AT = Achilles tendon.

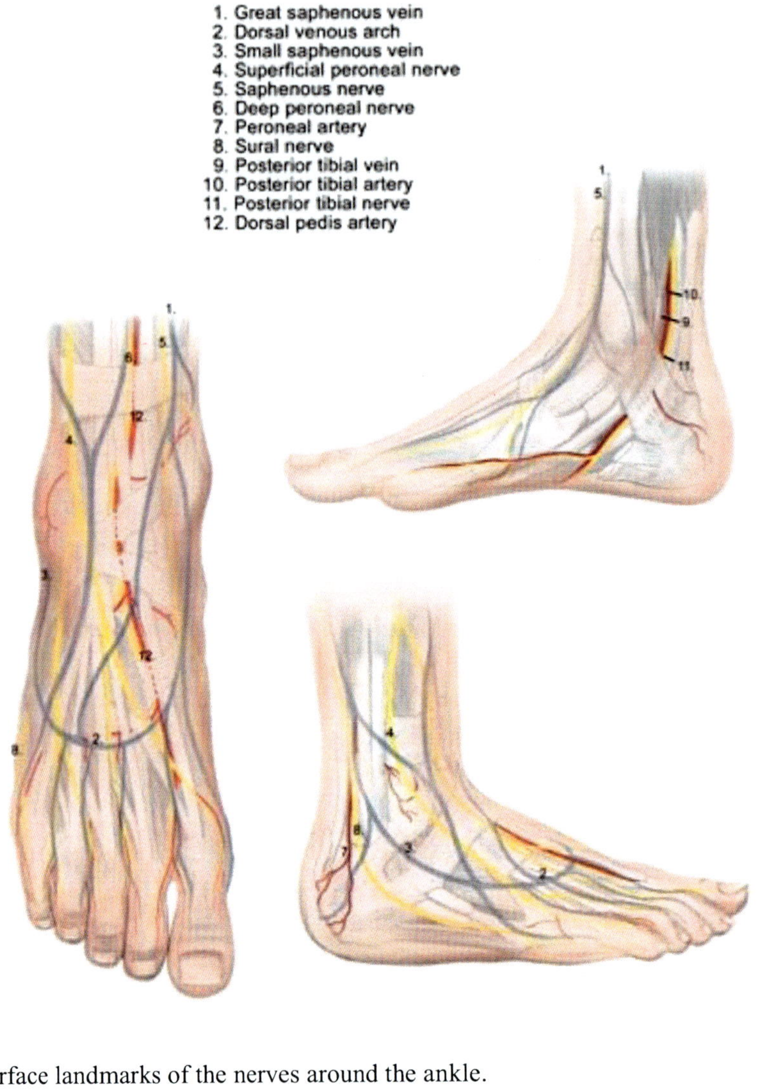

Figure 7: Surface landmarks of the nerves around the ankle.

- *The posterior tibial nerve is 2/3 the distance from the Achilles tendon to the lateral malleolus on the lateral side of the ankle – deep to the fascia.*
- *The deep peroneal nerve is between the tendons of the tibialis anterior and extensor hallucis longus muscles – deep to the fascia.*
- *The superficial peroneal nerve is situated lateral of the tendon of the extensor digitorum longus muscle – superficial to the fascia.*
- *The saphenous nerve runs with the great saphenous vein on the anterior aspect of the medial malleolus – superficial to the fascia.*
- *The sural nerve is situated half way between the Achilles tendon and lateral malleolus on the lateral side of the ankle.*

SONOANATOMY OF THE NERVES AROUND THE ANKLE

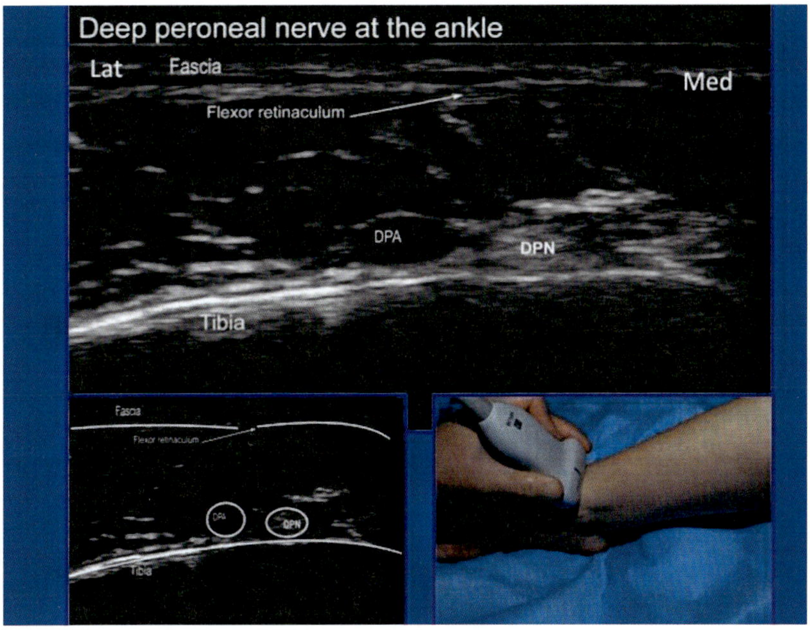

Figure 8: Sonoanatomy of the deep peroneal nerve at the ankle.
DPA = deep peroneal artery, DPN = deep peroneal nerve.

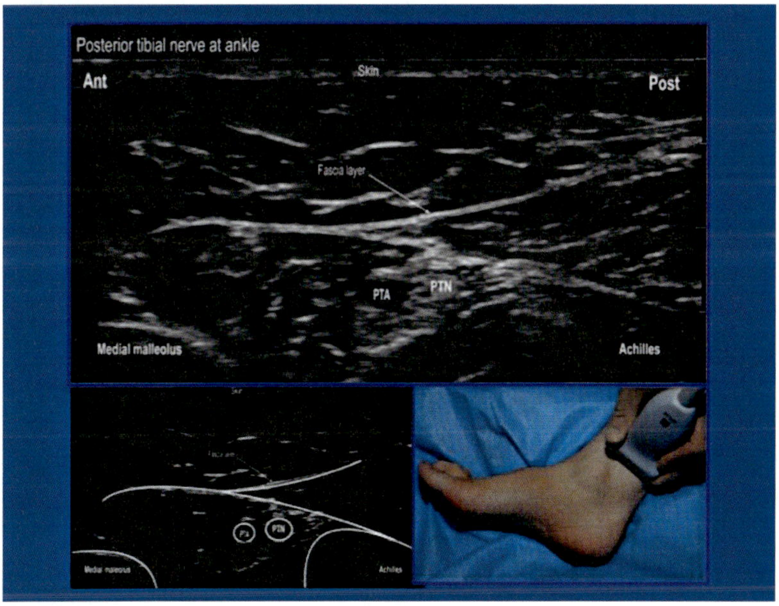

Figure 9: Sonoanatomy of the posterior tibial nerve at the ankle.
PTA = posterior tibial artery, PTN = posterior tibial nerve.

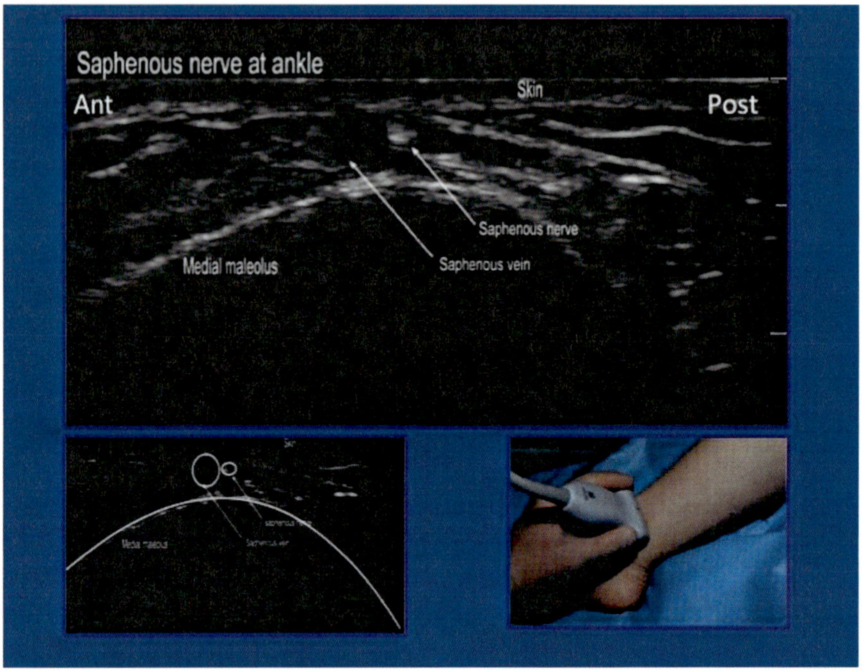

Figure 10: Sonoanatomy of the saphenous nerve at the ankle.

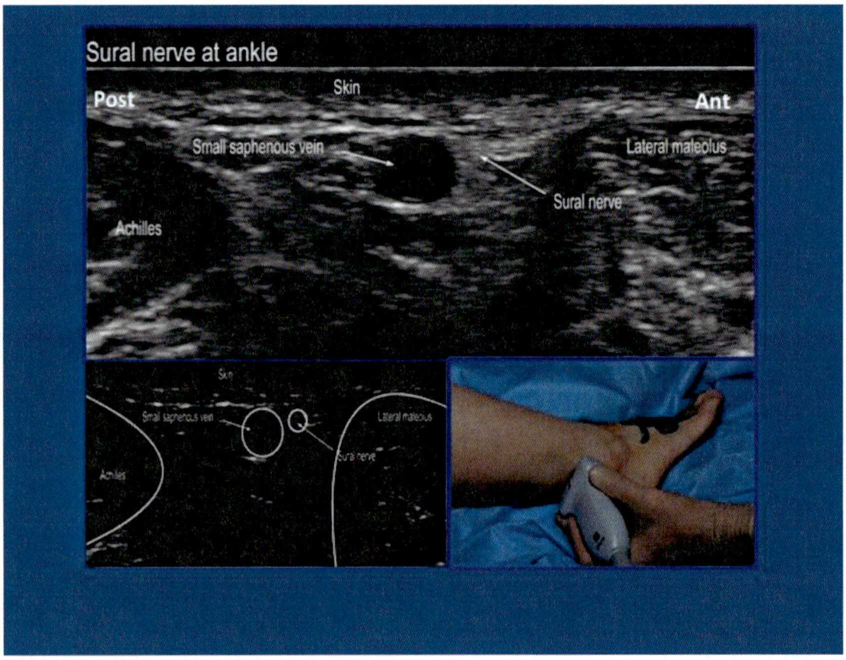

Figure 11: Sonoanatomy of the sural nerve at the ankle.
Achilles = Achilles tendon.

FUNCTIONAL ANATOMY

Electrical stimulation of the posterior tibial nerve causes unmistakable plantar flexion of the toes. This is often not present in diabetic patients (Movie **1**).

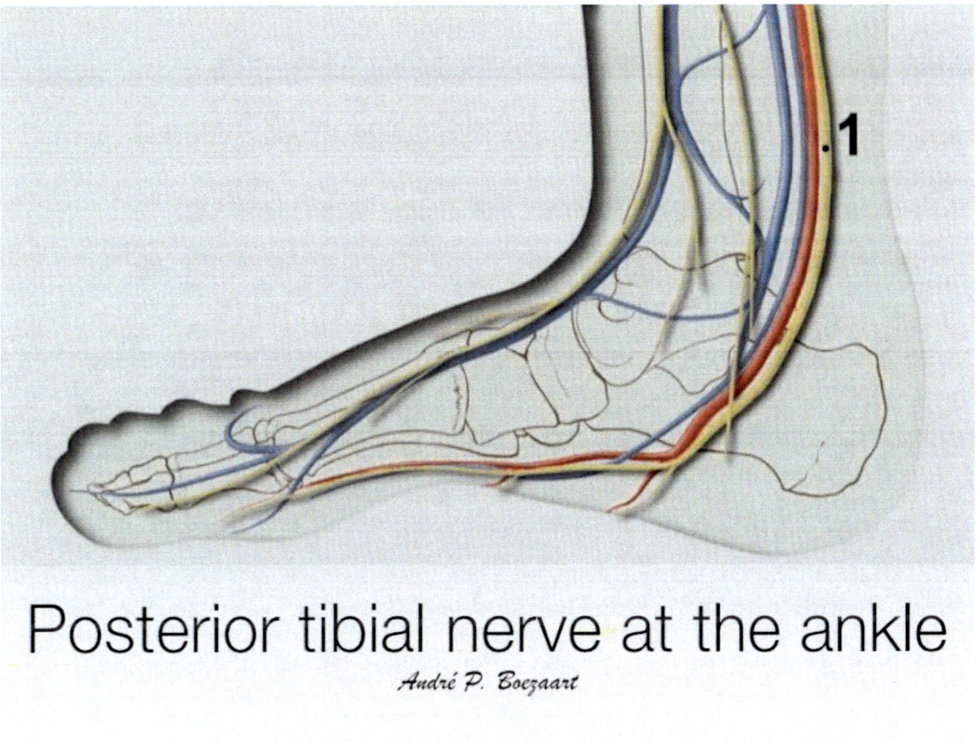

To view this movie click on this link:
https://raeducation.com/ebook

Movie 1: Percutaneous nerve stimulation of the posterior tibial nerve

INNERVATION OF THE ANKLE JOINT

All the nerves that cross the ankle joint innervate the joint. The more important contributions come from the deep nerves, but the innervation seems to be variable. Three to five articular branches from the ***deep peroneal nerve*** arise at the level of the articular interline. They innervate the anterior aspect of the capsule of the ankle joint, the anterior and inferior tibiofibular ligament, and the anterior talofibular ligament.

The ***posterior tibial nerve*** provides three to five articular branches and innervates the entire medial aspect of the articulation and the posterior and anterior aspect of the medial malleolus. It also innervates the anterior and posterior aspects of the ankle joint.

The ***saphenous nerve***, although being thought of as a pure cutaneous nerve, has a modest but important contribution to the innervation of the ankle joint through its two short articular branches to the anterior medial malleolus and the corresponding capsuloligamentous plane at that level (Fig. **15** of chapter 13).

The ***sural nerve*** provides articular branches to the perilateral malleolar capsule and ligament. The superficial peroneal nerve provides inconsistent innervation; it may provide anterolateral and anteromedial branches to the ankle joint.

The talotarsal joint receives nerve supply from the posterior tibial nerve, the ***medial plantar nerve***, and ***accessory deep peroneal nerve*** when present, whereas the cuneonavicular, the intercuneiform, and the cuneometatarsal joints are all innervated on the dorsum by the ***deep peroneal nerve*** and on the plantar side by the medial plantar nerve. The joints of the lateral cuneiform are exceptions in that the ***lateral plantar nerve*** innervates their plantar aspects.

ACKNOWLEDGEMENTS

The authors gratefully acknowledge the following people:

- The Head of the Department of Anesthesiology of the College of Medicine of the University of Florida, Dr. Tim Morey, and his department for their moral support and continuous encouragement.
- The faculty and fellows of the Division of Acute and Perioperative Pain Medicine of the above Department of Anesthesiology for affording the authors the time to produce this work by covering their clinical duties.
- Mary K. Bryson for her illustrations of Figs. (**1** – **3**).
- Corey Astrom of the Department of Anesthesiology of the College of Medicine of the University of Florida for her professional and high quality text editing.
- Dr. Anastacia Munro for her help with the preparation of this chapter and the ultrasound images.

- Raeducation.com LLC for their financial support.

CONFLICT OF INTEREST

The authors confirm that this chapter contents have no conflict of Interest.

ABBREVIATIONS

Achilles	=	Achilles tendon
AT	=	Achilles tendon
DP	=	deep peroneal nerve
DPA	=	deep peroneal artery
DPN	=	deep peroneal nerve
MM	=	medial malleolus
PT	=	posterior tibial nerve
PTA	=	posterior tibial artery
PTN	=	posterior tibial nerve
SA	=	saphenous nerve
SN	=	saphenous nerve
SU	=	sural nerve
Tib	=	tibia

SUGGESTED FURTHER READING

[1] Rickelman T, Boezaart AP: Ankle block. In Boezaart AP (ed): Anesthesia and Orthopaedic Surgery. New York, McGraw-Hill, 2006, pp. 253–7

[2] Boezaart AP. Atlas of Peripheral Nerve Block and Anatomy for Orthopaedic Anesthesia. Philadelphia, PA, Saunders Elsevier, 2008, pp. 197–210

[3] Sarrafian SK. Anatomy of the foot and ankle: Descriptive, topographic, functional. Philadelphia: J.B. Lippincott Company, 1993; pp. 356-90.

Chapter 17:
Functional Anatomy of the Nerves of the Lower Extremity

CHAPTER 17

Functional Anatomy of the Nerves of the Lower Extremity

André P. Boezaart*

Departments of Anesthesiology and Orthopaedic Surgery and Rehabilitation, Division of Acute and Perioperative Pain Medicine, University of Florida College of Medicine, Gainesville, Florida, USA

Abstract: All or most of the nerves of interest to regional anesthesiologists or acute pain physicians are mixed nerves with autonomic, sensory, motor, and proprioception functions. Each function is conducted by a specific type of nerve axon. We provided an overview of these axons and their functions in Chapter 2 (Table **1** of Chapter 2). For the purposes of this chapter, the authors focus on the sensory and motor function of each of the nerves. To create the video productions that accompany this chapter, Mary Bryson painted the muscles and nerves on a model and we used percutaneous nerve mapping as described by Bösenberg and his colleagues to illustrate the motor function of each nerve (Movies **1** to **6**). With the aid of a peripheral nerve stimulator, the path of many superficial peripheral nerves can be "mapped" prior to skin penetration by stimulating the motor component of the peripheral nerve percutaneously with 1.5- to 2.5-mA current output.

Keywords: Acute pain medicine, Autonomic function, Body painting, Common peroneal nerve function, Femoral nerve function, Motor function, nerve axon, Nerve functions, Nerve to sartorius function, percutaneous nerve mapping, peripheral nerve stimulator, Posterior tibial nerve function, proprioception function, Regional anesthesia, Sciatic nerve function, Sensory function, Surface anatomy, Tibial nerve function.

THE LUMBAR PLEXUS (AND LUMBOSACRAL TRUNK)

The ventral rami of the first three (L1-L3) and most of the 4th lumbar nerve roots (L4) form the lumbar plexus. A branch of L4 joins the 5th lumbar nerve root (L5) to form the lumbosacral trunk. These ventral rami descend laterally into the psoas major muscle and in its most common arrangement; a branch from the 12th thoracic root joins the L1 spinal root. After dividing, the upper part divides into the ilioinguinal and iliohypogastric nerves. The remainder of the lumbar plexus divides into the ventral and dorsal divisions, of which the dorsal divisions continue caudad as the femoral nerve and the lateral cutaneous nerve of the thigh. The ventral divisions continue caudad as the obturator nerve (see Chapters 11, 12, and 20).

***Corresponding author André P. Boezaart:** Departments of Anesthesiology and Orthopaedic Surgery, Division of Acute and Peri-operative Pain Medicine, University of Florida College of Medicine, 1600 SW Archer Road, Gainesville, Florida 32610, USA; Tel: 352-846-0913 (Work); Fax: 352-392-7029; E-mail: aboezaart@anest.ufl.edu

The dermatomal and osteotomal innervations of these lumbar roots are depicted in Figs. (**2, 3, 11** and **12**) of chapter 10.

Electrical stimulation [1, 2] of the lumbar plexus may result in motor responses of the iliopsoas, pectinius, Sartorius, or quadriceps muscles, the latter being most prominent. If the lumbosacral trunk is electrically stimulated, there will additionally be hamstring muscle twitches. This is often sought where the entire lumbosacral plexus needs to be blocked, as in surgery for acetabular fractures or other hip surgery where the joint capsule is not destroyed (see Chapters 10 and 13). The sensory neurotomal innervation in the lower extremity of the lumbar plexus is shown in Fig. (**1**).

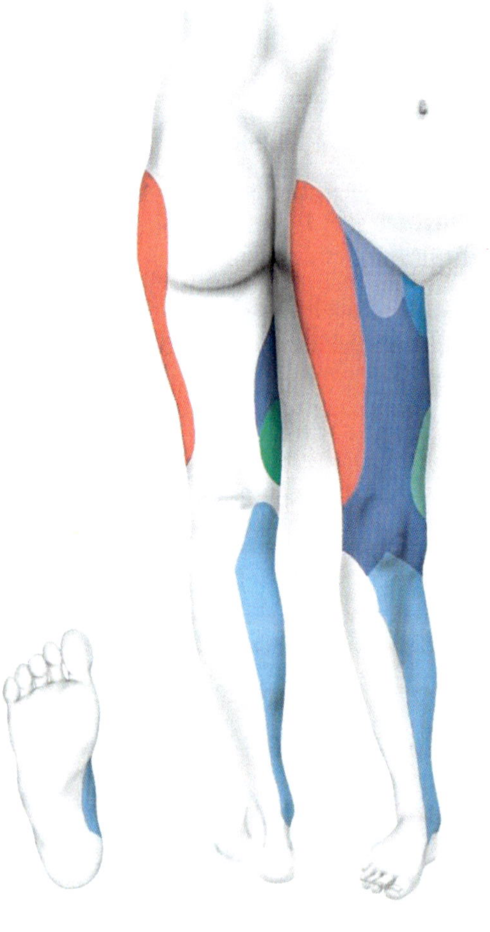

Figure 1: Schematic representation of the sensory neurotomes innervated by nerves of the lumbar plexus. *(These demarcations are not distinct segments as depicted here because there is significant overlap between adjacent neurotomes).*

THE SACRAL PLEXUS (AND LUMBOSACRAL TRUNK)

A small branch from L4 joins the 5th lumbar spinal root (L5) to form the lumbosacral trunk. This trunk, together with the ventral rami of the first three sacral roots (S1, S2, and S3), forms the sacral plexus. All the roots converge toward the greater sciatic foramen and form two cords, the larger upper cord that continues as the sciatic nerve, and the smaller lower cord that continues as the pudendal nerve. The sacral plexus is also divided into anterior and posterior divisions, of which the anterior division continues as the tibial nerve and the posterior division as the common peroneal nerve (see Chapter 13). Except for the hamstring muscles and posterior muscles of the lower limb, the smaller muscles innervated by the sacral plexus are usually not accessible for clinical observation. They include the quadratus femoris, the inferior and superior gemellus, and the obturator internus and piriformis muscles. (The other short muscles around the hip joint, the obturator externus and pectinius muscles, are innervated by the lumbar plexus *via* the obturator and femoral nerves, respectively). Electrical nerve stimulation of the sacral plexus, for example, during sacral paravertebral block [3] will thus result in contractions of the hamstring muscles (*via* the nerves to the hamstring muscles), dorsi and plantar flexion of the foot (*via* the tibial and common peroneal nerves), and levator ani, coccygeus, and sphincter ani externus contractions (*via* the pudendal nerve). The sacral plexus also gives rise to the superior gluteal nerve, which innervates the gluteus maximus muscle, the medial gluteus muscle, and the gluteus minimus and tensor fascia lata muscles. The inferior gluteal nerve also innervates the gluteus maximus muscle, and electrical stimulation of the sacral plexus will cause contractions of all these muscles. The sacral plexus also gives rise to the posterior cutaneous nerve of the thigh, which is a sensory nerve.

The sensory neurotomal innervation of the sacral plexus is depicted in Fig. (**2**). Because of the potential complications presented by the intimate relationship the sciatic plexus has with the neurovascular, genitourinal, and intestinal structures in the pelvis, there is a lack of specific data of sacral plexus information in human subjects.

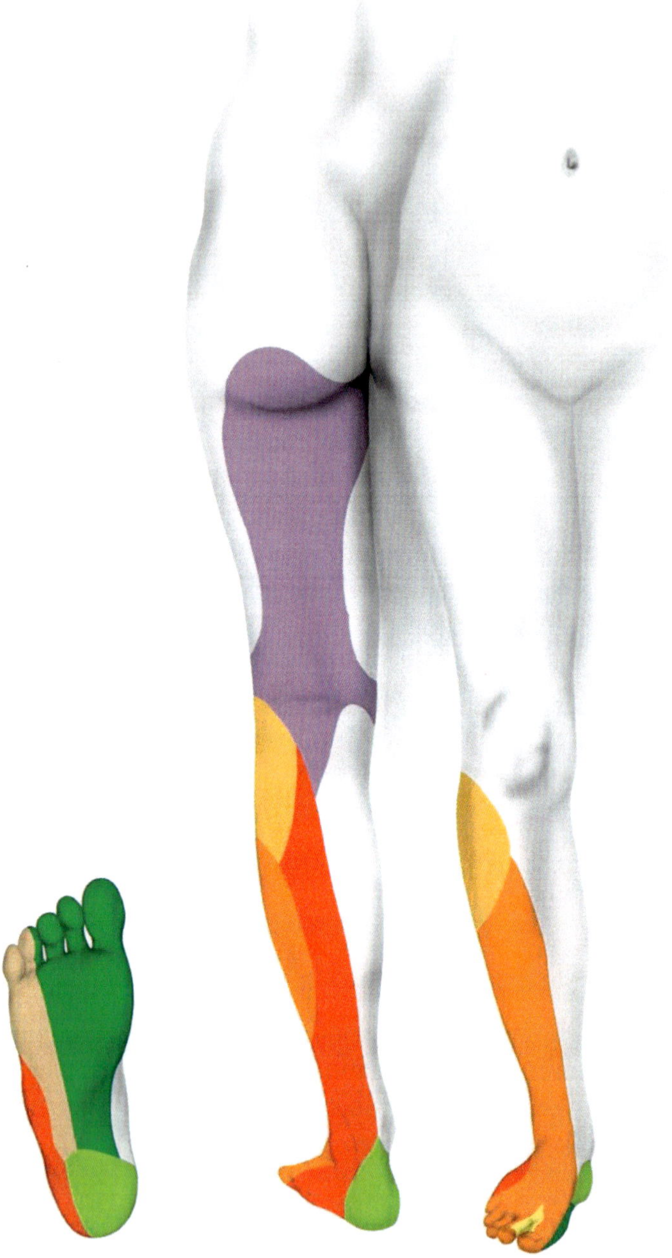

Figure 2: Schematic representation of the sensory neurotomes innervated by nerves of the sciatic plexus.
(These demarcations are not distinct segments as depicted here because there is significant overlap between adjacent neurotomes).

THE FEMORAL NERVE AND NERVE TO THE SARTORIUS MUSCLE

Please refer to Chapter 10 for an account of the macroanatomy of the femoral nerve. The femoral nerve is the largest branch of the lumbar plexus and it innervates the iliopsoas and sartorius pectinius muscles in the pelvis. Below the inguinal ligament, it innervates the four parts of the quadriceps muscle, the rectus femoris, the vastus lateralis, the vastus intermedius, and the vastus medialis muscles. Electrical stimulation of the femoral nerve will cause a motor response in these muscles with distinct movements of the patella (Movie **1**). These should not be confused with the motor response elicited from electrical stimulation of the nerve to sartorius, which is in close relationship to the femoral nerve and even a part of it [1] (see Chapter 10) (Movie **2**).

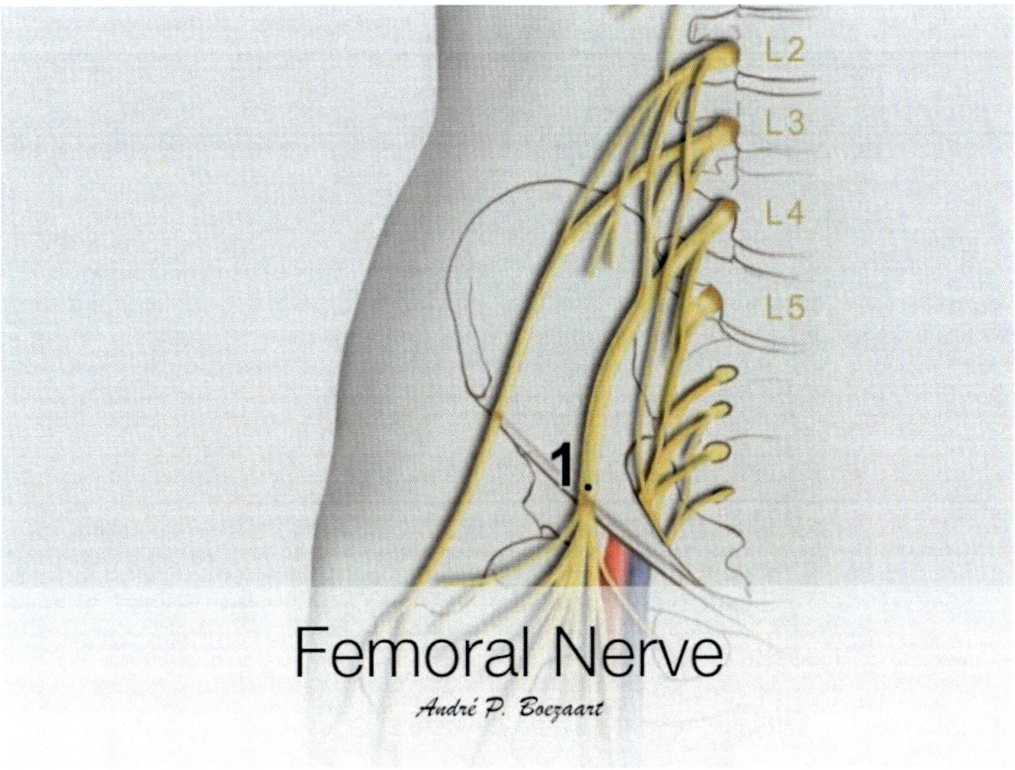

To view this movie click on this link:
https://raeducation.com/ebook

Movie 1: Percutaneous electrical stimulation of the femoral nerve.

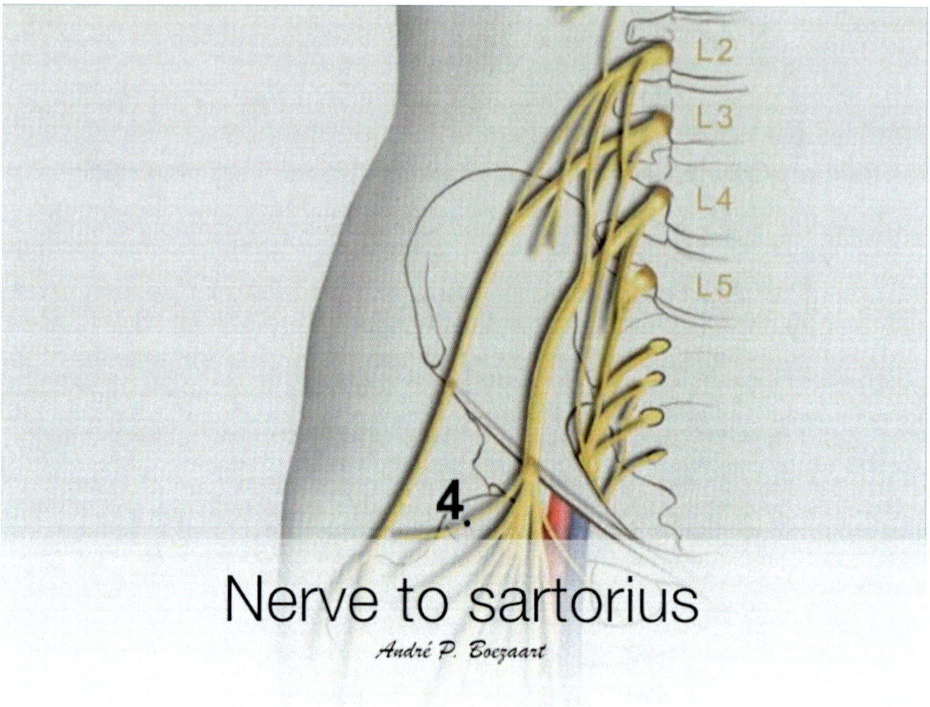

To view this movie click on this link:
https://raeducation.com/ebook

Movie 2: Percutaneous electrical stimulation of the nerve to sartorius muscle.

The sensory neurotomal innervation of the femoral nerve is depicted in Fig. **10** of Chapter 10.

THE OBTURATOR NERVE

The obturator nerve stems from the ventral rami of the lumbar plexus and exits the pelvis through the obturator foramen (see Chapter 10). After exiting the obturator foramen, it splits into anterior and posterior divisions that both innervate the adductor muscles of the thigh. Electrical stimulation of the obturator nerve will result in contractions of the adductor muscles of the thigh. The obturator nerve has a small area of sensory innervation to the skin on the medial side of the lower thigh [1] (see Fig **14**).

THE SCIATIC, TIBIAL, AND COMMON PERONEAL NERVES

The sciatic nerve is not only the largest branch of the sacral plexus; it is also the largest and longest nerve in the human body. The applied macroanatomy of the nerve is discussed in Chapter 13. In the subgluteal area where a sciatic nerve block is commonly performed, it is a bundle of three nerves (see Chapter 14): the tibial nerve, the common peroneal nerve, and the nerve to the hamstring muscles. The latter splits off medially in the mid-femoral region, thus, if a hamstring motor response is elicited during an attempted subgluteal nerve block, the stimulating needle tip is probably too medial and must be moved laterally. Electrical nerve stimulation of the tibial component, which is usually medial in the subgluteal area, will result in plantar flexion of the foot, while stimulation of the more lateral common peroneal component will result in eversion and dorsi flexion of the foot (Movies **3**, **4**, and **5**). The same motor responses are evoked if the tibial and common peroneal nerves are stimulated in the popliteal fossa. The posterior tibial nerve can also be stimulated percutaneously at the ankle (Movie **6**).

The sensory neurotomal innervation of the sciatic nerve and its branches are outlined in Fig. (**14**) of chapter 13.

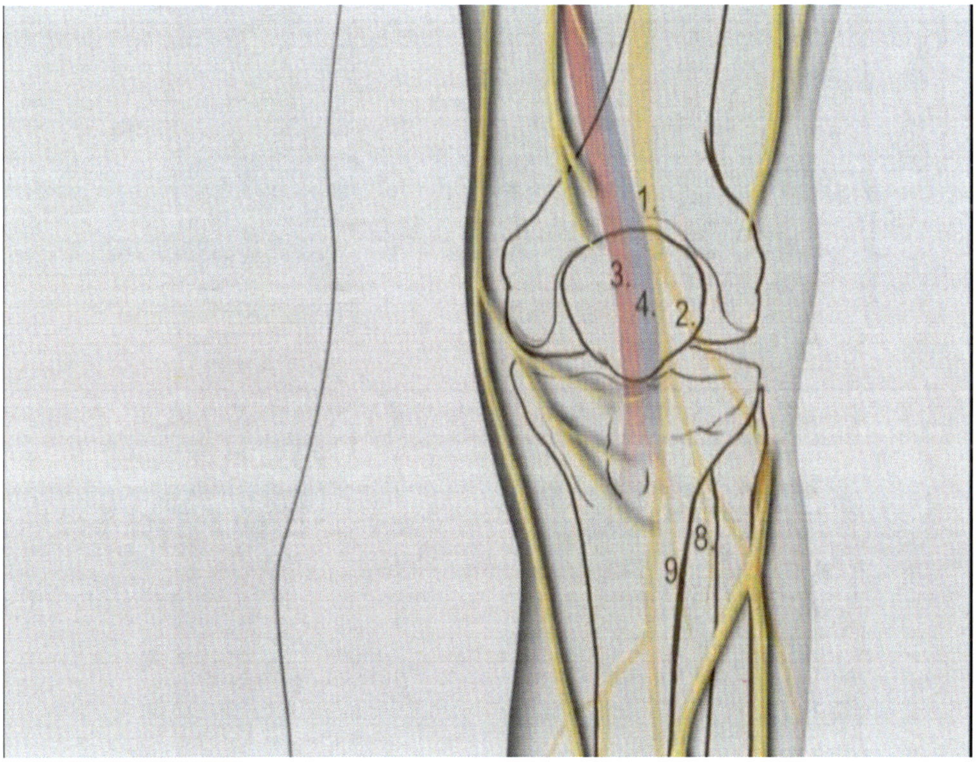

To view this movie click on this link:
https://raeducation.com/ebook

Movie 3: Direct electrical stimulation of the sciatic nerve in the subgluteal area.

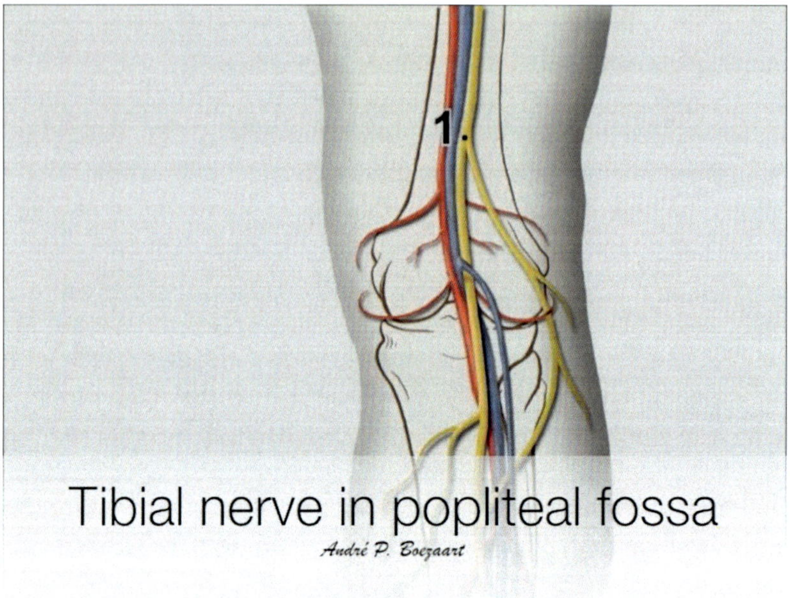

To view this movie click on this link:
https://raeducation.com/ebook

Movie 4: Percutaneous electrical stimulation of the tibial nerve.

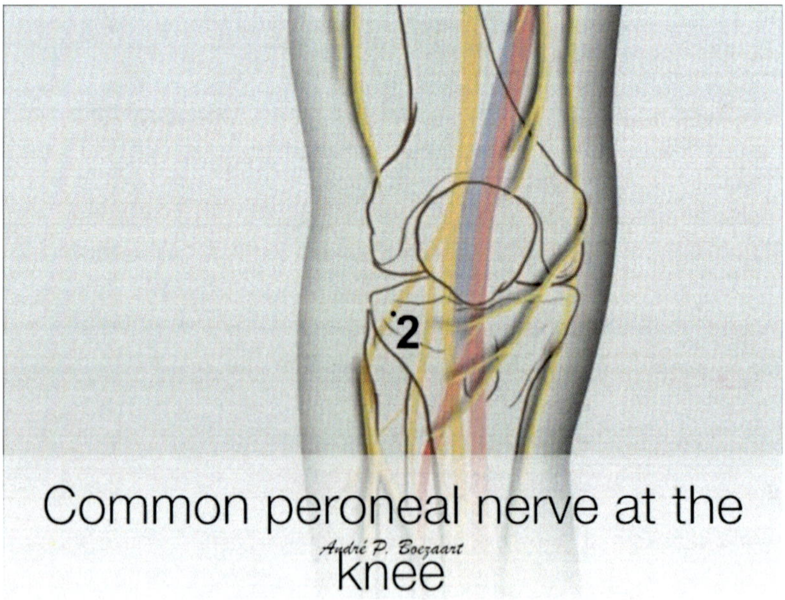

To view this movie click on this link:
https://raeducation.com/ebook

Movie 5: Percutaneous electrical stimulation of the common peroneal nerve.

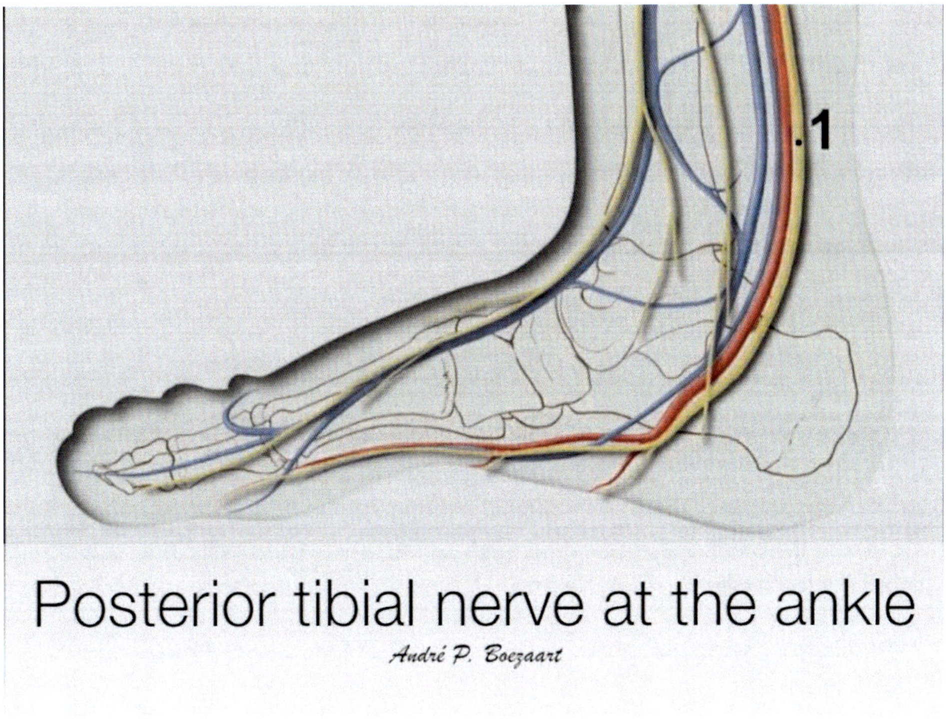

To view this movie click on this link:
https://raeducation.com/ebook

Movie 6: Percutaneous electrical stimulation of the posterior tibial nerve.

ACKNOWLEDGEMENTS

The author gratefully acknowledge the following people:

- The Head of the Department of Anesthesiology of the College of Medicine of the University of Florida, Dr. Tim Morey, and his department for their moral support and continuous encouragement.

- The faculty and fellows of the Division of Acute and Perioperative Pain Medicine of the above Department of Anesthesiology for affording the author the time to produce this work by covering his clinical duties.

- Corey Astrom of the Department of Anesthesiology of the College of Medicine of the University of Florida for her professional and high quality text editing.

- Mary K. Bryson for the body painting of the model, Kathy Fear CRNA (Iowa City).
- Nancy Hagen of the Iowa Public Radio for her narration of the movies.
- Raeducation.com LLC for their financial support.

CONFLICT OF INTEREST

The author confirms that this chapter contents have no conflict of Interest.

REFERENCES

[1] Salinas FV. Femoral nerve block. In: Boezaart AP, Ed. Anesthesia and orthopaedic surgery. New York: McGraw-Hill, 2006; 331-70

[2] Bösenberg AT, Raw R, Boezaart AP. Surface mapping of peripheral nerves in children with a nerve stimulator. Paediatr Anaesth 2002; 12: 398-403.

[3] Boezaart AP, Lucas SD, Elliott CE. Paravertebral block: cervical, thoracic, lumbar, and sacral. Curr Opin Anesthesiol 2009; 22: 637-43.

CHAPTER 18

Applied Anatomy of the Nerves of the Abdominal Wall and the Transversus Abdominis Plane (TAP)

Linda Le-Wendling[1] and André P. Boezaart[2,*]

[1]Department of Anesthesiology, Division of Acute and Perioperative Pain Medicine, University of Florida College of Medicine, Gainesville, Florida, USA and [2]Departments of Anesthesiology and Orthopaedic Surgery and Rehabilitation, Division of Acute and Perioperative Pain Medicine, University of Florida College of Medicine, Gainesville, Florida, USA

Abstract: From superficial to deep, the external oblique, internal oblique, and transversus abdominis muscles anterolaterally and the rectus abdominis muscles medially form the abdominal wall. Deep to these muscles, the transversalis fascia separates the abdominal visceral contents from the muscles that form the abdominal wall. The nerves that innervate the abdominal wall musculature and supply sensory innervation to its overlying skin and peritoneum are derived from the ventral rami of the intercostal nerves from the 6th to 12th thoracic spinal nerves (T6 to T12) and the 1st lumbar spinal root (L1). The anterior and lateral cutaneous branches of the ventral rami of the intercostal nerves travel in the plane between the internal oblique muscle and the transversus abdominis muscle (known as the TA plane - TAP). There is a thin fascial sheet between the internal oblique muscle and transversus abdominis muscle in which the nerves lay between the fascia and the transversus abdominis muscle. The cutaneous branches of the T6 to T12 nerves branch and communicate with adjacent nerves within the TA plane, forming an extensive network that results in three plexuses: the intercostal plexus anterolaterally, the TAP plexus running with the deep circumflex iliac artery, and the rectus sheath plexus running with the deep inferior epigastric artery. The macroanatomy and sonoanatomy (static and dynamic) of these muscles and nerves are discussed in this chapter.

Keywords: Acute pain medicine, Anterior rectus sheath, Arcuate line, Cutaneous branches of ventral rami, External oblique muscle, Iliohypgastric nerve, Ilioinguinal nerve, Intercostal nerves, Internal oblique muscle, Lumbar spinal roots, Peritoneum, Posterior rectus sheath, Regional anesthesia, TA plane, TAP, Transversalis fascia, Transversus abdominis muscle Rectus abdominis muscle, Ventral rami of the intercostal nerves.

***Corresponding author André P. Boezaart:** Departments of Anesthesiology and Orthopaedic Surgery, Division of Acute and Peri-operative Pain Medicine, University of Florida College of Medicine, 1600 SW Archer Road, Gainesville, Florida 32610, USA; Tel: 352-846-0913 (Work); Fax: 352-392-7029;
E-mail: aboezaart@anest.ufl.edu

MACROANATOMY

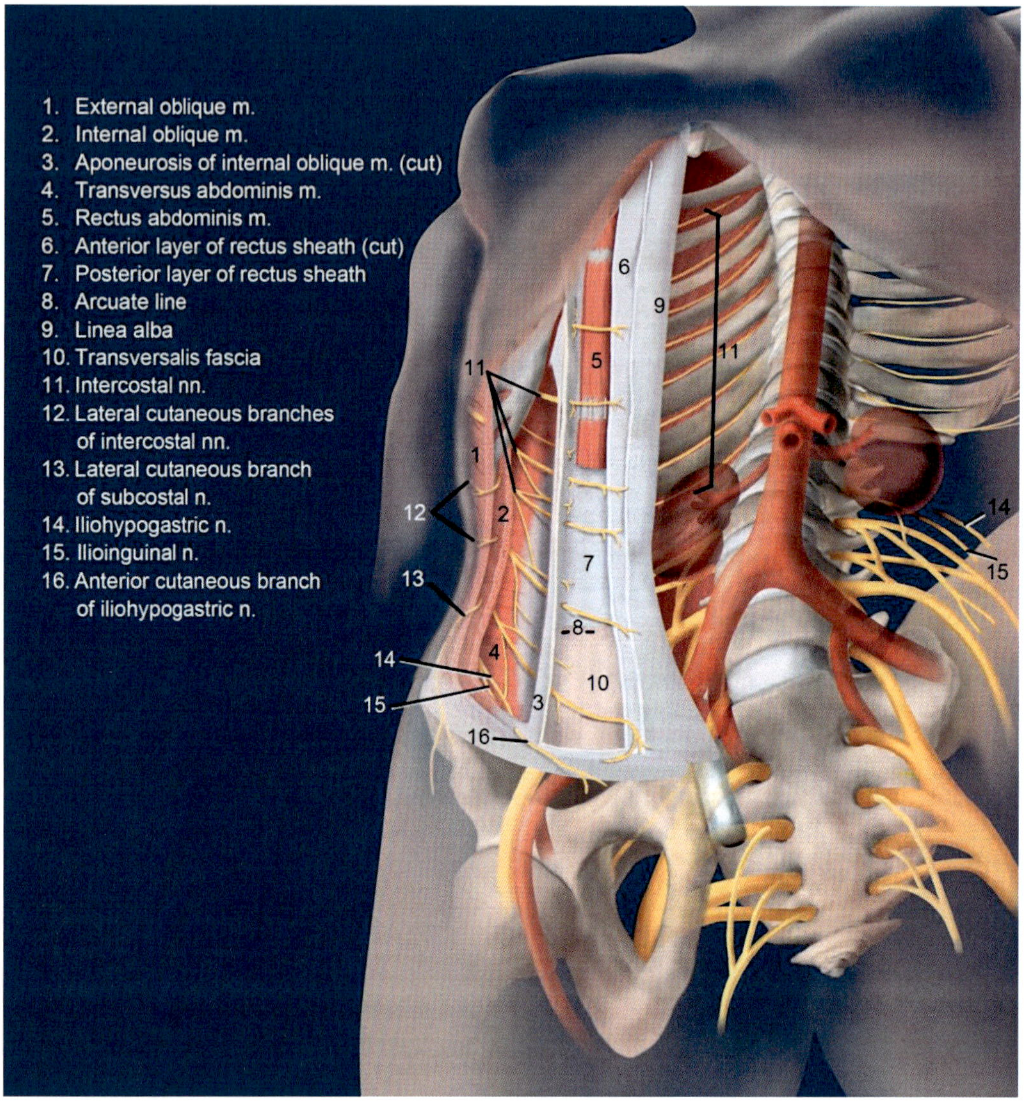

Figure 1: Abdominal wall muscles and nerves.
Transversus abdominis plane (TAP) is between numbers 2 and 4.

The segmental nerves T6 through T9 enter the abdominal wall along the costal margin at increasingly lateral positions to innervate the upper abdominal wall. Therefore, for analgesia of the abdominal wall above the umbilicus, the local anesthetic needs to be targeted along the subcostal margin. (The deposition of local anesthetic along the subcostal margin has been described as the subcostal

TAP block). Laterally, the segmental nerves lie between the internal oblique and transversus abdominis muscles. Medially, the external oblique and internal oblique muscles taper off and become aponeurotic, and the rectus abdominis muscle appears. Here, the nerves lie in the plane between the rectus abdominis and transversus abdominis muscles.

The T10 segmental nerve consistently innervates the abdominal wall at the level of the umbilicus and the T11 and T12 nerves innervate the abdominal wall below the umbilicus. These nerves lie in the TA plane between the mid-axillary and anterior axillary line above the iliac crest. Therefore, deposition of local anesthetic in the TAP plane just above the iliac crest, usually termed the "posterior TAP approach", generally results in analgesia of the lower abdominal wall.

The L1 nerve usually travels through the TA plane at the mid- to anterior axillary line. The L1 nerve innervates the musculature of the rectus abdominis muscle and the skin at the inferior aspect of the abdominal wall immediately above the inguinal ligament and the pubic symphysis. The divisions of the L1 nerve root are the ilioinguinal and iliohypogastric nerves [1-6]. In the posterior abdominal wall, these nerves emerge from the superolateral border of the psoas muscle, running anteriorly to the quadratus lumborum muscle as they head toward the iliac crest. They exist as a common trunk until dividing near the iliac crest or the ilioinguinal nerve courses through the posterior abdominal wall just inferior to the iliohypogastric nerve. At approximately 2.5 cm medial and 2.4 cm inferior to the anterior superior iliac spine (ASIS), the ilioinguinal nerve travels through the TA plane to the anterior surface of the internal oblique muscle. Roughly 0.5 cm cephalad, the iliohypogastric nerve pierces the anterior surface of the internal oblique muscle. These two nerves are less than 2 mm in width [3].

As the T6 to L1 nerves travel distally, they eventually innervate the rectus muscle, mostly penetrating its posterior surface. The nerves can be anesthetized just shallow to the posterior rectus sheath (known as a rectus sheath block). A few centimeters below the umbilicus lies the arcuate ligament. At this point, there is no posterior rectus sheath to provide a safe barrier or reduce the possibility of needle entry into the peritoneum during a nerve block. Here, the peritoneum is only separated from the rectus abdominis muscle by the thin transversalis fascia. Above the arcuate line, the posterior rectus sheath is formed by the aponeurosis of the internal oblique and transversus abdominis muscles, providing a more solid barrier between the rectus abdominis muscle and the peritoneum with its visceral components.

The TA plane contains not only the cutaneous branches of the intercostal nerve, but a rich network of vascular structures as well. Medially, the superior and inferior epigastric vessels provide blood flow to the rectus abdominis muscle and lie in the plane between the rectus abdominis muscle and the posterior rectus sheath. The subcostal, superficial epigastric, and deep circumflex iliac vessels provide vascular flow to the muscles of the anterolateral abdominal wall. Deposition of local anesthetic in the TA plane, therefore, results in systemic absorption with peak plasma concentrations within 30 minutes of injection [4].

SONOANATOMY

Ultrasound is a dynamic process whereby structures can and should be followed to their origins and destinations for optimal identification [6]. It is therefore not always satisfactory to study static ultrasound images. When studying the sonoanatomy of the abdominal wall, the authors strongly advise readers to study the macroanatomy first and then to view the accompanying video (Movie **1**) that illustrates the dynamic sonoanatomy of the abdominal wall and transversus abdominis space.

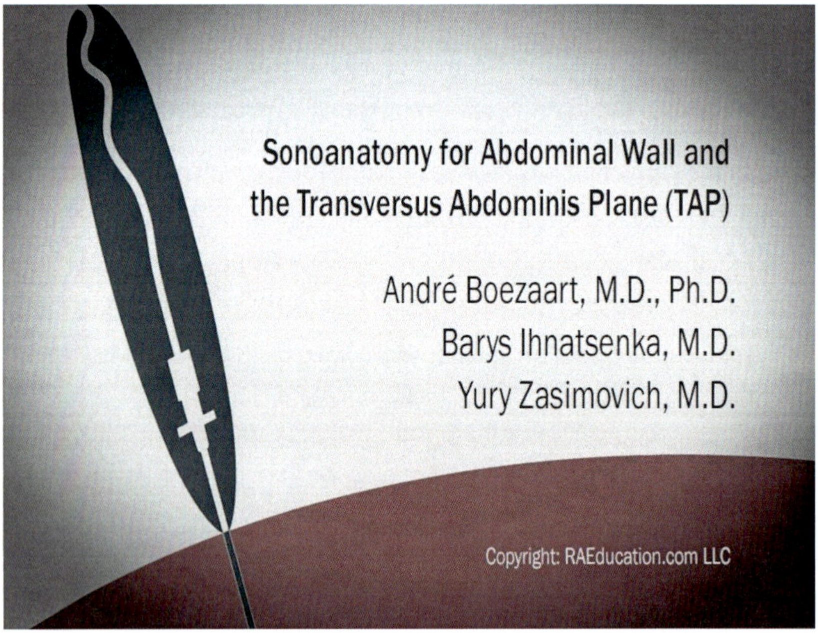

To view this movie click on this link:
https://raeducation.com/ebook

Movie 1: Dynamic sonoanatomy of the abdominal muscles and transversus abdominis plane (TAP).

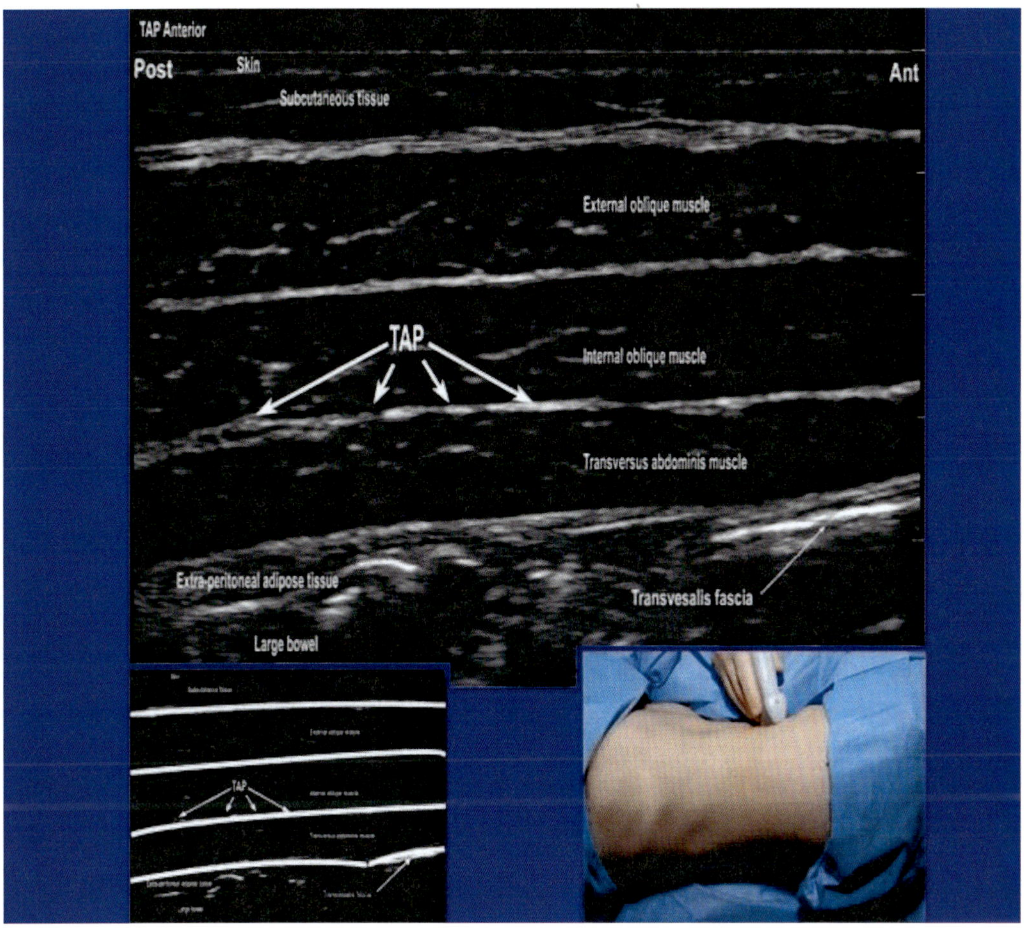

Figure 2: Anterior transversus abdominis plane
Anterior, between the iliac crest and the rib cage, there are three abdominal muscles. From superficial to deep they are the external oblique, internal oblique, and transversus abdominis muscles. The TAP is the fascia layer between the latter two. An anterior TAP block splits this layer to block the nerves situated here.

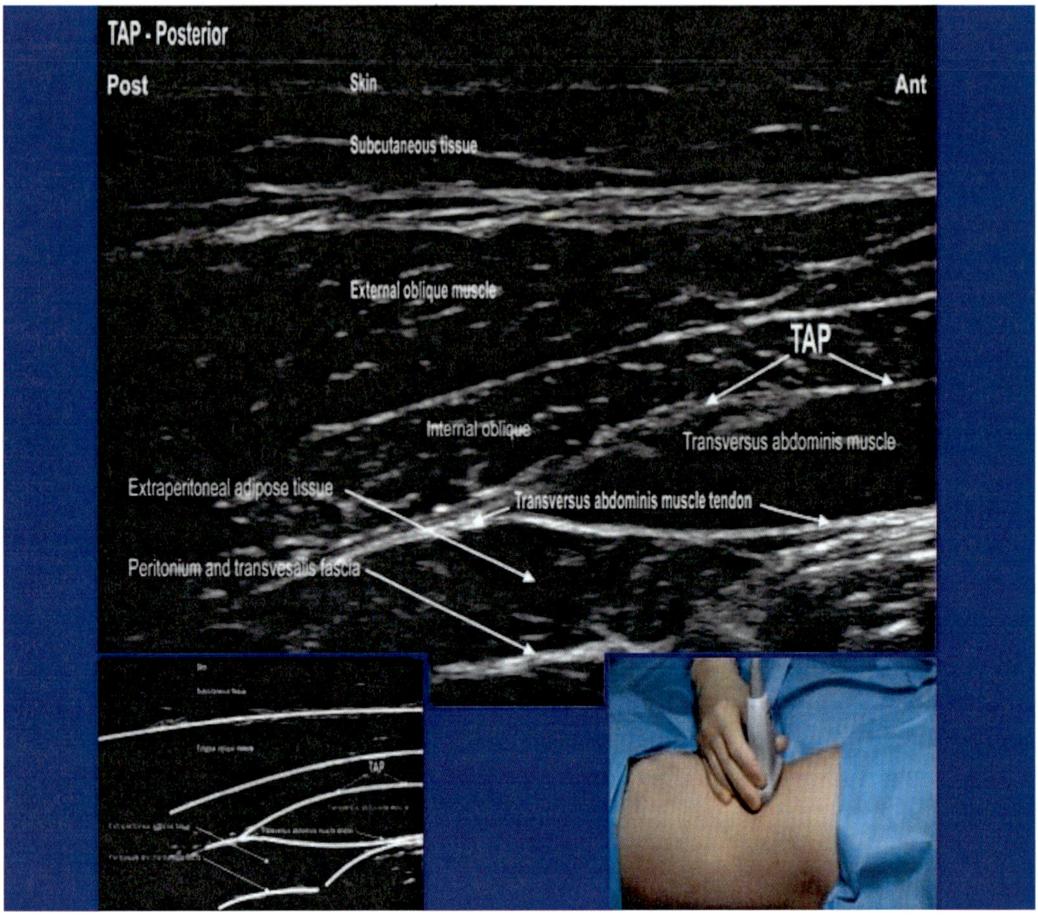

Figure 3: Posterior transversus abdominis plane
Ant = anterior; Post = posterior; TAP = transversus abdominis plane.
The transversus abdominis muscle becomes aponeurotic posterior. Note the TAP again between the internal oblique and transversus abdominis muscles. Also note the extraperitoneal adipose tissue and the transversalis fascia deep to the transversus abdominis muscle and the bowel deep to these structures.

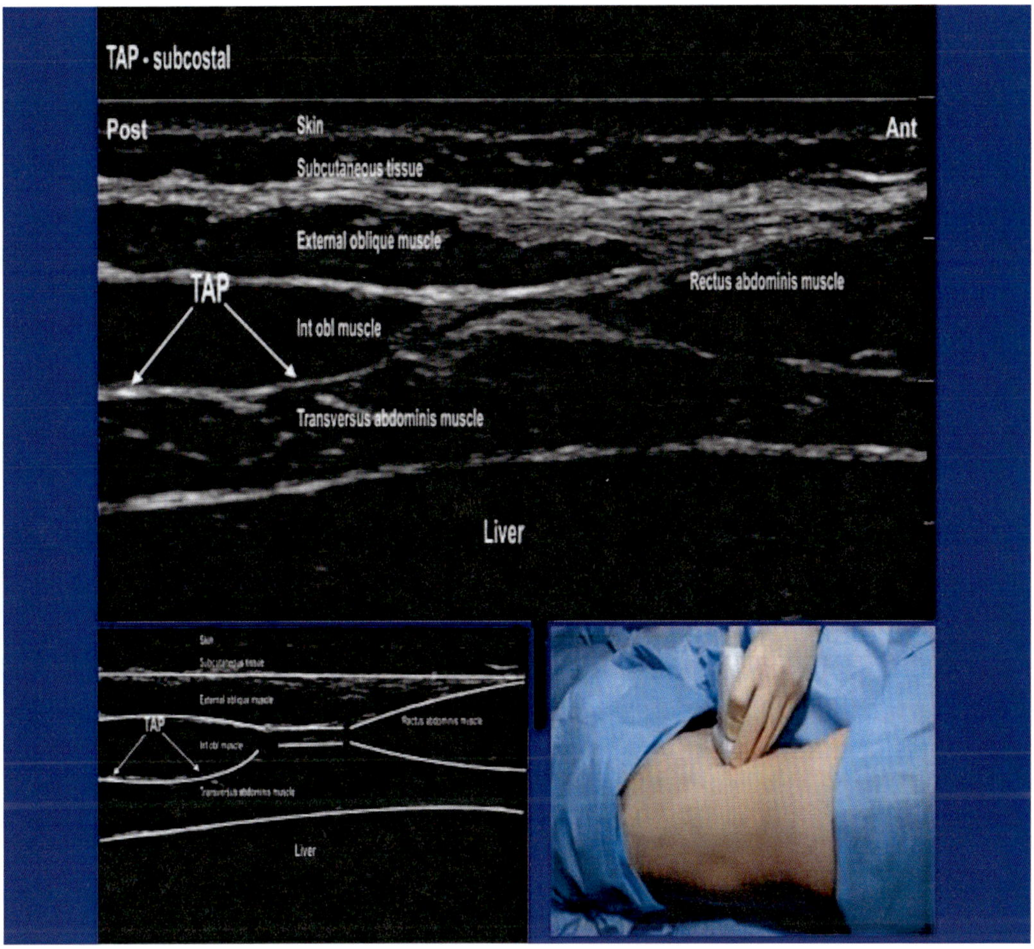

Figure 4: Subcostal transversus abdominis plane
Ant = anterior; Post = posterior; TAP = transversus abdominis plane
The tendons of all three abdominal muscles merge to form the anterior and posterior rectus sheath, which hosts the rectus abdominis muscle. Note the presence of the liver deep to the transversus abdominis muscle. Above the arcuate line (see text), the rectus sheath consists of the merged tendons of the abdominal muscles. Below this line, it consists of the transversalis fascia.

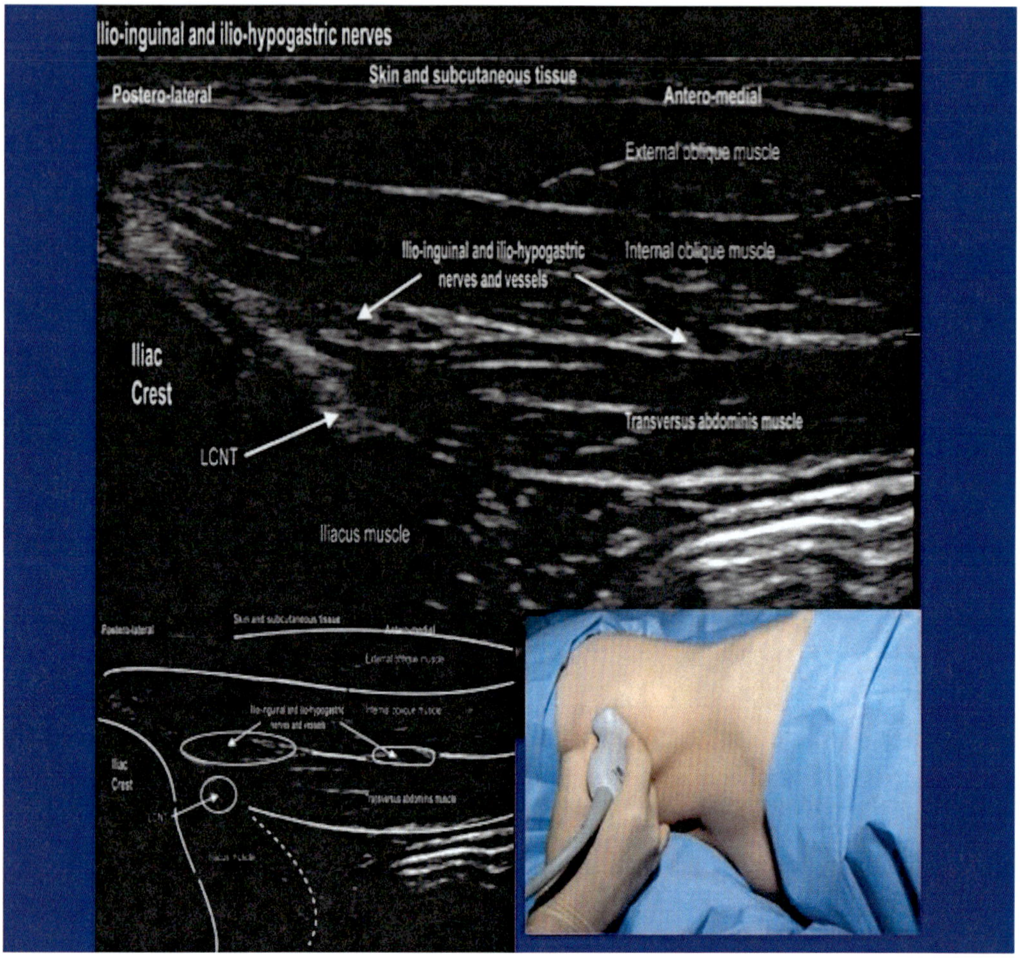

Figure 5: Ilioinguinal and iliohypogastric nerves
LCNT = lateral cutaneous nerve of the thigh.
Note the angle of the ultrasound probe. The abdominal muscles implant on the iliac crest, and the presence of the ilioinguinal and iliohypogastric nerve, arteries, and veins are situated in the fascia layer between the internal oblique and transversus abdominis muscles. The lateral cutaneous nerve of the thigh is on the anterior border of the iliacus muscle, which can be seen anterolateral to the iliac crest.

ACKNOWLEDGEMENTS

The authors gratefully acknowledge the following people:

- The Head of the Department of Anesthesiology of the College of Medicine of the University of Florida, Dr. Tim Morey, and his department for their moral support and continuous encouragement.

- The faculty and fellows of the Division of Acute and Perioperative Pain Medicine of the above Department of Anesthesiology for affording the authors the time to produce this work by covering their clinical duties.
- Dr. Anastacia Munro for her help with the preparation of the chapter and ultrasound images.
- Dr. Barys V. Ihnatsenka for his help with the preparation of the chapter and ultrasound images.
- Mary K. Bryson for her illustrations of Fig. (**1**).
- Corey Astrom of the Department of Anesthesiology of the College of Medicine of the University of Florida for her professional and high quality text editing.
- Nancy Hagen of the Iowa Public Radio for her narration of the movies.
- Raeducation.com LLC for their financial support.

CONFLICT OF INTEREST

The authors confirm that this chapter contents have no conflict of Interest.

ABBREVIATIONS

LCNT = lateral cutaneous nerve of the thigh

TAP = transversus abdominis plane

REFERENCES

[1] Rozen WM, Ashton MW, Barringon MJ, Ivanusic JJ, Taylor GI: Refining the course of the thoracolumbar nerves: a new understanding of the innervation of the anterior abdominal wall. Clin Anat 2008;21:325-33.

[2] Johnson TG, Von SJ, Hope WW: Clinical Anatomy of the abdominal wall: hernia surgery. OA Anatomy 2014;2:3.

[3] DD Rahn: Anterior abdominal wall nerve and vessel anatomy: clinical implications for gynecologic surgery. Am J Obstet Gynecol 2010;202:234.e1-5.

[4] Latzke D: Pharmacokinetics of the local anesthetic ropivacaine after transversus abdominis plane block in halthy volunteer. Eur J Clin Pharmacol 2012;68:419-25.

[5] JD Griffiths: Symptomatic local anesthetic toxicity and plasma ropivacaine concentrations after transversus abdominis plane block for Caesarean section. Br J Anaesthesia 2013;110:996-1000.

[6] Ihnatsenka BV, Boezaart AP: Ultrasound: Basic understanding and learning the language. Int J Shoulder Surg 2010;4:55-62.

Chapter 19:
Applied Macro-, Micro-, and Sonoanatomy of the Thoracic Paravertebral Space

CHAPTER 19

Applied Macro-, Micro-, and Sonoanatomy of the Thoracic Paravertebral Space

Barys V. Ihnatsenka[1], André P. Boezaart[2,*] and Yury Zasimovich[1]

[1]*Department of Anesthesiology, Division of Acute and Perioperative Pain Medicine, University of Florida College of Medicine, Gainesville, Florida, USA and* [2]*Departments of Anesthesiology and Orthopaedic Surgery and Rehabilitation, Division of Acute and Perioperative Pain Medicine, University of Florida College of Medicine, Gainesville, Florida, USA*

Abstract: The thoracic paravertebral space (TPVS) is a wedge-shaped space of which the anterior boundary is the parietal pleura of the lung. The superior costotransverse ligament (SCTL) and the internal intercostal membrane (IIM) form the posterior boundary, while the posterolateral aspect of the vertebra, the intervertebral disc, and the intervertebral foramen form the medial border. Superior and inferior the boundaries are the heads and necks of the ribs. The TPVS contains spinal nerve roots, the posterior rami of the thoracic nerves, the anterior rami, which comprises the intercostal nerves, the gray and white rami communicantes to the sympathetic chain and the sympathetic chain itself, the spinal rami from the aorta, and an intervertebral veins that form a vascular plexus. The TPVS communicates superiorly and inferiorly with the adjacent TPVS above and below, medially with the spinal epidural space, and laterally with the intercostal space. The macro- and microanatomy and sonoanatomy (static and dynamic) of these spaces and its nerve roots and relationships to other structures are discussed in this chapter.

Keywords: Acute pain medicine, Anterior rami, Gray rami communicantes, Intercostal nerves, Intercostal space, Internal intercostal membrane, Intervertebral artery, Intervertebral disc, Intervertebral foramen, Intervertebral vein, Macroanatomy, Microanatomy, Parietal pleura, Posterior rami, Regional anesthesia, Sonoanatomy, Spinal epidural, Spinal nerve roots, Superior costotransverse ligament, Sympathetic chain, Thoracic paravertebral block, Thoracic paravertebral space, White rami communicantes.

***Corresponding author André P. Boezaart:** Departments of Anesthesiology and Orthopaedic Surgery, Division of Acute and Peri-operative Pain Medicine, University of Florida College of Medicine, 1600 SW Archer Road, Gainesville, Florida 32610, USA; Tel: 352-846-0913 (Work); Fax: 352-392-7029;
E-mail: aboezaart@anest.ufl.edu

MACROANATOMY

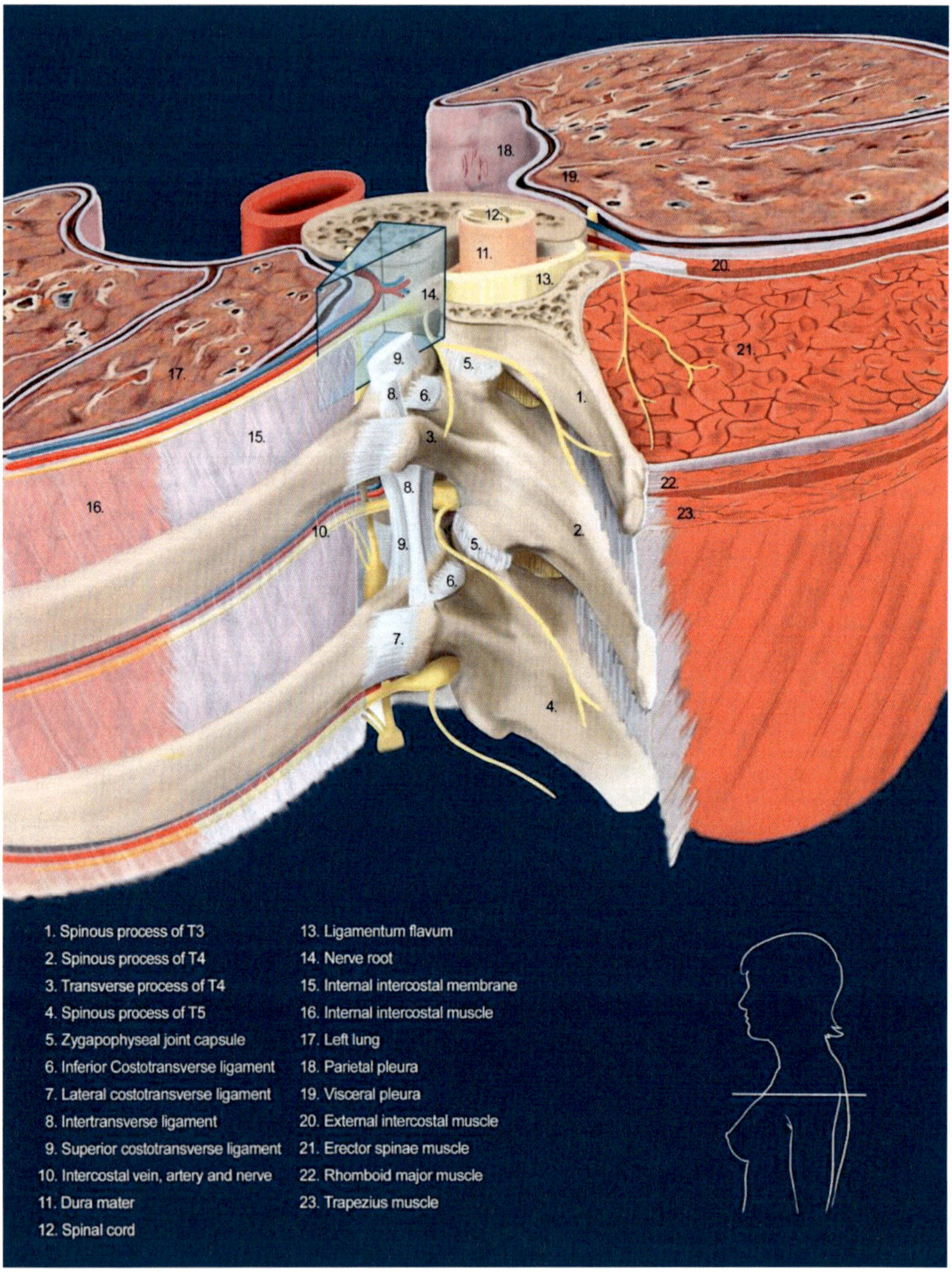

Figure 1: Macroanatomy of the thoracic paravertebral space viewed from the posterior at the level of the 4th thoracic vertebra.

Blue wedge-shaped area represents thoracic paravertebral space.

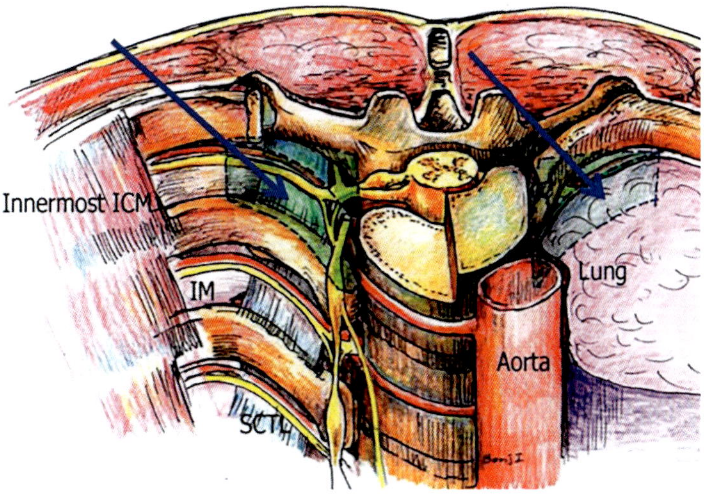

Figure 2: Anterior view of the wedge-shaped space that forms the thoracic paravertebral space. *Arrows point to thoracic paravertebral spaces bilateral. Innermost ICM = innermost intercostal muscle; IM = internal intercostal muscle; SCTL = superior costotransverse ligament. The lung and parietal pleura have been removed on the right side.*

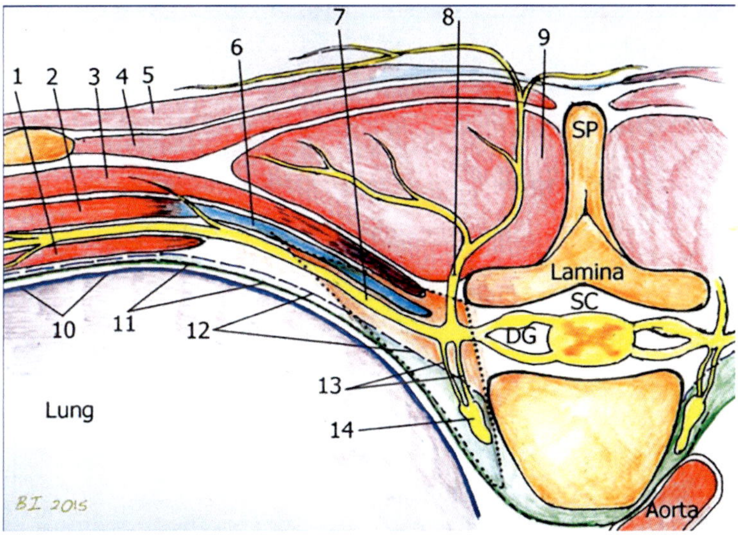

Figure 3: Schematic representation of the wedge-shaped thoracic paravertebral space. *1 = innermost intercostal muscle; 2 = internal intercostal muscle; 3 = external intercostal muscle, which fuses with the SCTL; 4 = rhomboid major muscle; 5 = trapezius muscle; 6 = internal intercostal membrane, which covers the external and internal intercostal muscles and fuses with superior costotransverse ligament; 7 = ventral ramus of thoracic spinal root (intercostal nerve); 8 = dorsal ramus of thoracic spinal root; 9 = erector spinae muscle; 10 = visceral pleura of the lung; 11 = parietal pleura of the lung; 12 = endothoracic fascia; 13 = gray and white rami communicantes; 14 = sympathetic trunk and ganglion; SP = spinous process of vertebra; SC = spinal cord; DG = dorsal root ganglion.*

Note that the spinal nerve is situated below the corresponding transverse process (TP) of that vertebra (Figs. **1-6**). Thus, the 4th thoracic spinal root (T4) is inferior (under) the transverse process of T4, and the nerve root is located in the middle or just above the middle of the interspace between two adjacent TPs. The ventral rami of each spinal nerve continue as intercostal nerves on the inferior border of the rib. The greater and lesser splanchnic nerves originate from the sympathetic ganglia of T5 to T9 and T10 and T11, respectively. These sympathetic nerves carry visceral pain impulses from the celiac ganglia and plexus and aorticorenal ganglia and superior mesenteric ganglia (see Chapter 22). Blocking these nerves with local anesthetic agents *via* a thoracic paravertebral block (TPVB) thus indirectly blocks these ganglia and could explain why a TPVB may provide excellent analgesia for pain originating from the upper abdominal viscera if performed on the appropriate level. Due to overlap in innervation of adjacent dermatomes, one should probably block three or more adjacent nerve roots to provide a reliable dense block of one single dermatome and also because longitudinal spread up and down the TPVB is not consistently reliable. This may well be related to the needle (or catheter) placement anterior (deep) to the endothoracic fascia, while the spinal root is posterior to it, but this notion awaits further clarification. The endothoracic fascia may also explain the inconsistent findings in longitudinal *versus* lateral (intercostal) spread of local anesthetic agent. Again, this notion awaits further scrutiny.

The ligaments bordering the TPVS have significant clinical implications. The SCTL forms the posterior boundary of the TPVS and runs obliquely from the TP above to the rib below. It is from 2 to 8 mm thick, and penetration of the ventral part of SCTL with a needle signifies the entrance into the TPVS. This needle penetration may produce a distinctive "pop" or "feel of give" with a short bevel or Tuohy needle, or a distinct loss of resistance (LOR) to air or fluid (5% dextrose in water, saline, or local anesthetic agent, for example) if this technique is used [1].

The SCTL has thinner areas or gaps where it is totally absent, especially medially. It is slightly more dense and thick laterally (around the tip of the TPs) and more superficially (closer to skin) at its' cephalad insertion point. It is deeper (anterior, closer to parietal pleura) at its' caudad insertion point. Consistent "pop." "give," or LOR may therefore not be encountered if the needle is too medial from the tip of the TP.

In the middle of the interspace between two TPs of adjacent vertebrae, the ventral part of SCTL is about 1 cm anterior (deep) to dorsal aspect of the TP and approximately 3 to 5 mm dorsal (superficial) to the parietal pleura.

Despite the gaps in the SCTL, deposition of local anesthetic agent dorsal (superficial, posterior) to it will be responsible for a suboptimal block or no block of the ventral rami of spinal nerve at all. This can generally be blamed on the fact that the internal intercostal membrane may cover the posterior parts of the ventral rami. Posterior rami of intercostal nerve, however, are dorsal (posterior, superficial, closer to the skin) to the SCTL and can be blocked if the local anesthetic is deposited superficial to the SCTL.

Finally, the spinal nerve root is situated ventrally (anterior) to the internal intercostal membrane, which is a continuation of the internal intercostal muscle and which fuses with the SCTL.

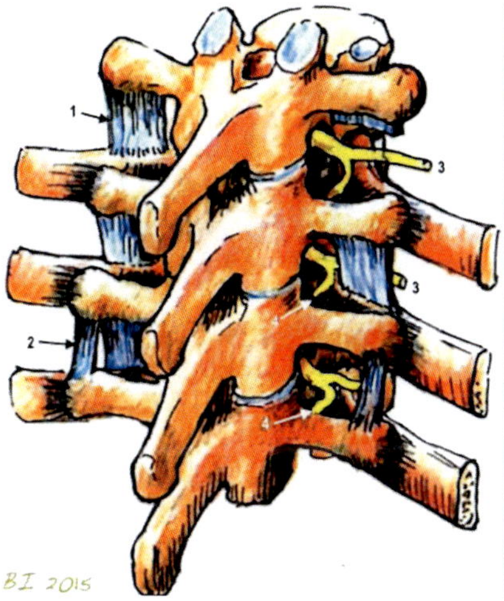

1. Superior costo-transverse ligament
2. Intertransverse ligament
3. Anterior ramus of spinal nerve
4. Posterior ramus of intercostal nerve

Figure 4: The relationships of the nerves and the ligaments in the thoracic paravertebral space viewed from posterior.

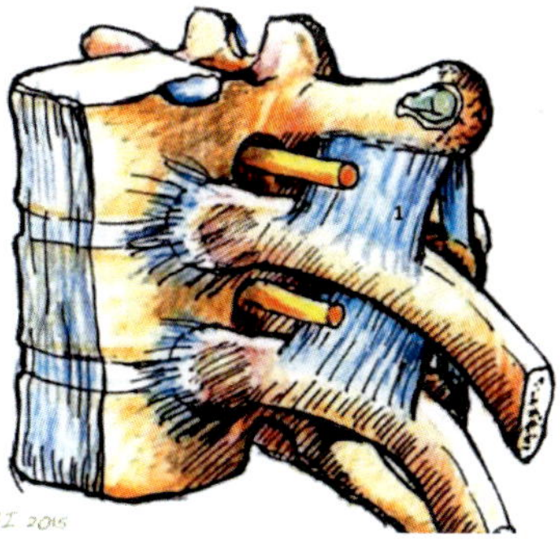

Figure 5: The relationship of the thoracic spinal root to the superior costotransverse ligament as viewed from anterior.
1 = costotransverse ligament.

Some important facts about the TP of the thoracic vertebrae:

- Because we cannot see or palpate the TPs, and yet they are is such vital landmarks for successful and safe TPVB, it is important to have an accurate gauge of their depth or distance from the skin where they should be encountered with a needle. If we enter below or above them and advance our needle too far anterior and we do not know the correct distance, we could enter the pleura and lung and cause pneumothorax (see Sonoanatomy section).

- Because of the acute caudad angulation in the thoracic vertebrae, the spinous process (SP) of a thoracic vertebra, which is most often palpable, is typically situated at the level of the vertebra and its' TP is below it. For example, the SP of the 4th vertebra is on the same axial level as the TP of the 5th thoracic vertebra (T5). This may be a useful fact if ultrasound is not used to perform TPVB.

- The TPs in the upper thoracic region (T1-T5) are slightly wider and pointed upward compared to those at lower thoracic levels.

- The TPs are more superficial (closer to the skin) in the mid-thoracic region.

- The lateral tip of the TP is, on average, 2.5 to 3 cm from midline. This may also be a useful fact when ultrasound guidance is not used when performing TPVB.

- The TP in the lower thoracic region do not completely overlap the ribs as they do in the upper thoracic region. The ribs are ventral and cephalad of the TPs. This is why most authors recommend "walking off" of the bony structure inferiorly (caudad) [1, 2].

- The TPs are angled such that they are shallower laterally (at their tips) and deeper medially where they are closer to the lamina (Fig. **6**).

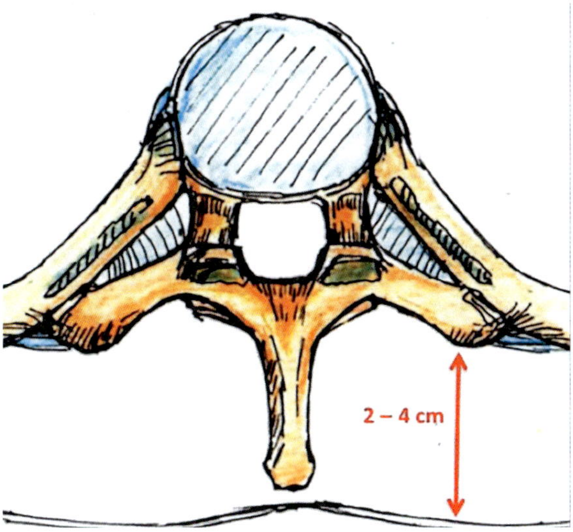

Figure 6: Typically, the tip of the transverse process is from 2 to 4 cm from the skin. This varies from patient to patient depending on the body habitus. Note the angle of the transverse process.

MICROANATOMY

The thoracic spinal roots, like all spinal roots, are covered by the meninges for undetermined distances that vary from one patient to another (Fig. **7**).

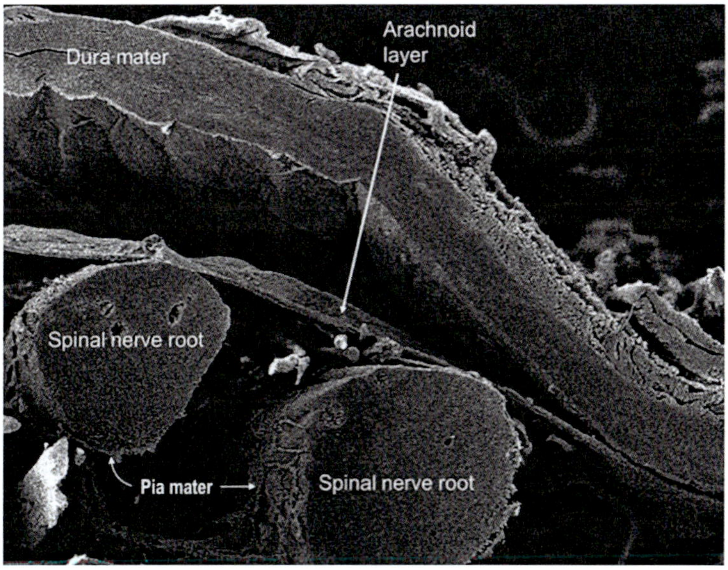

Figure 7: Ultrastructure of the meninges (dura, arachnoid, and pia maters) surrounding nerve root. Scanning electron microscopy - magnification ×20. (*Reprinted from Reina [10] with permission*).

Daniel Moore [3] has conclusively shown that ink injected into the intercostal nerves of animals consistently spreads to the spinal cord.

Postdural puncture headache has been described after TPVB [4], and numerous cases of severe central (spinal) neurological deficits and total spinal block have also been described that resulted from paravertebral block - cervical, thoracic, and lumbar [5-8]. The anatomical basis for this [9] is depicted in Fig. (**8a**). Injecting local anesthetic deep into the dura but outside the arachnoid [10] may result in the so-called "massive epidural" [11], whereas subdural and subarachnoid injection will result in subarachnoid block - the extent depending on the volume of local anesthetic injected.

Perineural cysts are well-recognized arachnoid cysts that are formed by degeneration and distention of the spinal root sheath arachnoid granulations. They are more prevalent in older people in the cervical region, but are found in all areas of the spine [12, 13]. They appear in approximately 9% to 18% of asymptomatic patients as saccular diverticula in the lumbar and sacral regions (Tarlov cysts; Fig. **8b**). Thirty percent of elderly people have these asymptomatic saccular diverticula of the lower cervical and thoracic spinal roots [11-13] (Fig. **8**, **a** and **b**). Injecting local anesthetic into a cyst represents a subarachnoid injection. They are filled with cerebrospinal fluid.

Finally, Dag Selander [14] and Daniel Moore [15] have demonstrated the presence of paraneural spaces (see Chapter 20, Fig. **6**) that provide a pathway for local anesthetic to reach the spinal cord if it is injected into the parenchyma (deep to the pia mater) of the spinal root, which is merely a branch or continuation of the spinal cord [16] (Fig. **8a**). Recently, Miguel Reina beautifully demonstrated these paraneural spaces with high magnification microscopy [9, 17].

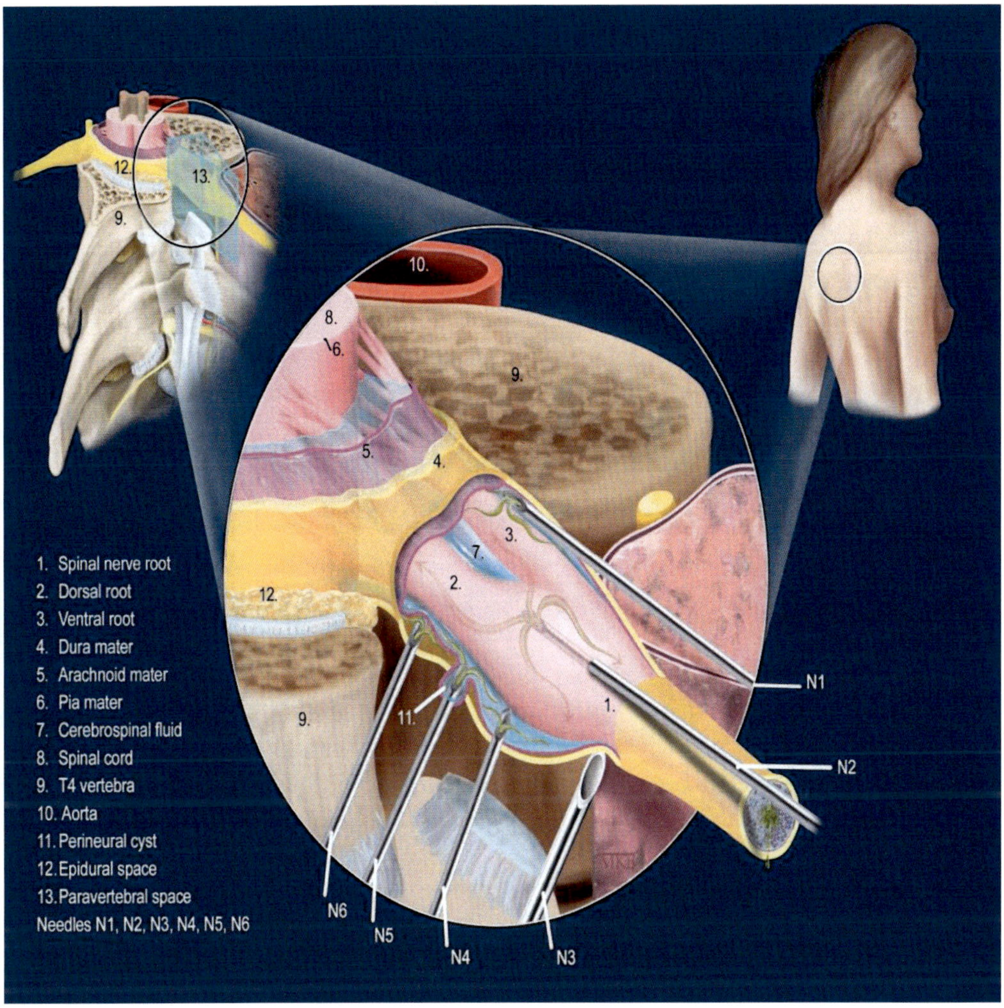

Figure 8a: Schematic representation of the thoracic paravertebral space and the meninges surrounding the spinal root.

The six possible needle placements are depicted:
Needle 1 (N1): Subarachnoid placement of relatively thin needle during trans-foraminal injection (usually steroids)
Needle 2 (N2): Intra-parenchymal placement of relatively this needle during nerve root block (e.g. interscalene block at cervical level) or intercostal nerve block [Moore]
Needle 3 (N3): Extradural needle of Tuohy needle during paravertebral block
Needle 4 (N4): Subarachnoid placement of relatively thin needle during paravertebral block
Needle 5 (N5): Needle placement into a perineural cyst during paravertebral block (See also Fig. **6** *of chapter 21)*
Needle 6 (N6): Subdural (extra-arachnoid) needle placement during paravertebral block

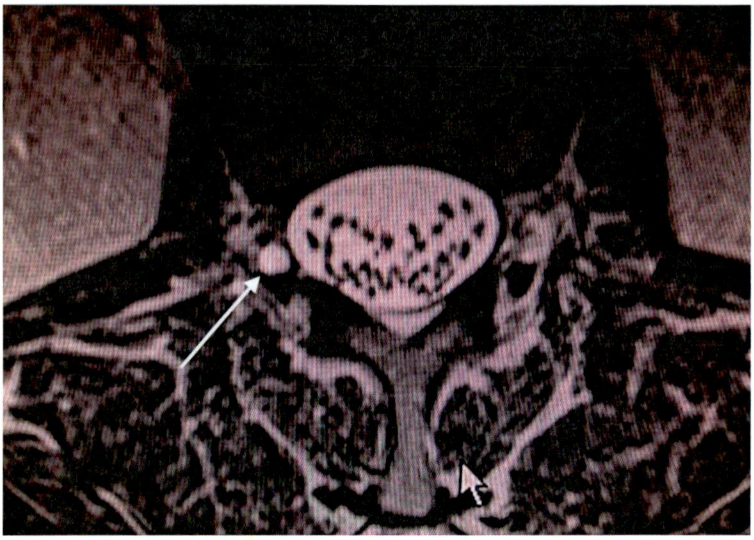

Figure 8b: Magnetic resonance image (MRI) of a paravertebral arachnoid cyst. Arrow points to paravertebral arachnoid cyst.

SURFACE ANATOMY

The patient can be positioned in the lateral or sitting position (Fig. **9**).

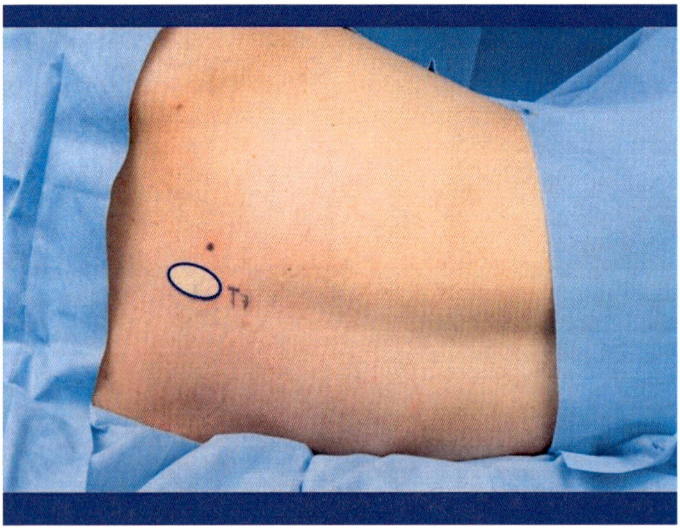

Figure 9: Surface landmarks for thoracic paravertebral space.
The spinous process of a vertebra, the 7th thoracic vertebra in this case (T7), is identified and marked. It is on the inferior margins of the scapulae. A point 2.5 to 3 cm lateral to the midpoint of the spinous process of T7 marks the position of the transverse process of the 8th thoracic vertebra (T8).

FUNCTIONAL ANATOMY

When the spinal roots are approached and the stimulating needle is posterior to the superior costotransverse ligament, a motor response of the intercostal muscle may be elicited, but with a nerve stimulator output that is set relatively high, around 5 mA. Once this ligament is penetrated, and the needle is on the spinal root, the same motor response may be obtained with lower nerves stimulator settings of the intercostal muscles. Approaching the spinal roots of the 7th root downwards will also elicit abdominal muscle motor responses. The patient will often report a "thumping" sensation in the area innervated by the specific thoracic nerve root or intercostal nerve. Electrical stimulation of the posterior rami of the intercostal nerves or spinal roots will result in twitches of the erector spinae muscles.

SONOANATOMY

Ultrasound is a dynamic process whereby structures can and should be followed to their origins and destinations for optimal identification [18]. Because of this, it is not always satisfactory to study static ultrasound images. When studying the sonoanatomy, the authors strongly advise readers to first study the macro- and microanatomy and then to view the accompanying video (Movie 1) that illustrates the dynamic sonoanatomy. After studying this text, it is advisable to recruit a model and reproduce the images depicted in this chapter.

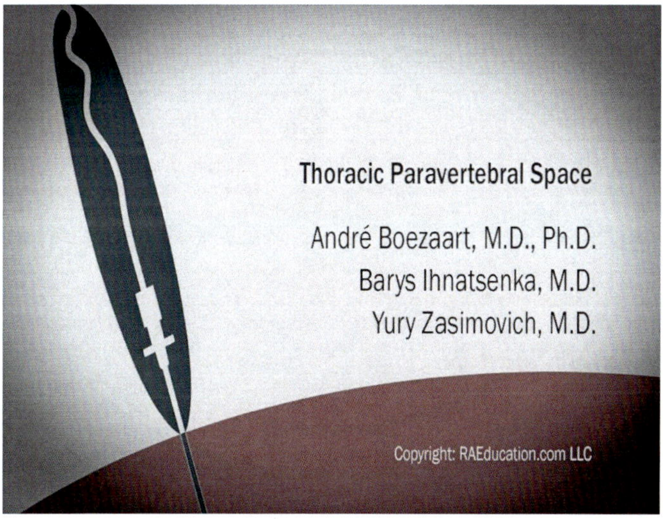

To view this movie click on this link:
https://raeducation.com/ebook

Movie 1: The dynamic sonoanatomy of the thoracic paravertebral space.

The ultrasound transducer probe that was used to prepare the images for this chapter was a 6- to 13-MHz linear probe with a 38-cm footprint (HFL - 38, SonoSite Fujifilm, Bothell, WA, USA).

As is the case with almost all sonoanatomy images, the finer and important ultrastructure of the membranes that surround the nerves [8] cannot be readily visualized with regular ultrasound technology. Please refer to the Microanatomy (Chapter 2) sections for an explanation of these membranes. This ultrastructure of the nerves is especially important when spinal nerve roots are concerned. All spinal nerve roots are covered by meninges for varying distances, and injecting deep to the meninges can have devastating effects. For example, injecting local anesthetic agents deep to the arachnoid mater renders the injection a subarachnoid injection, which has effects similar to that of a spinal subarachnoid injection. Injecting into the parenchyma of a nerve root or deep to the pia mater may have effects similar to injecting into the spinal cord, of which the spinal roots are merely branches (see Microanatomy Chapter 2).

We placed the model in the prone position with her back exposed to obtain the ultrasound images used for this section, but patients may typically be placed in a lateral or sitting position depending on the clinical situation.

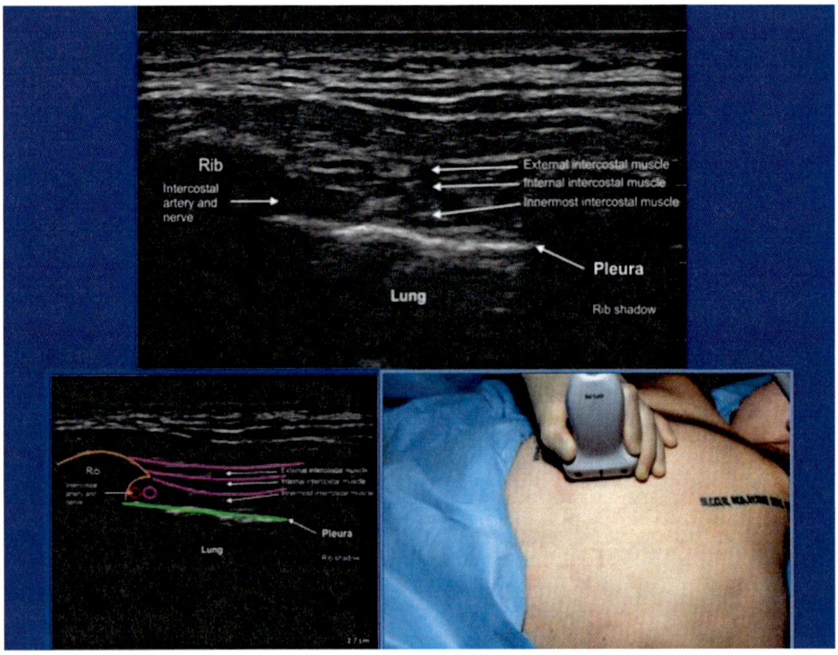

Figure 10a: Sonoanatomy of the thoracic paravertebral space - intercostal.
The left side of the image is cephalad and the right side is caudad.

We start the scanning (Figs. **10a** and **b** and Fig. **11**) lateral in the sagittal plane where there is no doubt that the image indicates the ribs. Note the position of the intercostal neurovascular bundle inferomedial to the ribs. With dynamic ultrasound, the shimmering and pulsation of the lung and the movement of the pleura can be visualized. The pulsation of the intercostal artery can also usually be seen, especially if the Doppler function of the ultrasound probe is used. (Conveniently, tattoo on the back of this model is in the midline.

We now slide the ultrasound transducer probe toward the midline, from the red line in Fig. (**10b**) to the blue line, and the transverse process of the vertebra comes into view. In this instance, it is the transverse process of the 4th thoracic vertebra (T4). (This is usually the main focus area of thoracic paravertebral blocks done for breast surgery [1]).

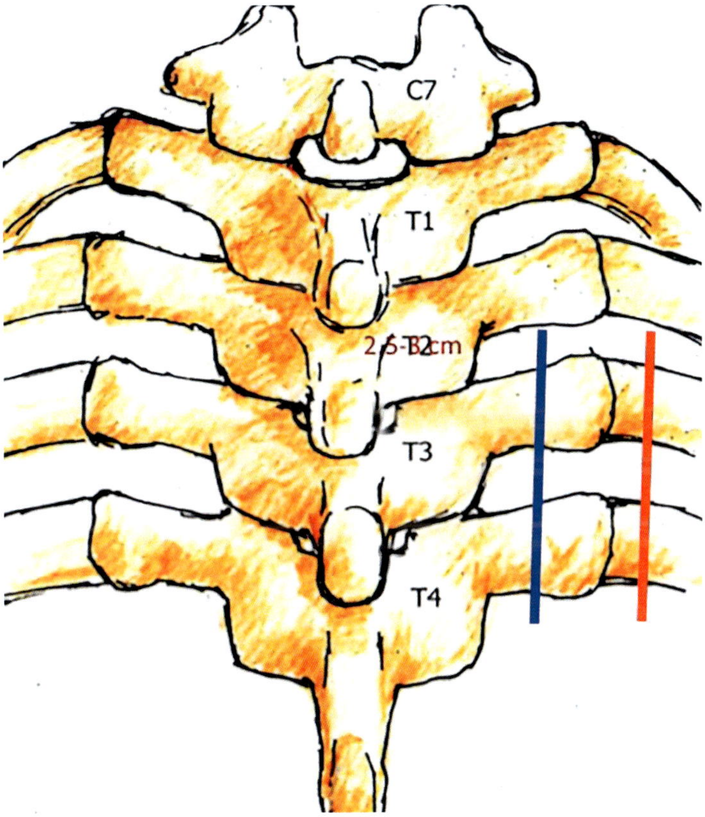

Figure 10b: Orientation of the ultrasound transducer probe from the ribs (Fig. **19b-1a**) to the rib below and the transverse process superior (Fig **19b-2**).
The red line indicates placement of the probe over the ribs in the sagittal plane. The blue line indicates placement of the probe over the rib and transverse process of T4 in the sagittal plane.

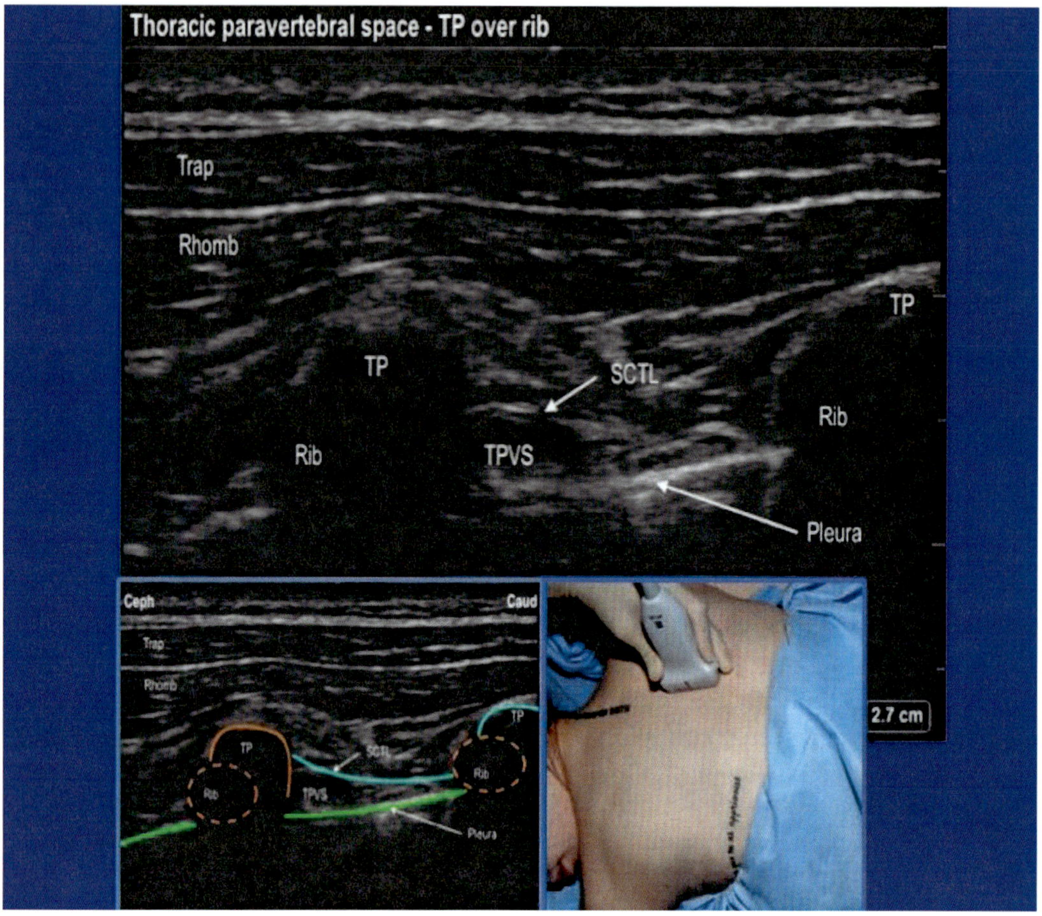

Figure 11: Sonoanatomy of the thoracic paravertebral space in the sagittal plane showing the superior transverse process and the rib below.
The probe is held slightly oblique here. The left side of the image is cephalad. Trap = trapezius muscle; Rhomb = rhomboid muscle; SCTL = superior costotransverse ligament; TP = transverse process of the 4th thoracic vertebra; TPVS = thoracic paravertebral space; 2.7 cm = distance from the skin in centimeters.

In the next image (Fig. **12a**), the ultrasound probe is turned slightly more oblique and this now clearly distinguishes the rib (inferior) from the transverse process. The rib underneath the transverse process of the 4th thoracic vertebra is obscured by the acoustic shadow of the transverse process.

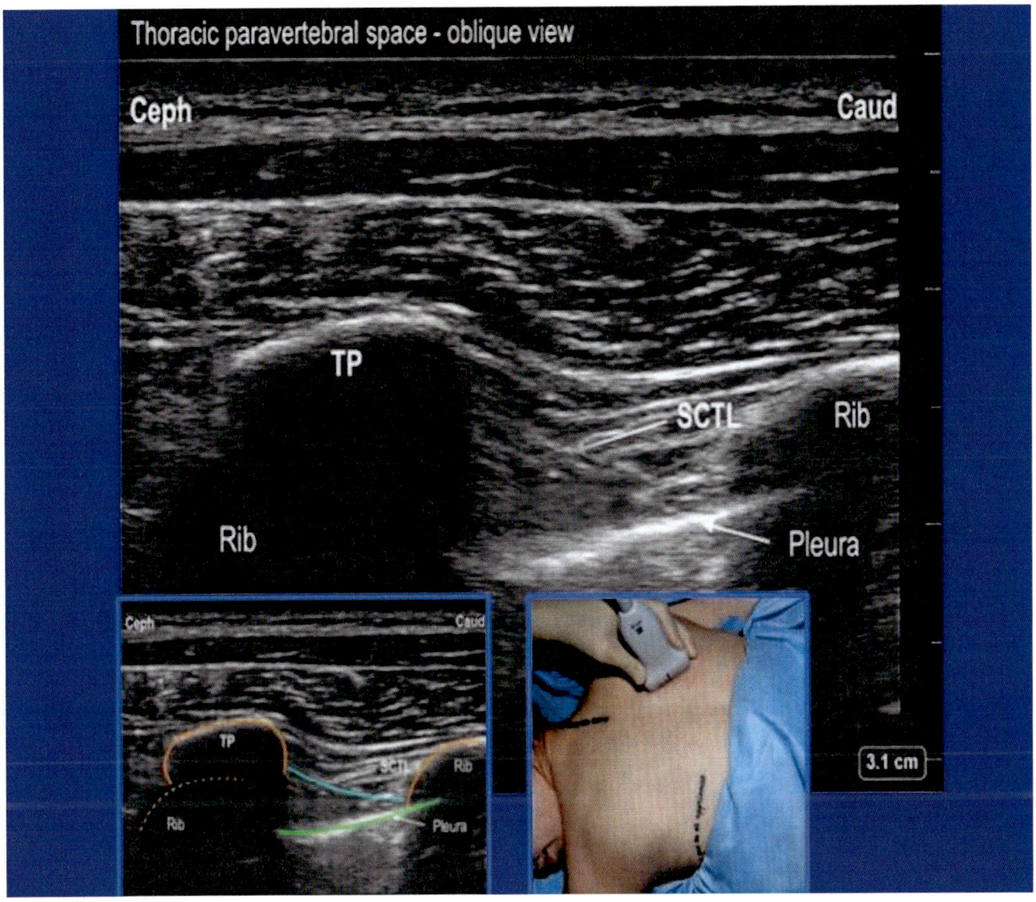

Figure 12a: Sonoanatomy of the thoracic paravertebral space in the sagittal plane. The probe is held more oblique than in the previous figure (Fig **11**).
Ceph = cephalad; Caud = caudad; SCTL = superior costotransverse ligament; TP T4 = transverse process of the 4th thoracic vertebra; PV Space = thoracic paravertebral space.

If the ultrasound probe is in the pure sagittal position as in Fig. (**12**, **a** and **b**), one can be see that the transverse process obscures the rib underneath it.

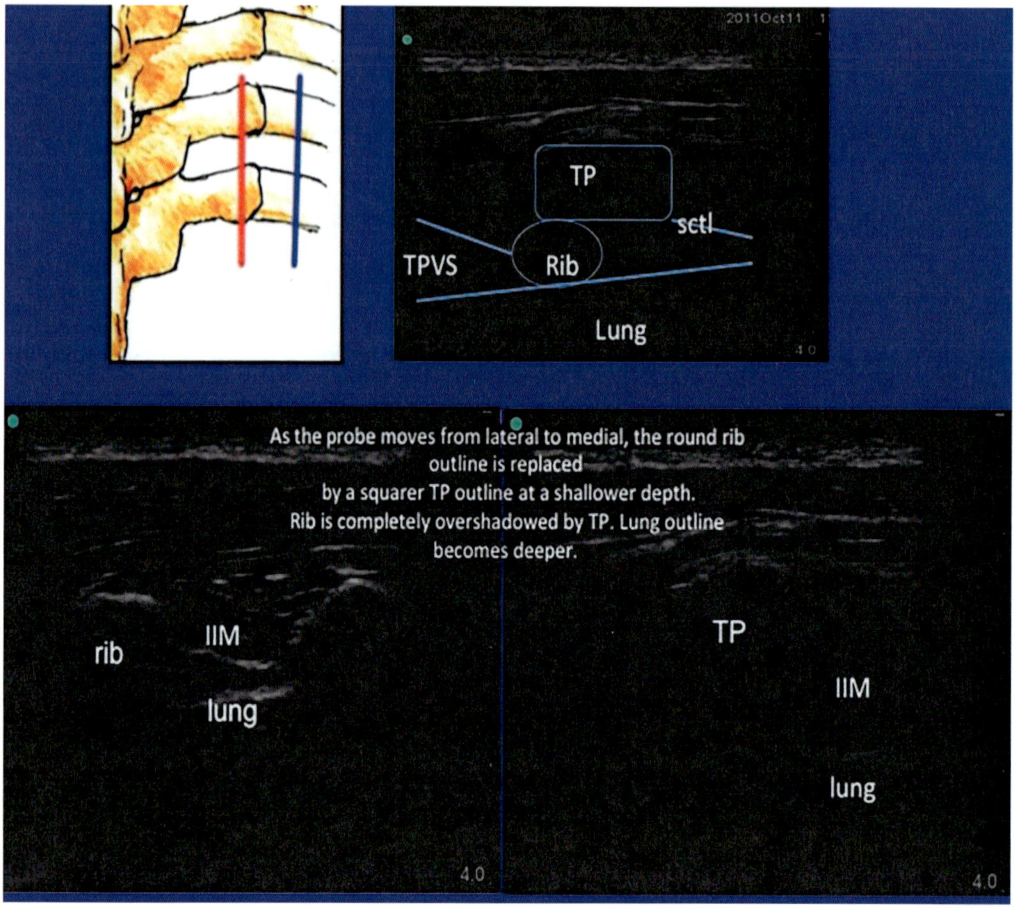

Figure 12b: Sonoanatomy of the thoracic paravertebral space with probe in the vertical sagittal place.

The ultrasound probe is on the blue line of the drawing on the top left and in the left-hand ultrasound image and moved to the red line in the right-hand ultrasound image. TP = transverse process; TPVS = thoracic paravertebral space; sctl = superior costotransverse ligament; IMM = internal intercostal membrane; 4.0 = depth in centimeters from the skin.

We now turn the ultrasound transducer probe axial, as shown in Fig. (**13a**). The probe is on the red line.

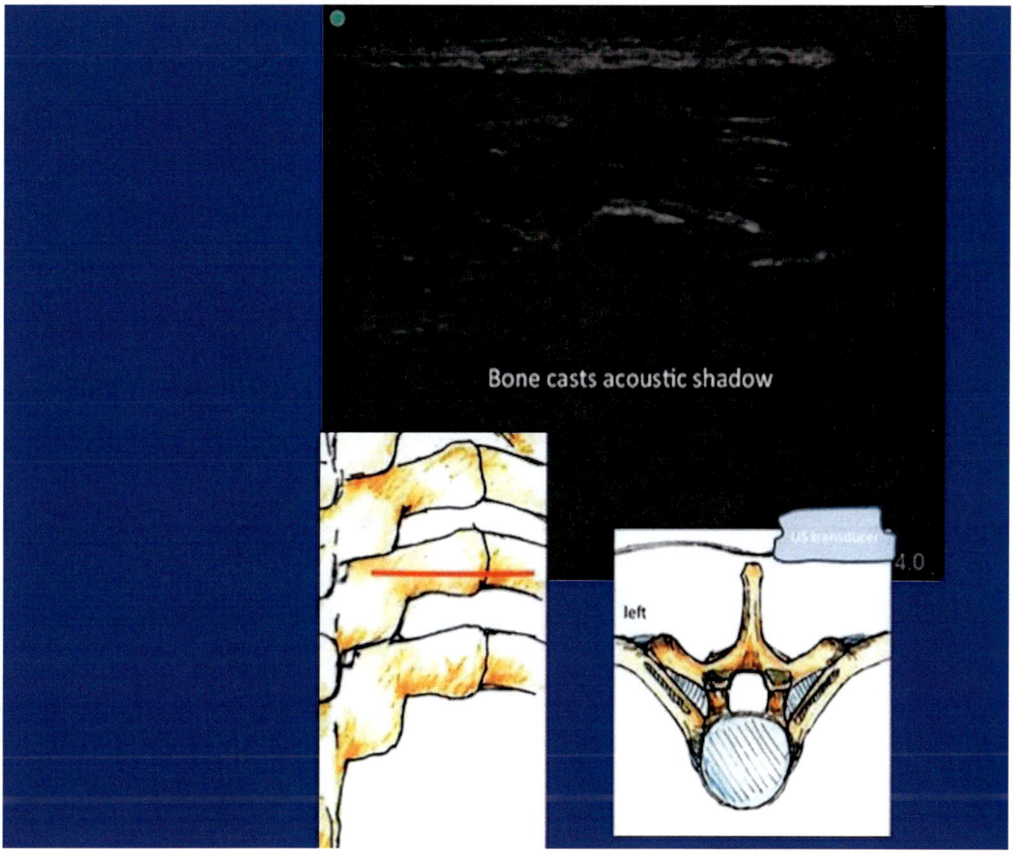

Figure 13a: Sonoanatomy of the thoracic paravertebral space in the axial view.
The top figure depicts the ultrasound image and the acoustic shadow cast by the transverse process and the rib seen when the ultrasound transducer is placed on the red line shown in the bottom left picture.

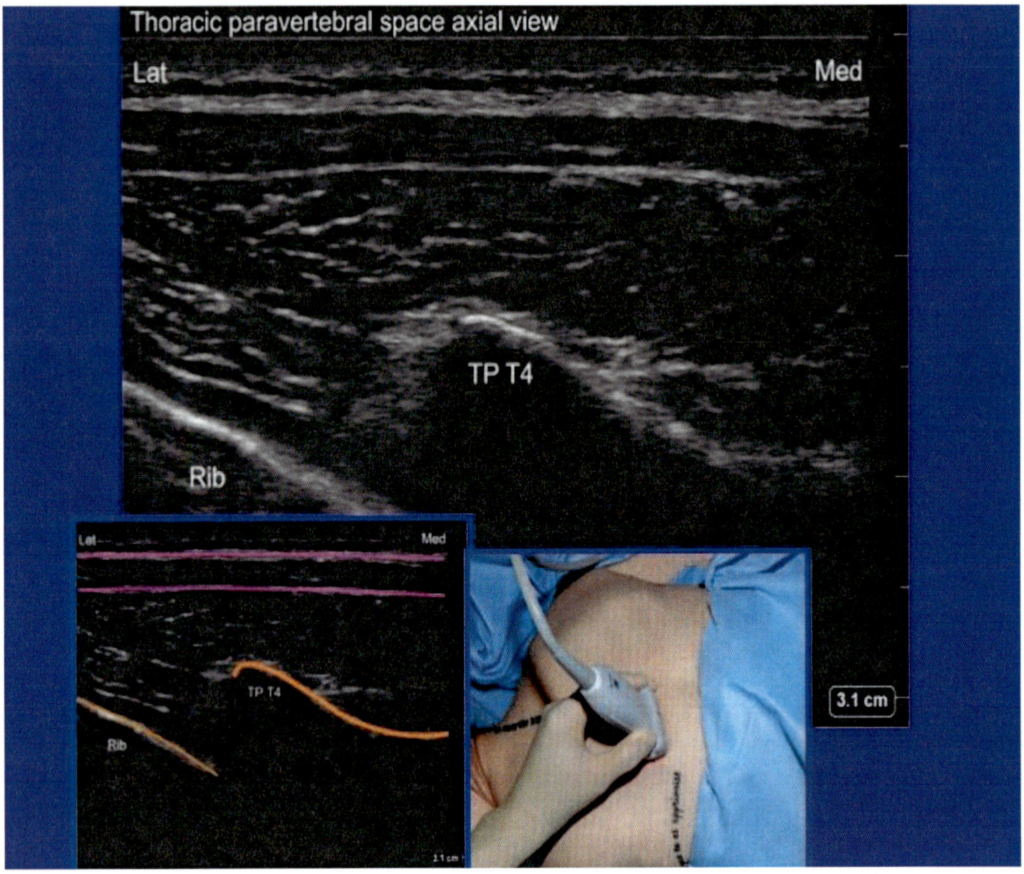

Figure 13b: Sonoanatomy of the thoracic paravertebral space in the axial paravertebral view.
The probe is placed over the transverse process and just below the rib the rib.
Lat = lateral; Med = medial; TP T4 = transverse process of the 4th thoracic vertebra; 3.1cm indicates distance from the skin in centimeters.

We now slide the probe down caudally and the acoustic shadow cast by the rib and transverse process disappears as the ultrasound beam moves off of the bone. The beam is moved from the red line in the bottom left inlay picture of Fig. (**14a**) and (**14b**) to the blue line.

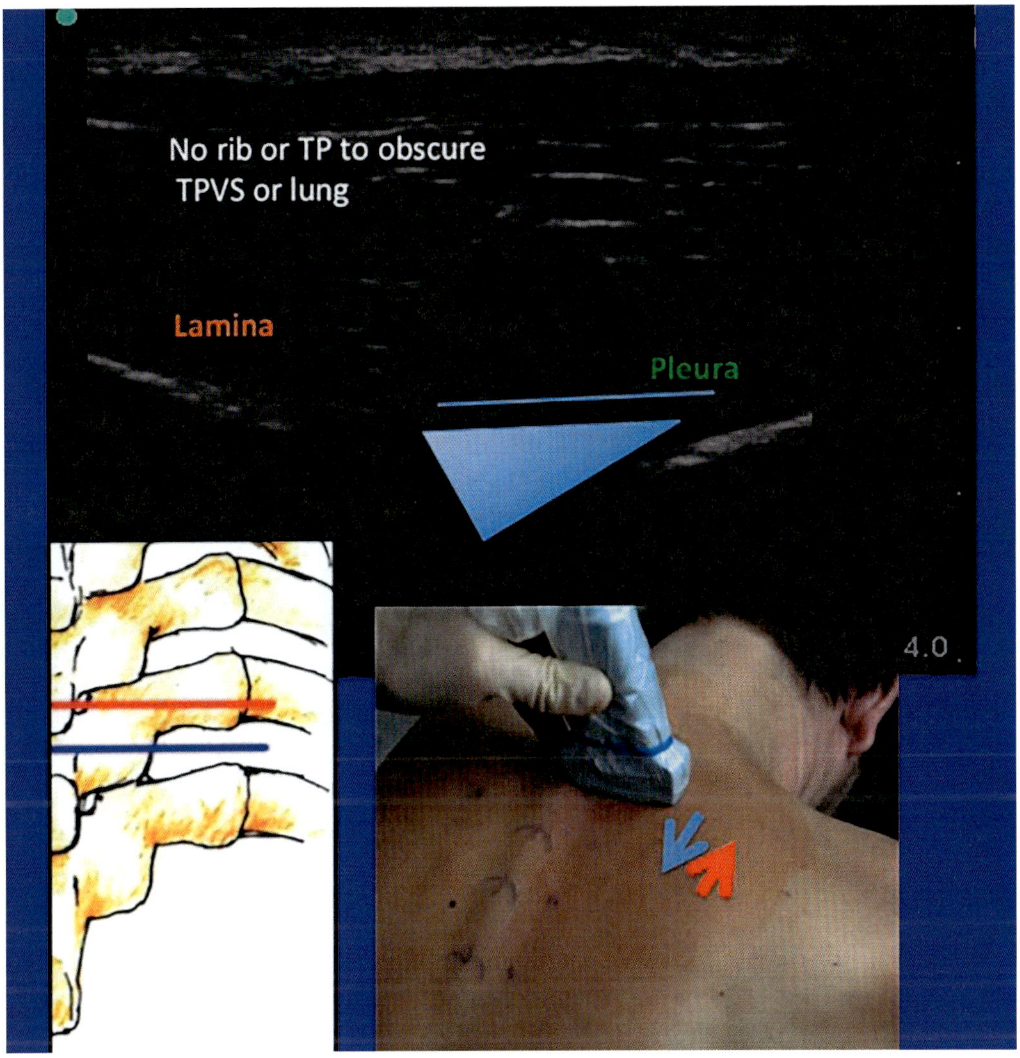

Figure 14a: Sonoanatomy of the thoracic paravertebral space in the axial view.
The ultrasound probe is moved from the red line position to that of the blue line. The thoracic paravertebral space is indicated by the blue triangle.
TP = transverse process; TPVS = thoracic paravertebral space.

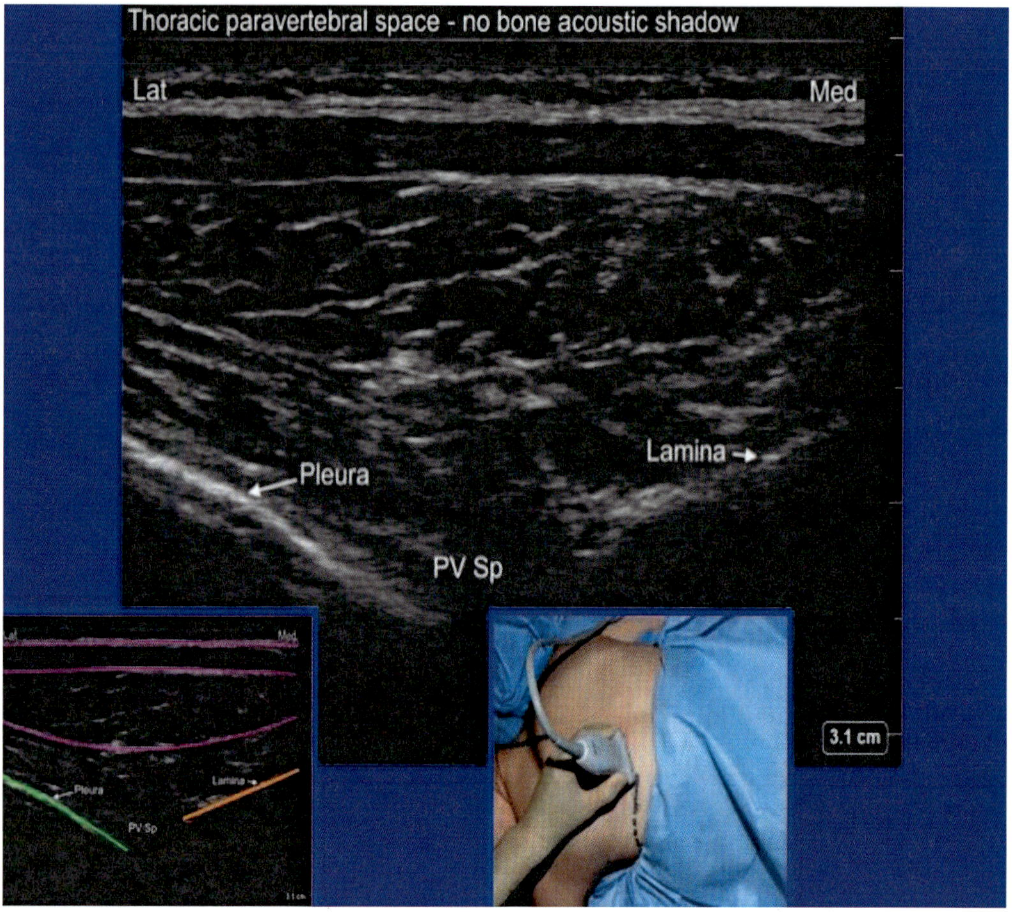

Figure 14b: Sonoanatomy of the thoracic paravertebral space in the axial view.
The acoustic shadow cast by the transverse process and rib disappears as the probe is moved caudad and the paravertebral space comes into view. Lat = lateral; Med = medial; PV Sp = thoracic paravertebral space; 3.1 cm = the depth in centimeters from the skin.

It is always easy to see the lung and pleura with dynamic ultrasound scanning because the lung has a typical and unmistakable shimmering and pulsating movement (See Video production, Movie 19-1), whereas the pleura is a white hyperechoic appearance that is differentiated from bone in that bone casts an acoustic shadow that is also unmistakable. In some images and at certain angles of the beam, the lung appears "deeper" or further anterior than in others, and in some images, it totally disappears. Fig. (**15**) may make understanding this phenomenon easier.

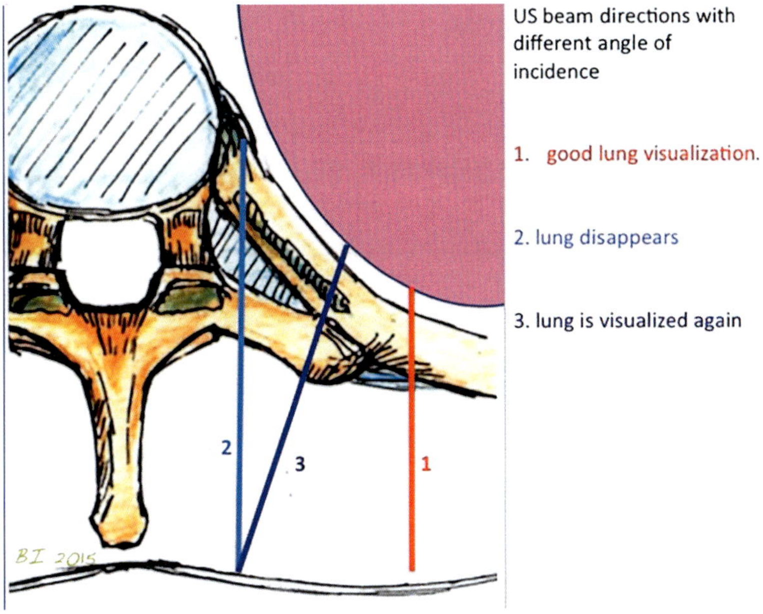

Figure 15: Lung visualization with the ultrasound beam at thoracic paravertebral area.
US beam = ultrasound beam; 1 = the lung is well visualized typically about 4 to 6 cm lateral of the spinous process of the vertebra; 2 = the lung is not visible because the ultrasound beam is directed between the lung and the vertebral body; 3 = tilting the beam laterally brings the lung into view again.

Thus, when probe is slid from lateral to medial in the sagittal plane, the lung outline becomes more ventral. To optimize the angle of incidence with the pleura, the ultrasound probe should be tilted laterally. If the probe is not tilted laterally and continuously scanning medially in the sagittal plane, the pleura line will disappear, which is an artifact secondary to an unfavorable angle of incidence.

ACKNOWLEDGEMENTS

The authors gratefully acknowledge the following people:

- The Head of the Department of Anesthesiology of the College of Medicine of the University of Florida, Dr. Tim Morey, and his department for their moral support and continuous encouragement.

- The faculty and fellows of the Division of Acute and Perioperative Pain Medicine of the above Department of Anesthesiology for affording the authors the time to produce this work by covering their clinical duties.

- Dr. Anastacia Munro for her help with the preparation of the chapter and ultrasound images.

- Corey Astrom of the Department of Anesthesiology of the College of Medicine of the University of Florida for her professional and high quality text editing.

- Nancy Hagen of the Iowa Public Radio for her narration of the movies.

- Raeducation.com LLC for their financial support.

CONFLICT OF INTEREST

The authors confirm that this chapter contents have no conflict of Interest.

ABBREVIATIONS

Caud	=	caudad
Ceph	=	cephalad
DG	=	dorsal root ganglion.
IM	=	internal intercostal muscle
IMM	=	internal intercostal membrane
Innermost ICM	=	innermost intercostal muscle
Lat	=	lateral
Med	=	medial
PV Space	=	thoracic paravertebral space
Rhomb	=	rhomboid muscle
SC	=	spinal cord
SCTL	=	superior costotransverse ligament

SP = spinous process of vertebra

TP = transverse process

TP T4 = transverse process of the 4th thoracic vertebra

TPVS = thoracic paravertebral space

Trap = trapezius muscle

REFERENCES

[1] Boezaart AP, Raw RM. Continuous thoracic paravertebral block for major breast surgery. Reg Anesth Pain Med 2006; 31:470-476.

[2] Klein SM, Bergh A, Steele SM, MD, Georgiade GS, Greengrass RA. Thoracic Paravertebral Block for Breast Surgery. Anesth Analg 2000; 90:1402-1405.

[3] Moore DC. Complications of Regional Anesthesia. Springfield: Illinois, Charles C. Thomas Publisher 1955; p. 52.

[4] Sharrock NE: Postdural headache following thoracic somatic paravertebral nerve block. Anesthesiology 1980; 52:360-362.

[5] Lekhak B, Bartley C, Conacher ID, Nouraei SM. Total spinal anaesthesia in association with insertion of a paravertebral catheter. Br J Anaesth 2001; 86:280-282.

[6] Benumof JL, Semenza J. Total spinal anesthesia following intrathoracic intercostal nerve blocks. Anesthesiology 1975; 43:124-125.

[7] Garutti I, Hervias M, Barrio JM, Fortea F, De La Torre J. Subdural spread of local anesthetic agent following thoracic paravertebral block and cannulation. Anesthesiology 2003; 98:1005-1007.

[8] Boezaart AP, Lucas SD, Elliott CE. Paravertebral block: cervical, thoracic, lumbar and sacral. Curr Opin Anaesthesiol 2009; 22:637-643.

[9] Reina MA, Colman LR, Peyrano EC. Ultrastructure of nerve root cuffs: Dura-epineurium transition tissue. In: Reina MA, ed. Atlas of functional anatomy for regional anesthesia and pain medicine. New York: Springer Science and Business Media 2015; pp. 705-747.

[10] Reina MA, Pulido P, De Sola RG. Ultrastructure of the spinal arachnoid layer. In: Reina MA, ed. Atlas of functional anatomy for regional anesthesia and pain medicine. New York: Springer Science and Business Media 2015; pp. 435-453.

[11] Boezaart AP, Kadieva VS. Inadvertent extra-arachnoid [subdural] injection of a local anaesthetic agent during epidural anaesthesia. S Afr Med J 1992; 81:325-326.

[12] Nabors M, Pait TG, Byrd EB. Updated assessment and current classification of spinal meningeal cysts. J Neurosurg 1988; 68: 366-377.

[13] Holt S, Yates PO. Cervical nerve root "cysts." Brain 1964; 87:481-490.

[14] Selander D, Sjöstrand J. Longitudinal spread of intraneurally injected local anesthetics. Acta Anaesth Scand 1978: 22:622-634.

[15] Moore DC, Hain RF Ward A, Bridenbaugh LD. Importance of the perineural spaces in nerve blocking. JAMA. 1954; 156:1050--1055.

[16] Hernández JM, Reina MA, De Andrés JA. Nerve root and type of needle used in transforaminal injection. In: Reina MA, ed. Atlas of functional anatomy for regional anesthesia and pain medicine. New York: Springer Science and Business Media 2015; pp. 813-826.

[17] Reina MA, Colman LR, Prats-Galino A. Ultrastructure of human spinal nerve roots, In: Reina MA, ed. Atlas of functional anatomy for regional anesthesia and pain medicine. New York: Springer Science and Business Media 2015; pp. 553-571.

[18] Ihnatsenka BV, Boezaart AP. Ultrasound: Basic understanding and learning the language. Int J Shoulder Surg. 2010; 4:55-62.

Chapter 20:
Applied Macro- and Sonoanatomy of the Lumbar Paravertebral Space

CHAPTER 20

Applied Macro- and Sonoanatomy of the Lumbar Paravertebral Space

André P. Boezaart[1,*] and Barys V. Ihnatsenka[2]

[1]Departments of Anesthesiology and Orthopaedic Surgery and Rehabilitation, Division of Acute and Perioperative Pain Medicine, University of Florida College of Medicine, Gainesville, Florida, USA and [2]Department of Anesthesiology, Division of Acute and Perioperative Pain Medicine, University of Florida College of Medicine, Gainesville, Florida, USA

Abstract: The positioning of the lumbar plexus within the psoas muscle is somewhat controversial. Winnie, for example, described the plexus as lying between the psoas and quadratus lumborum muscles. From this description, "psoas compartment block" was termed for the lumbar plexus block. Other names for the same thing are "lumbar plexus block", "lumbar paravertebral block", "quadratus lumborum block" and "fascia iliaca block" to name a few. Most authors described the plexus and its nerve branches within the psoas muscle between its anterior and posterior masses. The ventral rami of the first three and the major part of the fourth lumbar spinal roots (L2, L3, and L4) form the lumbar plexus. A contribution from the 1st lumbar nerve (L1) is common. As soon as the ventral rami of these spinal nerve roots exit the intervertebral foramina, they become embedded in the psoas muscle, anterior to the transverse processes. At the L4 to L5 level, however, the lumbar plexus branches are still medial and close to the transverse processes. The distance of the lumbar plexus to the skin varies with body habitus and gender. Capdevila and his colleagues described the distances as varying from 57 to 93 mm in women and from 61 to 101 mm in men.

The macro-, microanatomy, and sonoanatomy (static) of the lumbar plexus, its nerve roots, and relationships to other structures are discussed in this chapter.

Keywords: Acute pain medicine, Fascia iliaca, Femoral nerve, Genitofemoral nerve, Iliohypogastirc nerve, Ilioinguinal nerve, Intervertebral foramina, Lumbar paravertebral block, Lumbar plexus, Lumbar plexus block, Lumbosacral trunk, Macroanatomy, Microanatomy, Obturator nerve, Psoas compartment block, Psoas muscle, Quadratus lumborum block, Quadratus lumborum muscle, Regional anesthesia, Sciatic nerve, Sonoanatomy, Spinal nerve roots, Transverse processes, Ventral rami.

***Corresponding author André P. Boezaart:** Departments of Anesthesiology and Orthopaedic Surgery, Division of Acute and Peri-operative Pain Medicine, University of Florida College of Medicine, 1600 SW Archer Road, Gainesville, Florida 32610, USA; Tel: 352-846-0913 (Work); Fax: 352-392-7029;
E-mail: aboezaart@anest.ufl.edu

MACROANATOMY

The positioning of the lumbar plexus within the psoas muscle is somewhat controversial. Winnie [1], for example, described the plexus between the psoas and quadratus lumborum muscles. From this description, "psoas compartment block" was termed for the lumbar plexus block. Other names for the same thing are "lumbar plexus block", "lumbar paravertebral block", "quadratus lumborum block" and "fascia iliaca block" to name a few. Authors described the plexus and its nerve branches within the psoas muscle [2-4] between its anterior and posterior masses (Figs. **4** and **8**).

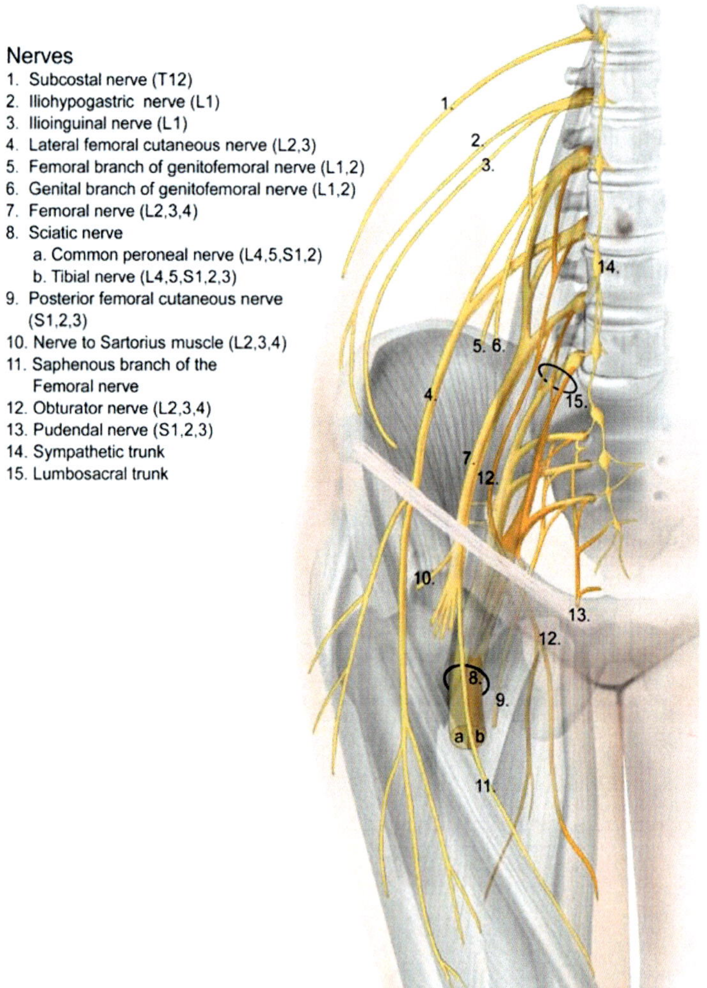

Figure 1: The lumbosacral plexus.

The ventral rami of the first three and the major part of the fourth lumbar spinal roots (L2, L3, and L4) form the lumbar plexus (Fig. **1**). A contribution of the 1st lumbar nerve (L1) is common (Fig. **1**). As soon as the ventral rami of these spinal nerve roots exit the intervertebral foramina, they become embedded in the psoas muscle, anterior to the transverse processes. At the L4 to L5 level, however, the lumbar plexus branches are still medial and close to the transverse processes. The distance of the lumbar plexus to the skin varies with body habitus [2, 5] and gender [2, 4]. Capdevila and his colleagues described the distances as varying from 57 to 93 mm in women and from 61 to 101 mm in men [2].

Within the psoas muscle, the first three and the greater part of the fourth lumbar ventral rami split into anterior and posterior divisions that form the individual branches of the lumbar plexus. The three superior branches are the iliohypogastric, ilioinguinal, and genitofemoral nerves, and the three caudal branches are, laterally, the femoral cutaneous nerve or lateral cutaneous nerve of the thigh; centrally, the femoral nerve; and, medially, the obturator nerve (Fig. **2**). The obturator nerve, however, is more variable [5]. The smaller part of the fourth lumbar ventral rami joins the fifth rami to form the lumbosacral trunk, the upper portion of the sacral plexus.

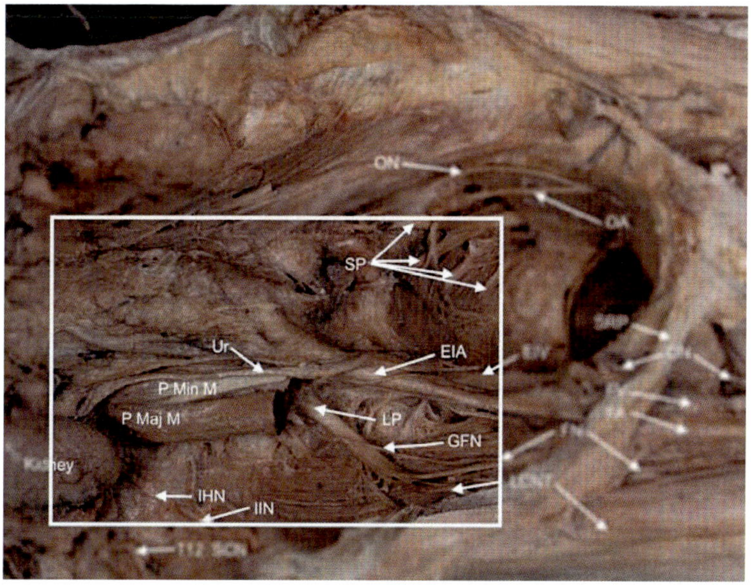

Figure 2: Macroanatomy of the posterior retroperitoneal space.
P Maj M = psoas major muscle; P min M = psoas minor muscle; Ur = ureter; IIN = ilioinguinal nerve; IHN = iliohypogastric nerve; LP = lumbar plexus; GFN = genitofemoral nerve; EIA = external iliac artery; SP = sacral plexus; ON = obturator nerve.

The iliohypogastric nerve is the more cephalad branch of the lumbar plexus originating from the superior division of the first lumbar (L1) ventral rami, and it often receives a contribution from the 12th thoracic nerve. The ilioinguinal nerve also arises from the superior division of the L1 ventral rami. It courses slightly more caudad to the iliohypogastric nerve. Both of these nerves course anterior and pass through the transversus abdominis plane at some point superomedial to the iliac crest (see Chapter 22).

The inferior division of the first lumbar ventral rami (L1) and the small superior division of L2 ventral rami fuse to form the genitofemoral nerve, which then usually crosses the psoas muscle obliquely, where it emerges at its medial border and courses caudad between the psoas muscle and the peritoneum in close proximity to the to the vertebral column. In the male, it supplies motor innervation to the cremaster muscle and to the skin over the femoral triangle, scrotum, major labia, and mons pubis.

The dorsal divisions of the L2 and L3 ventral rami form the lateral femoral cutaneous nerve or lateral cutaneous nerve of the thigh (Fig. **1**). It exits from underneath the lateral part of the psoas muscle at the L4 level and passes under the lateral part of the inguinal ligament to supply sensory innervation to the skin of the lateral part of the thigh.

The largest branch of the lumbar plexus is the femoral nerve. It forms from the union of the large dorsal divisions of the L2, L3, and L4 ventral rami and emerges from the posterolateral border of the psoas muscle at the junction of the muscle's upper two-thirds and lower one-third. After emerging, it runs caudally in the groove between the psoas and iliacus muscles, behind the fascia iliaca, and continues below the inguinal ligament, lateral to the femoral artery. The psoas and iliacus muscles are covered by the fascia iliaca, which is a continuation of the fascia covering the front of the quadratus lumborum muscle. This fascia separate the femoral nerve from the femoral vessels (Fig. **2**).

The smaller anterior divisions of the L2, L3, and L4 ventral rami form the obturator nerve, which leaves the psoas muscle at its internal and posterior border between L5 and S1. At this point, the fascia iliaca and the psoas muscle separate the obturator nerve from the femoral nerve. (Fig. **1** of chapter 10) illustrates the innervation by peripheral nerves of the lower extremity.

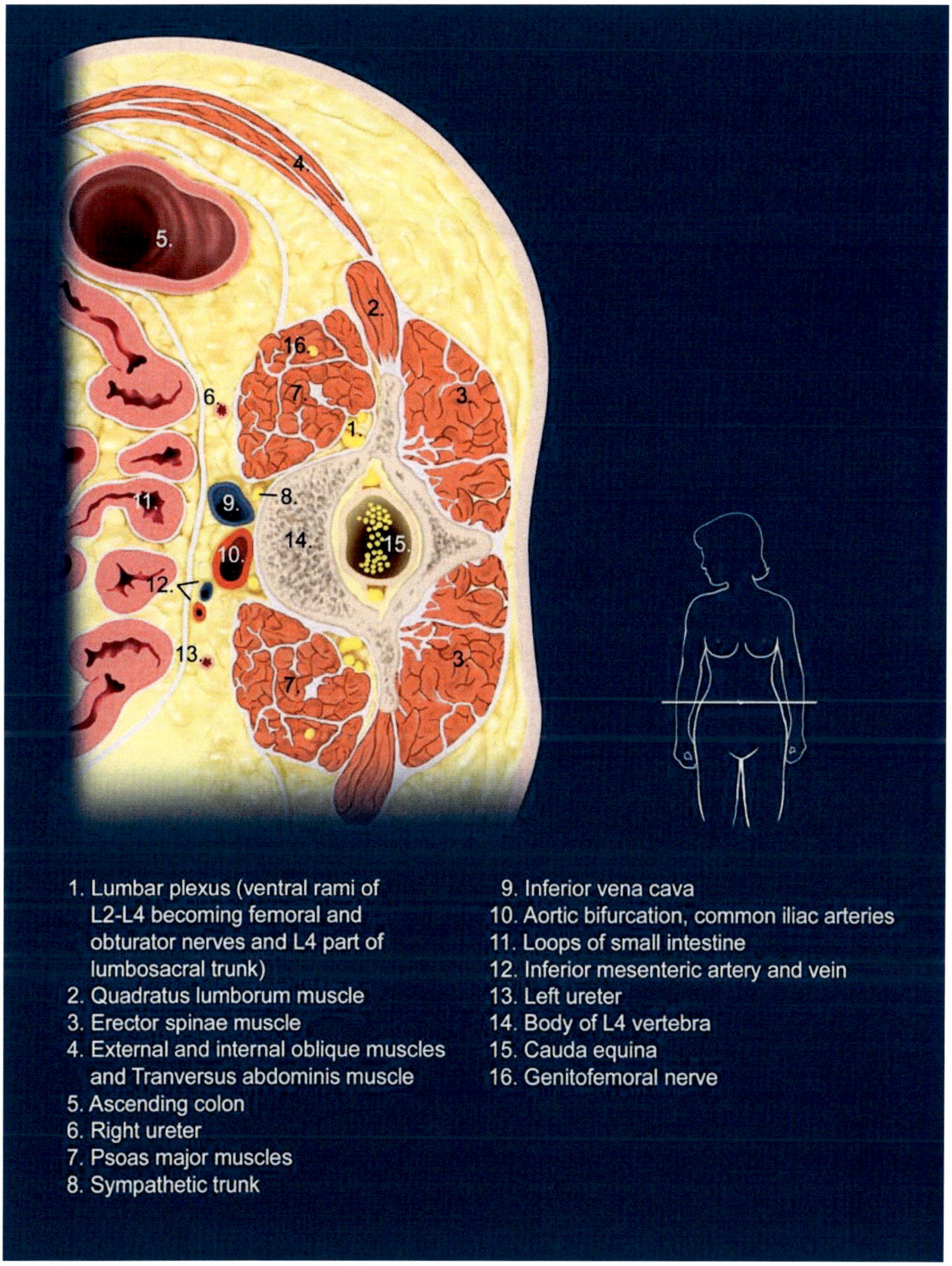

Figure 3: Relative positioning of lumbar plexus, genitofemoral nerve, and lumbar sympathetic chain at the level of the 4th lumbar vertebra.

Note the loosely packed fibers of the vascular psoas muscle and the position of the quadratus lumborum muscle and the lumbar plexus is usually between the anterior and posterior masses of the psoas major masses. At the level of the 4th lumbar vertebra the nerves are more lateral and anterior (inside the psoas major muscle) than higher up at the level of the second lumbar vertebra for example. At the latter level the lumbar nerve roots are directly below the transverse process and medial in the paravertebral space.

MICROANATOMY

As with all spinal nerve roots, the lumbar plexus spinal roots are surrounded by meninges for undetermined distances that vary from one patient to another (please also refer to Chapter 2).

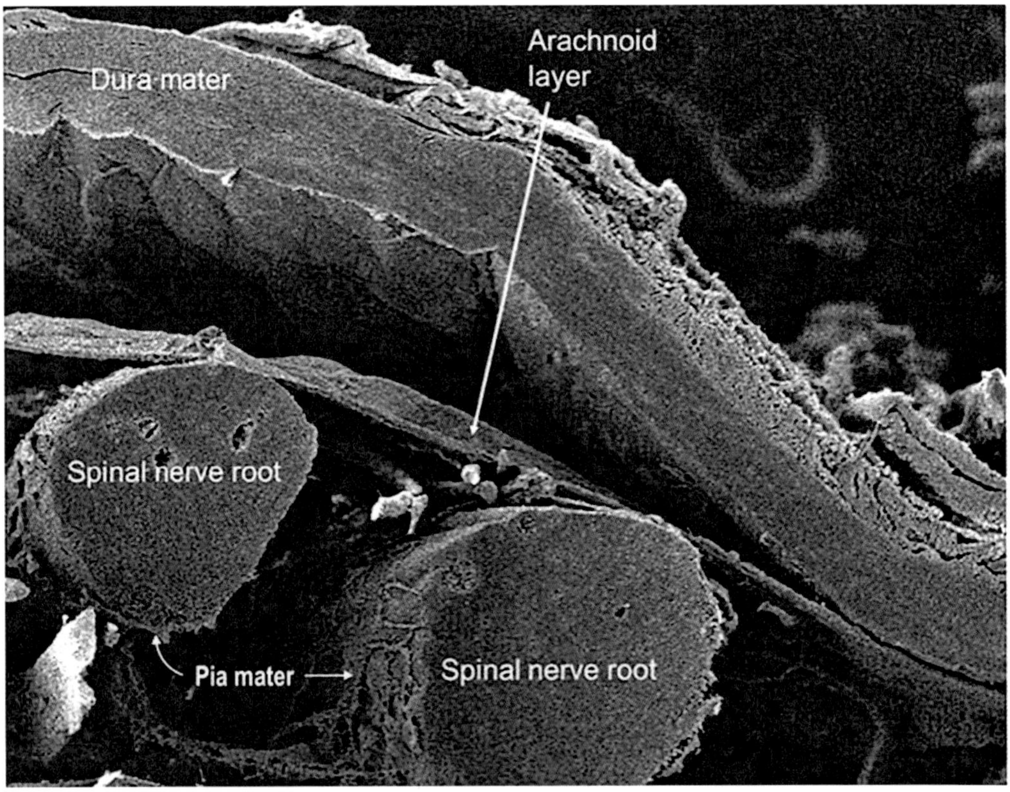

Figure 4: Ultrastructure of the meninges (dura, arachnoid, and pia maters) surrounding nerve root. Scanning electron microscopy - magnification ×20 (*Reprinted from Reina [10] with permission*).

Numerous cases of severe central (spinal) neurological deficits and total spinal block have also been described that resulted from paravertebral block - cervical, thoracic, lumbar, and sacral [6-9]. The anatomical basis for this [10] is depicted in Figs. (**5**) and (**8a** of Chapter 19). Injecting local anesthetic deep to the dura, but outside the arachnoid, may result in a so-called "massive epidural" [11], whereas subarachnoid injection will result in a subarachnoid block - the extent and spread depending on the volume of local anesthetic injected [6, 8] (Fig. **5**).

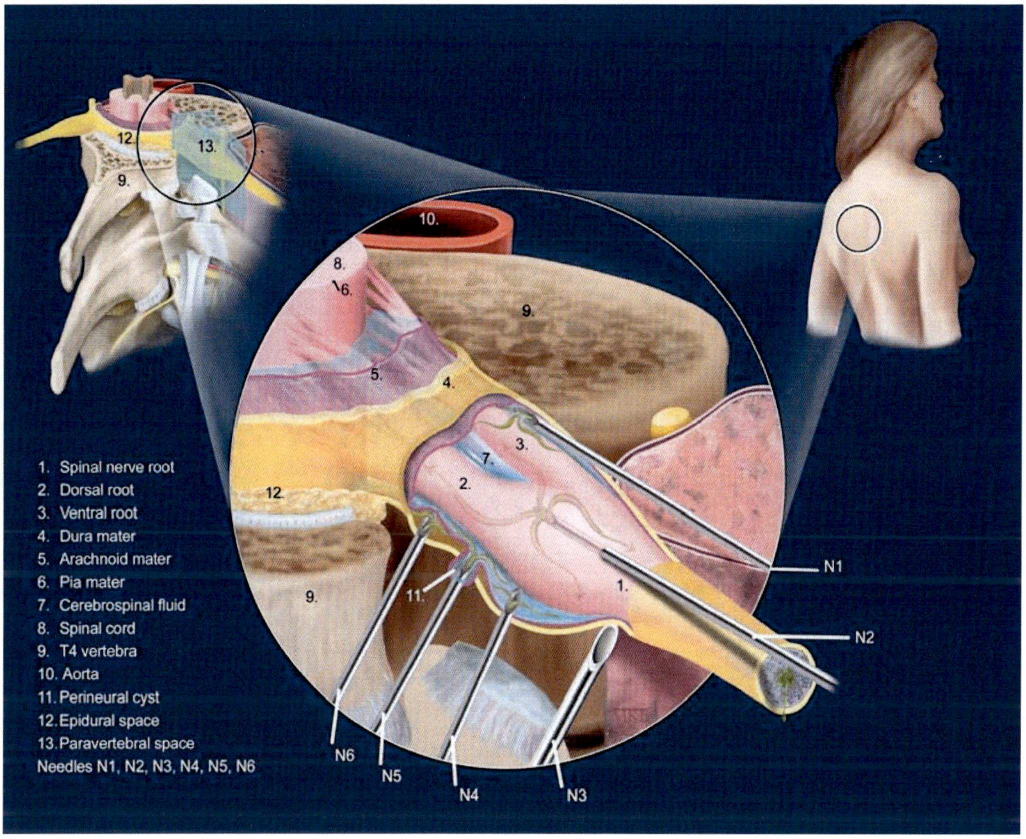

Figure 5: Schematic representation of the thoracic paravertebral space and the meninges surrounding the spinal root.
The six possible needle placements are depicted:
Needle 1 (N1): Subarachnoid placement of relatively thin needle during trans-foraminal injection (usually steroids)
Needle 2 (N2): Intra-parenchymal placement of relatively this needle during nerve root block (e.g. interscalene block at cervical level) or intercostal nerve block [Moore]
Needle 3 (N3): Extradural needle of Tuohy needle during paravertebral block
Needle 4 (N4): Subarachnoid placement of relatively thin needle during paravertebral block
Needle 5 (N5): Needle placement into a perineural cyst during paravertebral block (See also Fig. **6***)*
Needle 6 (N6): Subdural (extra-arachnoid) needle placement during paravertebral block

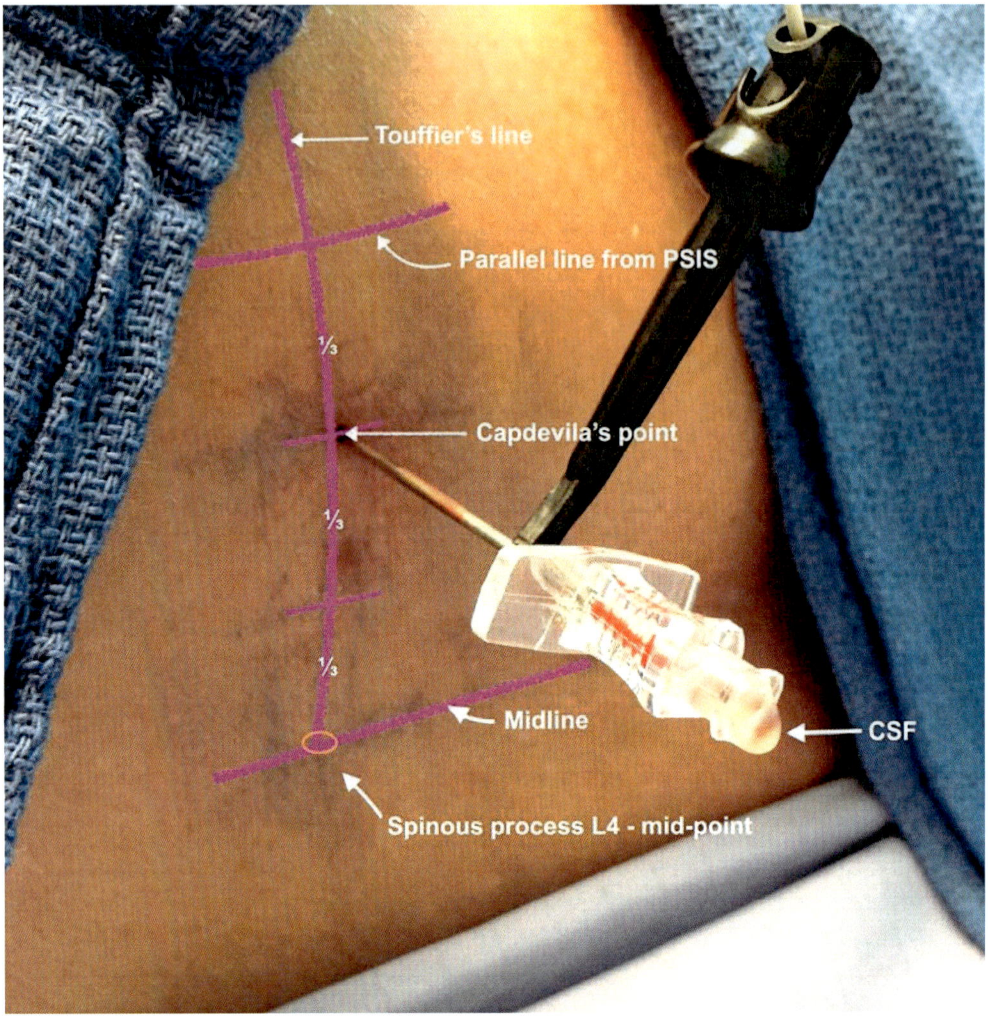

Figure 6: Accidental dural puncture during attempted lumbar plexus block.
Touffier's line is line connecting two iliac crests; PSIS = posterior superior iliac spine; Midline is line on spinous processes of vertebrae; L4 = 4th lumbar vertebra, CSF = cerebrospinal fluid; Capdevila's point = Two-thirds the distance from the parallel line from PSIS and midline.

Furthermore, perineural cysts are well-recognized arachnoid cysts that are formed by the degeneration and distention of spinal root sheath arachnoid granulations [12, 13]. They are more prevalent in the cervical region of the elderly, but are found in all areas of the spine [12, 13]. (See Chapter 21, Fig. **6**). They appear in approximately 9% to 18% of asymptomatic patients as saccular diverticula in the lumbar and sacral regions (Tarlov cysts; Fig. **8** of chapter 19). Thirty percent of elderly people have these asymptomatic saccular diverticula of the lower cervical and thoracic spinal roots (Fig. **7**, **a** and **b** of chapter 19) [11-13]. Injecting local anesthetic into a cyst represents a subarachnoid injection. They are filled with cerebrospinal fluid.

Finally, Dag Selander [14] and Daniel Moore [15] have demonstrated the presence of paraneural spaces that provide a pathway for local anesthetic to reach the spinal cord if it is injected into the parenchyma (deep to the pia mater) of the spinal root, which is merely a branch or continuation of the spinal cord (Fig. **8a** of chapter 19) [16]. Recently, Miguel Reina beautifully demonstrated these paraneural spaces with high-magnification microscopy [17].

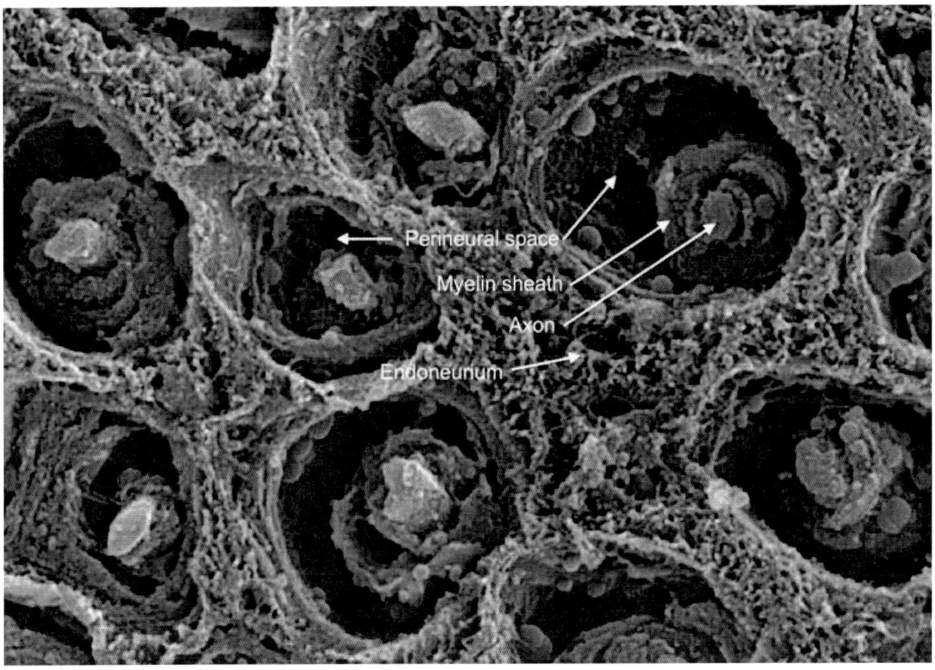

Figure 7: Perineural spaces.
Scanning electron microscopy, magnification ×2,000. (Reprinted from Reina [17] with permission)

Surface Anatomy

Capdevila described the surface landmarks of the lumbar plexus from a posterior approach [2] (Fig. **8**), which are commonly used today. He drew a line, Tuffier's line, between the left and right iliac crests, which passes over the spinous process of the fourth lumbar vertebra (T4). The posterior superior iliac spine (PSIS) is then identified at the posterior end of the iliac crest. Depending on body habitus, it can usually be palpated by following the iliac crest to its posterior end. A line parallel to the midline is then drawn from the PSIS and the Tuffier's line is divided into thirds between the midline and the parallel line from the PSIS. According to Capdevila's technique, needle entry is at the junction of the lateral and middle thirds of this line.

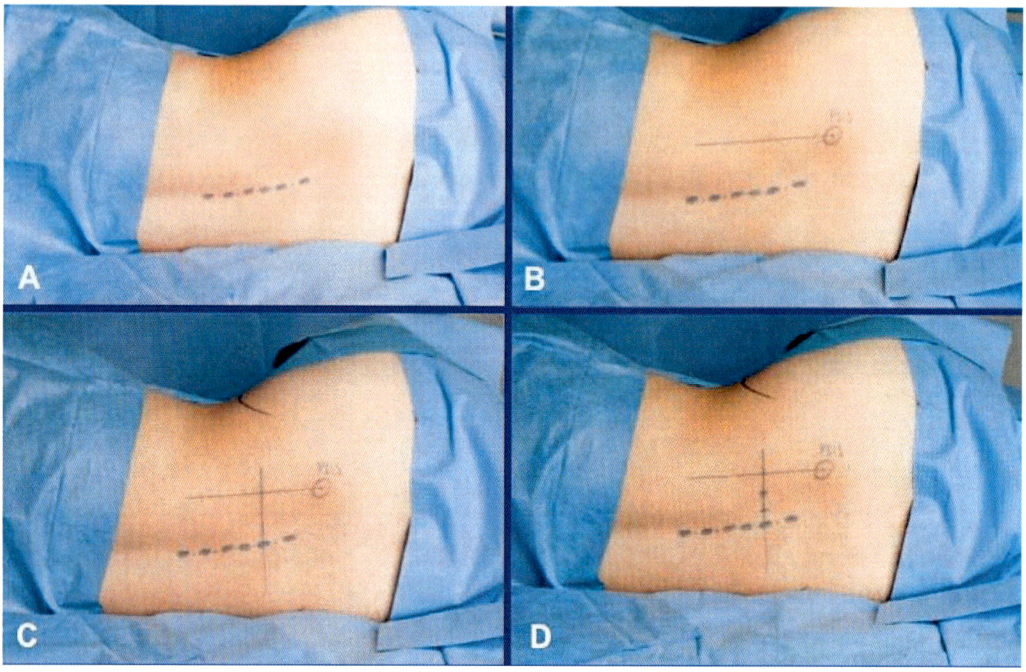

Figure 8: Surface anatomy of the lumbar plexus.
A. The patient is in the lateral (or sitting) position and a line is drawn to indicate the midline over the spinous processes of the lumbar vertebrae.
B. The posterior iliac spine (PSIS) is identified and a line parallel to the one in A is drawn from the PSIS.
C. The line joining the left and right iliac crests is drawn; this is the so-called "Tuffier's line".
D. The distance from the lines in A and B is divided into three equal parts and needle entry is at the junction of the lateral and middle thirds.

It is often desirable to place a lumbar paravertebral block such that the lumbar and the sacral plexus are involved, as in hip arthroplasty surgery and acetabular fracture internal reduction and internal fixation surgery. The spinous process of the 5th lumbar vertebra is identified and used. The transverse processes of the lumbar vertebrae are usually directly lateral to the midpoint of the particular spinous processes of the same vertebrae. This is different in the thoracic region (see Chapter 19), where the spinous process of a particular vertebra overlies the body of the subsequent vertebra because of the acute downward angulation of the spinous processes in the thoracic region.

SONOANATOMY

Although we describe the sonoanatomy of the lumbar plexus in this section, its value in a lumbar plexus block has not yet been fully described or appreciated. The basic principles of ultrasound technique apply [18], and in some patients, the clinical situation and the patient's body habitus dictate that the correct lumbar spinal level be identified. Ultrasound is invaluable for this purpose.

To obtain the images in this section, we placed the model in the lateral position and used a 2 - 5 MHz curvilinear ultrasound transducer probe with a 60 mm footprint (C-60, SonoSite Fujifilm, Bothell, WA, USA).

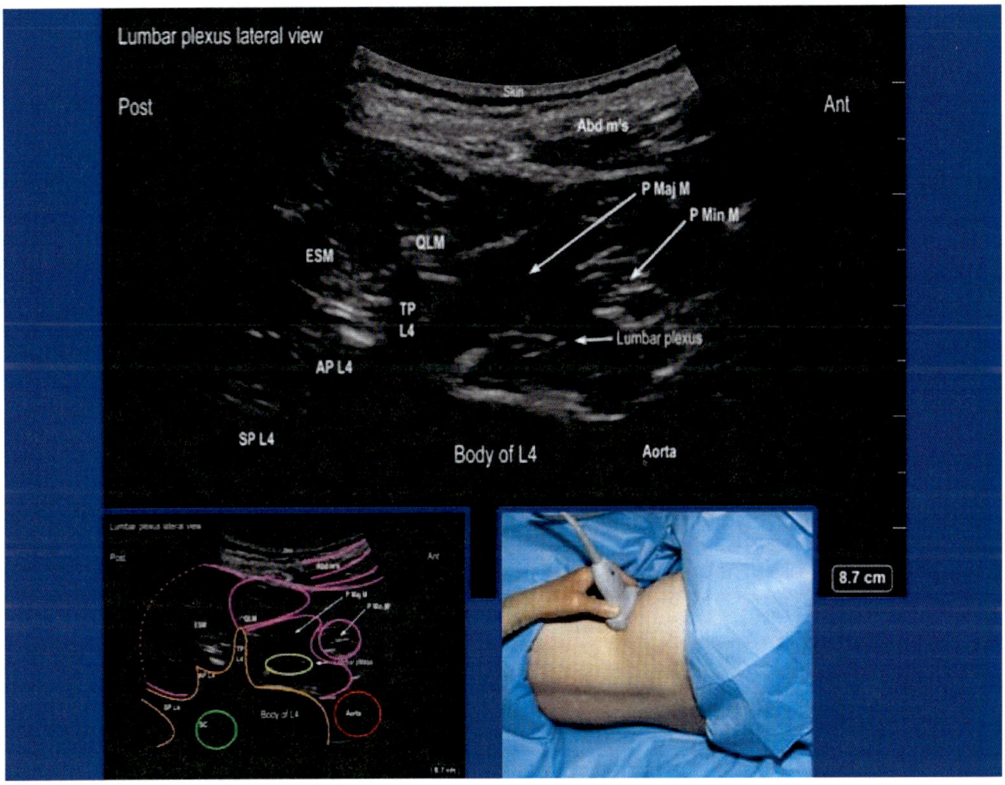

Figure 9: Sonoanatomy of the lumbar plexus as viewed laterally with the ultrasound probe in an axial plane.
Post = posterior; Ant = anterior; Abd m's = abdominal muscles; ESM = erector spinae muscle; QLM = quadratus lumborum muscle; P Maj M = psoas major muscle; P Min M = psoas minor muscle; TP L4 = transverse process of the 4th lumbar vertebra; AP L4 = articular process of the 4th lumbar vertebra; SP L4 = spinous process of the 4th lumbar vertebra; Body of L4 = body of the 4th lumbar vertebra; 8.7 cm = distance in centimeters from the skin or ultrasound probe.

We now slide the ultrasound transducer probe to a more posterolateral position to obtain the next image (Fig. **9**).

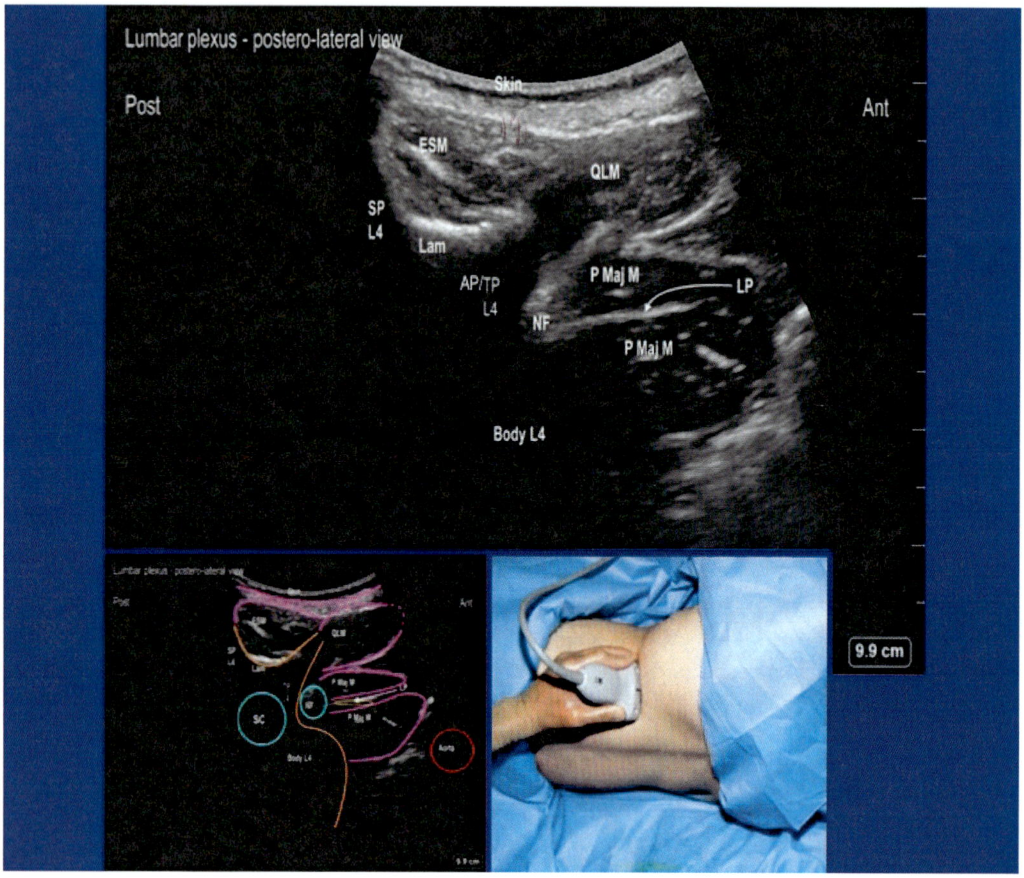

Figure 10: Sonoanatomy of the lumbar plexus from a posterolateral view with the ultrasound probe in an axial plane.
Post = posterior; Ant = anterior; ESM = erector spinae muscle; QLM = quadratus lumborum muscle; SP L4 = spinous process of the 4th lumbar vertebra; Lam = lamina of the 4th lumbar vertebra; AP/TP L4 = transverse process to articular process transition area of the 4th lumbar vertebra; NF = neuroforamen; P Maj M = psoas major muscle; LP = lumbar plexus; Body L4 = body of the 4th lumbar vertebra; 9.9 cm = the distance in centimeters from the skin to the ultrasound transducer probe.

Note the position of the lumbar plexus inside the body of the psoas major muscle.

To prepare the next image (Fig. **10**), the model remained in the lateral position and we placed the ultrasound transducer probe in the sagittal plane a few centimeters (3 - 4 cm) lateral to the spinous processes of the lumbar vertebrae.

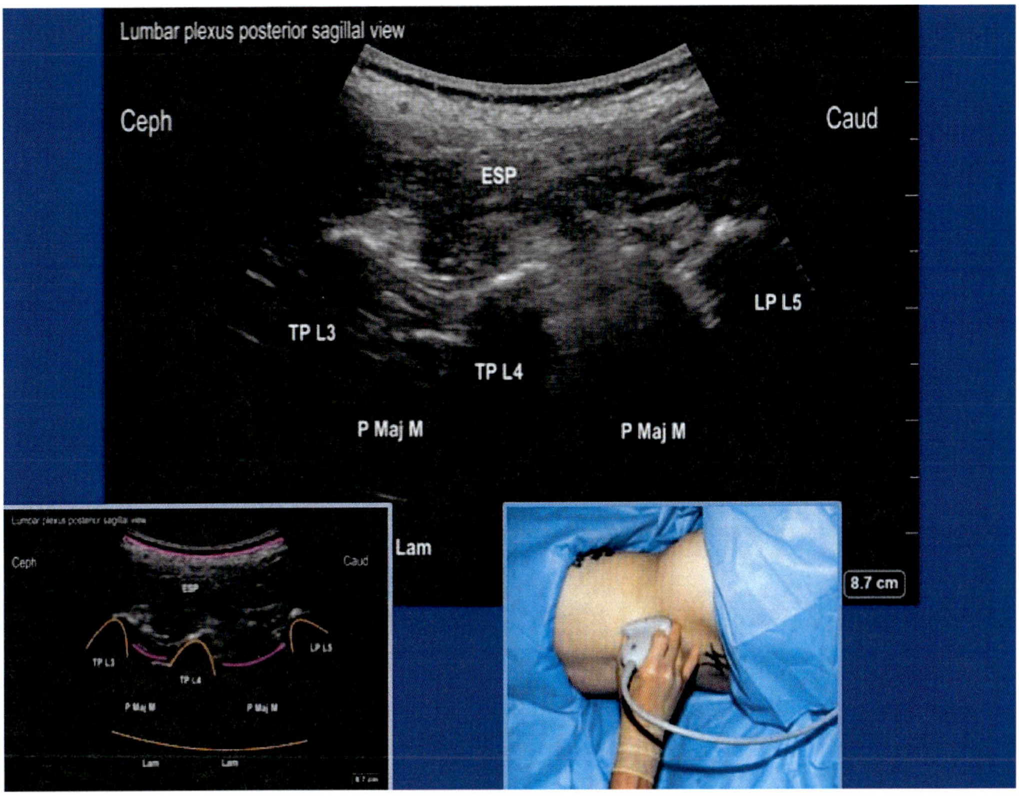

Figure 11: Sonoanatomy of the lumbar plexus viewed from a posterior position with the ultrasound probe in the paramedian sagittal plane.
Ceph = cephalad; ESP erector spinae muscle; TP L3 = transverse process of the 3rd lumbar vertebra; TP L4 = transverse process of the 4th lumbar vertebra; TP L5 = transverse process of the 5th lumbar vertebra; P Maj M = psoas major muscle; Lam = lamina of the 3rd lumbar vertebra; 8.7 cm = distance in centimeters from the skin or ultrasound probe.

FUNCTIONAL ANATOMY

Electrical stimulation of the lumbar plexus will result in an unmistakable motor response in the ipsilateral quadriceps muscle similar to femoral nerve stimulation (see Movie 20-1). Stimulation of the obturator nerve would cause twitching of the adductor muscles of the thigh. Because the obturator nerve is more anterior than the lumbar plexus, it is rare to encounter this. If the stimulating needle enters on the level of the 5th lumbar vertebra, we usually encounter the lumbosacral trunk and electrical nerve stimulation of this causes unmistakable ipsilateral quadriceps and hamstring muscle contractions. On rare occasions motor responses from the thigh adduction muscles (obturator nerve), lower abdominal muscles (ilioinguinal nerve), psoas muscle and cremaster muscles may be encountered.

ACKNOWLEDGEMENTS

The authors gratefully acknowledge the following people:

- The Head of the Department of Anesthesiology of the College of Medicine of the University of Florida, Dr. Tim Morey, and his department for their moral support and continuous encouragement.
- The faculty and fellows of the Division of Acute and Perioperative Pain Medicine of the above Department of Anesthesiology for affording the authors the time to produce this work by covering their clinical duties.
- Dr. Anastacia Munro for her help with the preparation of the chapter and ultrasound images.
- Corey Astrom of the Department of Anesthesiology of the College of Medicine of the University of Florida for her professional and high quality text editing.
- Nancy Hagen of the Iowa Public Radio for her narration of the movies.
- Raeducation.com LLC for their financial support.

CONFLICT OF INTEREST

The authors confirm that this chapter contents have no conflict of Interest.

ABBREVIATIONS

Abd m's	=	abdominal muscles
Ant	=	anterior
AP L4	=	articular process of the 4th lumbar vertebra
AP/TP L4	=	transverse process to articular process transition area of the 4th lumbar vertebra
Body L4	=	body of the 4th lumbar vertebra

Ceph	=	cephalad
CSF	=	cerebrospinal fluid
EIA	=	external iliac artery
ESM	=	erector spinae muscle
ESP	=	erector spinae muscle
GFN	=	genitofemoral nerve
IHN	=	iliohypogastric nerve
IIN	=	ilioinguinal nerve
L4	=	4th lumbar vertebra
Lam	=	lamina of the 3rd lumbar vertebra
Lam	=	lamina of the 4th lumbar vertebra
LP	=	lumbar plexus
NF	=	neuroforamen
ON	=	obturator nerve
P Maj M	=	psoas major muscle
P min M	=	psoas minor muscl
Post	=	posterior
PSIS	=	posterior superior iliac spine
QLM	=	quadratus lumborum muscle
SP	=	sacral plexus
SP L4	=	spinous process of the 4th lumbar vertebra

TP L3 = transverse process of the 3rd lumbar vertebra

TP L4 = transverse process of the 4th lumbar vertebra

TP L5 = transverse process of the 5th lumbar vertebra

Ur = urete

REFERENCES

[1] Winnie AP, Ramamurthy S, Durrani Z, *et al.* Plexus blocks for lower extremity surgery: New answers to old problems. Anesth Rev 1974; 1:1-6.

[2] Capdevila X, Macaire P, Dadure C, *et al.* Continuous psoas compartment block for postoperative analgesia after total hip arthroplasty: New landmarks, technical guidelines, and clinical evaluation. Anesth Analg 2002: 94:1606-1613.

[3] Hanna MH, Peat SJ, D'Costa F. Lumbar plexus block: an anatomical study. Anaesthesia 1993; 48:675-678.

[4] Farny J, Drolet P, Girard M. Anatomy of the posterior approach to the lumbar plexus block. Can J Anaesth 1994; 41:480-485.

[5] Kirchmair L, Entner T, Wissel J, *et al.* A study of the anatomy for ultrasound-guided posterior lumbar plexus block. Anesth Analg 2001; 93:477-481.

[6] Gentili M, Aveline C, Bonnet F. Total spinal anesthesia after posterior lumbar plexus block. Ann Fr Anesth Reanim 1998; 17:740-742.

[7] Houten J. Paraplegia after lumbosacral nerve root block, report of three cases. The Spine J 2002; 2:70-75.

[8] Pousman RM, Mansoor Z, Sciard D. Total spinal after continuous posterior lumbar plexus block. Anesthesiology 2003; 98:1281-1282.

[9] Boezaart AP, Lucas SD, Elliott CE. Paravertebral block: cervical, thoracic, lumbar and sacral. Curr Opin Anaesthesiol 2009; 22: 637-643.

[10] Reina MA, Pulido P, De Sola RG. Ultrastructure of the spinal arachnoid layer. In: Reina MA, ed. Atlas of functional anatomy for regional anesthesia and pain medicine. New York: Springer Science and Business Media 2015; pp. 435-453.

[11] Boezaart AP, Kadieva VS. Inadvertent extra-arachnoid [subdural] injection of a local anaesthetic agent during epidural anaesthesia. S Afr Med J 1992; 81:325-326.

[12] Nabors M, Pait TG, Byrd EB. Updated assessment and current classification of spinal meningeal cysts. J Neurosurg 1988; 68:366-377.

[13] Holt S, Yates PO. Cervical nerve root "cysts". Brain 1964; 87:481-490.

[14] Selander D, Sjöstrand J. Longitudinal spread of intraneurally injected local anesthetics. Acta Anaesth Scand 1978: 22:622-634.

[15] Moore DC, Hain RF Ward A, Bridenbaugh LD. Importance of the perineural spaces in nerve blocking. JAMA 1954; 156:1050-1055.

[16] Hernández JM, Reina MA, De Andrés JA. Nerve root and type of needle used in transforaminal injection. In: Reina MA, Ed. Atlas of functional anatomy for regional anesthesia and pain medicine. New York, Springer Science and Business Media 2015; pp. 813-826.

[17] Reina MA, Navarro RA, Matos EMD. Ultrastructure of myelenated and unmyelinated axons. In: Reina MA, ed. Atlas of functional anatomy for regional anesthesia and pain medicine. New York: Springer Science and Business Media 2015; pp. 3-18.

[18] Ihnatsenka BV, Boezaart AP. Ultrasound: Basic understanding and learning the language. Int J Shoulder Surg 2010; 4:55-62.

CHAPTER 21

Applied Macro-, Micro-, and Sonoanatomy of the Neuraxium

André P. Boezaart[1,*] and Barys V. Ihnatsenka[2]

[1]Departments of Anesthesiology and Orthopaedic Surgery and Rehabilitation, Division of Acute and Perioperative Pain Medicine, University of Florida College of Medicine, Gainesville, Florida, USA and [2]Department of Anesthesiology, Division of Acute and Perioperative Pain Medicine, University of Florida College of Medicine, Gainesville, Florida, USA

Abstract: The spinal column has 33 vertebrae: seven cervical, twelve thoracic, five lumbar, five sacral (fused), and four coccygeal. There are four curves in the spinal column: the cervical and lumbar curve convex anteriorly, whereas the thoracic and sacral curves convex posteriorly. The macro-, microanatomy, and sonoanatomy (static) of neuraxium, its content and relationships to other structures are discussed in this chapter. Special attention is given to the ligaments of the spine, and the ligamentum flavum in particular, paying special attention to the shapes that the spinal canal takes in certain regions, and the structure and consistency of the ligamentum flavum. Two further questions are specifically addressed in detail in this chapter. The first questions are why an epidural block is "segmental" and does not, like subarachnoid anesthesia, block the entire spinal cord distal to the site of injection. The second question answered in this chapter is why elderly people are less prone than their younger counterparts to developing postdural puncture headache following accidental dural puncture during attempted epidural block. Both of these questions are comprehensively addressed in this chapter on microanatomical grounds.

Keywords: Acute pain medicine, Arachnoid mater, Arachnoid villi, Arachnoid villus, Coccygeal, Dura mater, Dural puncture, Epidural anesthesia, Epidural block, Ligamentum flavum, Lumbar, Meninges, Neuraxium, Pia mater, Postdural puncture headache, Regional anesthesia, Sacral, Segmental, Spinal column, Spinal cord, Spinal ligaments, Spinal roots, Subarachnoid anesthesia, Thoracic, Vertebrae Cervical.

MACROANATOMY

The spinal column has 33 vertebrae: seven cervical, twelve thoracic, five lumbar, five sacral (fused), and four coccygeal. There are four curves in the spinal

***Corresponding author André P. Boezaart:** Departments of Anesthesiology and Orthopaedic Surgery, Division of Acute and Peri-operative Pain Medicine, University of Florida College of Medicine, 1600 SW Archer Road, Gainesville, Florida 32610, USA; Tel: 352-846-0913 (Work); Tel: 352-213-3272 (Mobile); Fax: 352-392-7029; E-mail: aboezaart@anest.ufl.edu

column: the cervical and lumbar curve convex anteriorly, whereas the thoracic and sacral curves convex posteriorly [1].

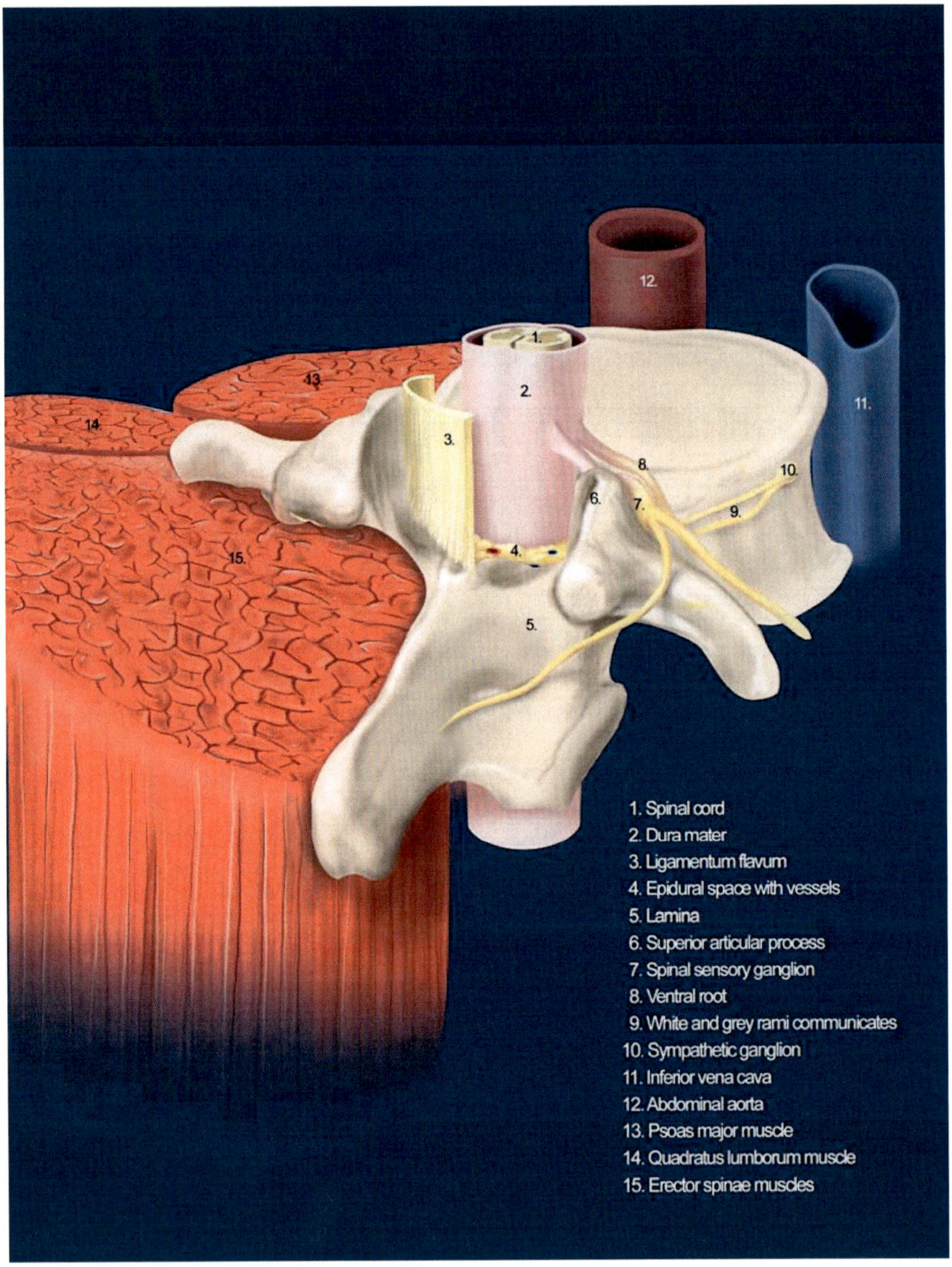

Figure 1: Schematic representation of the epidural space.

All vertebrae have a similar structure consisting of a vertebral body anterior and an arch of bone posteriorly that surrounds the spinal canal. This arch comprises two pedicles that accommodate the articular processes of the facet joints anteriorly and two laminae posteriorly. The transverse processes are situated at the junction of the pedicles and the laminae meet at the spinous process of each vertebra. The caudal angulations of these spinous processes vary. Except for the thoracic region where they are steeply angulated caudally, they are almost horizontal in the cervical and lumbar regions. The spinous processes are rudimentary in the sacral area.

Four important ligaments support the spine [1, 2]. These are the supraspinous, interspinous, and longitudinal ligaments, and the ligamentum flavum.

The supraspinous ligament is a strong structure that connects the apices of the spinous processes. It is present from the sacrum to 7th cervical vertebra (C7). From here it continues cephalad to the external occipital protuberance as the ligamentum nuchae. The thickness of this ligament varies, but it is thickest and broadest in the lumbar region. It tends to keep the spinous processes of the vertebrae in the midline and, in case of spinal scoliosis, causes the vertebrae to rotate as their bodies curve laterally. This is an important consideration when performing neuraxial procedures on patients with scoliosis.

The interspinous ligament is a thin membranous structure that connects the adjacent spinous processes. Because it is so thin, when performing a midline approach to an epidural block, one can experience a distinct but false loss of resistance to air when moving slightly out of the midline and thus out of this ligament. Posteriorly, it blends with the supraspinous ligaments and anteriorly with the ligamentum flavum. Similar to the supraspinous ligament, it is also thickest in the lumbar region, which perhaps is one possible explanation why midline lumbar epidural approaches are more successful than midline thoracic epidural approaches for novices where false positive loss of resistance to air or saline is common.

The longitudinal ligaments bind the vertebral bodies together anteriorly and posteriorly to the bodies of the vertebrae; the posterior one inside the spinal canal, whereas the ligamentum flavum (LF) fibers connect the adjacent laminae at the anterior aspect of the spinal canal. It gets its name from the fact that it consists of yellow elastic fibers. Laterally, the ligament begins at the root of the articular process and extends medially and posteriorly to the junction of the lamina and the spinous process. The LF consist of two disk-shaped halves and these two components fuse loosely in the midline thus covering the entire interlaminar space, but this fusion is incomplete in most instances, which renders the LF thin or absent in the midline and therefore relatively easy to penetrate or relatively difficult to "feel" with a needle in the midline. Just lateral from the midline, it is thick and dense and it gets thinner again further lateral (Figs. **2** and **3**).

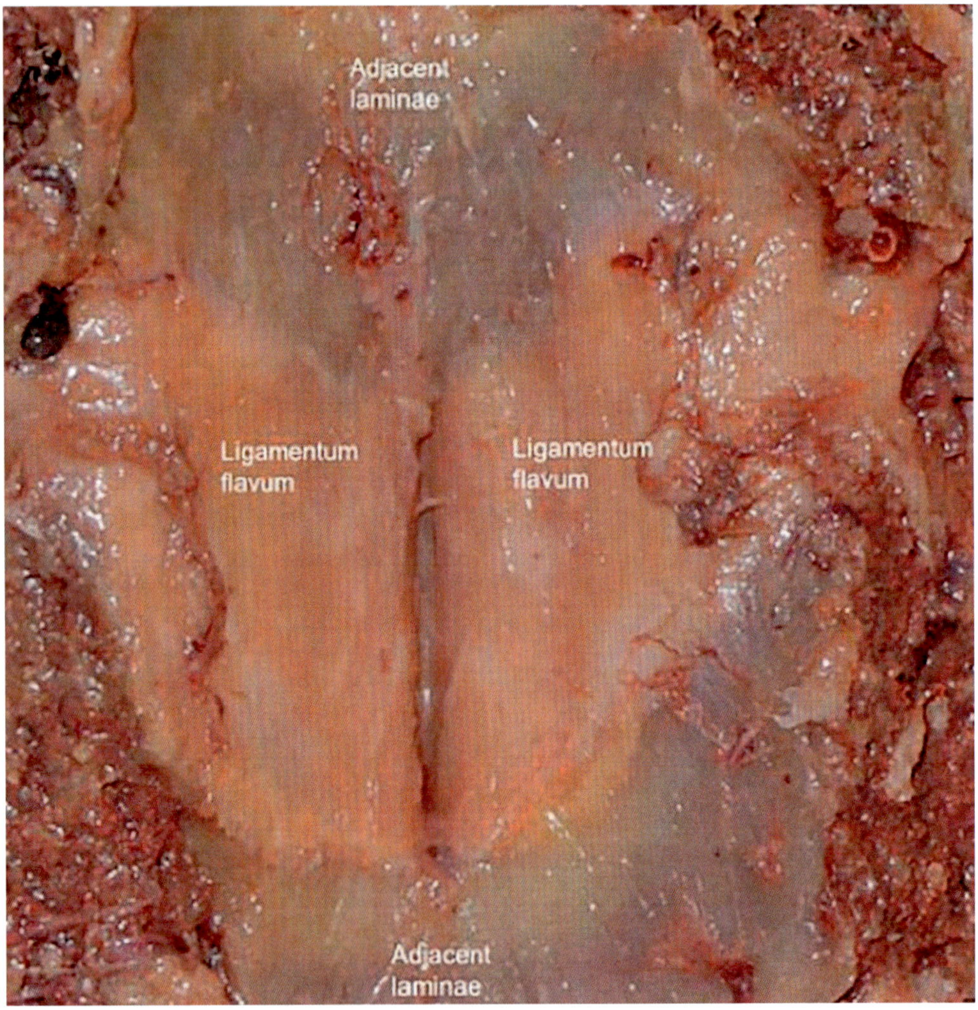

Figure 2: The ligamentum flavum as viewed from anterior.
It consists of a pair of disk-shaped halves that span two adjacent laminae. They loosely meet in the midline, often leaving a gap between the two dense and thick lateral parts (Reprinted from Reina with permission [3]).

In the lumbar region, the angle formed by the two disks of the LF is acute, as can be seen in Figs. **3** and **5**. This leaves a relatively large triangular posterior epidural space, which is filled with adipose tissue and loose connective tissue and more laterally contains the epidural venous plexus (as does the rest of the epidural space [4]).

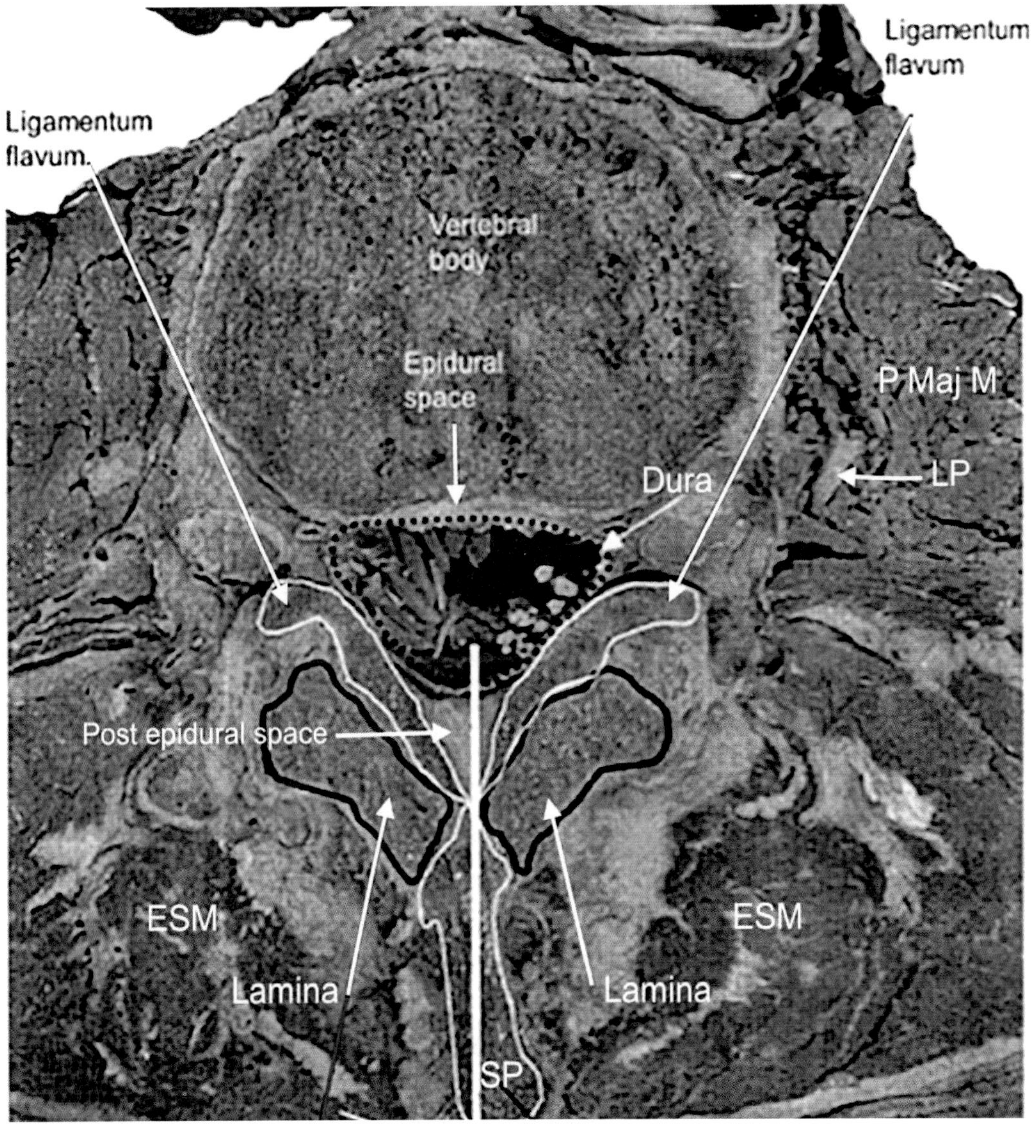

Figure 3a: Transection through the 4th lumbar vertebra to illustrate the ligamentum flavum and its relationships with the epidural space, dura mater, and the laminae of the vertebra.
In this case there is a subtle midline gap. ESM = erector spinae muscle; P Maj M = psoas major muscle; LP = lumbar plexus; Lamina = lamina of the 4th thoracic vertebra. (Reprinted from Reina with permission [5]).

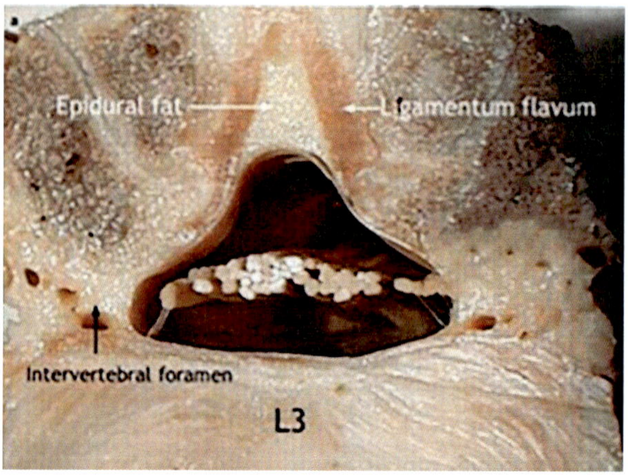

Figure 3b: Transverse section of the spinal canal at the level of L3 showing ligamentum flavum (Reprinted from Reina with permission [5]).

On rare occasions, there are congenital septae in the posterior epidural space, which may be responsible for a unilateral epidural [6]. In advanced age, the LF can also calcify and form bone [7], which can make penetration with a needle difficult.

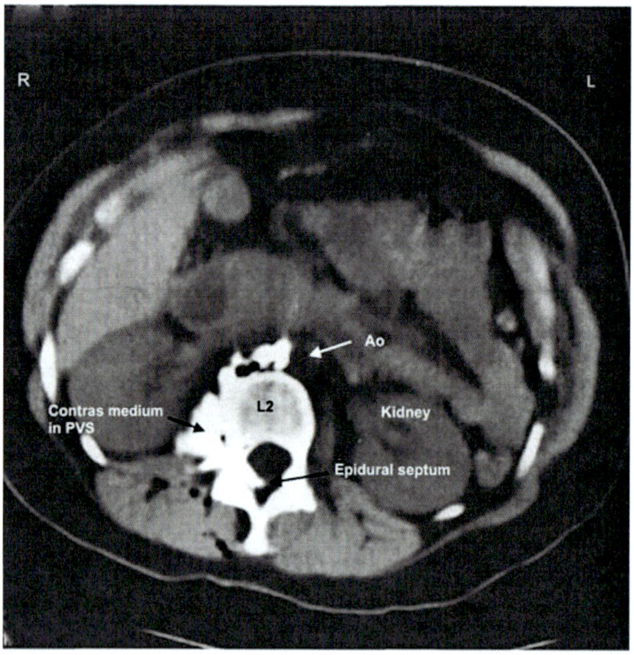

Figure 4: Computerized axial temo-epidurographic (CAT scan) documentation following unilateral epidural due to congenital epidural septum.
R = right; L = left; PVS = paravertebral space; Ao = abdominal aorta; L2 = body of 2nd lumbar vertebra.

Note the position of the kidneys and the contrast medium spreading laterally and anteriorly in the paravertebral space and around the body of the vertebra. Also note the clear epidural septum impeding contralateral spread of contrast medium.

The shape of the spinal canal differs in the different regions of the spine [8].

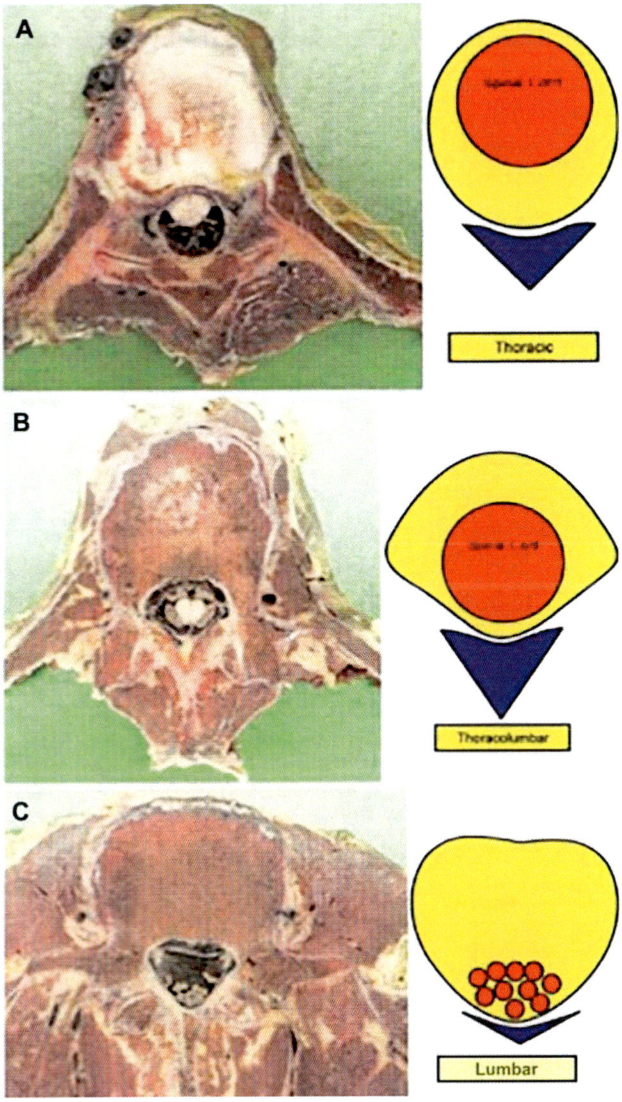

Figure 5: Anatomic axial sections at the (A) mid-thoracic region, (B) thoracolumbar region, and (C) lower lumbar regions, showing the respective relationships in the spinal canal.
Blue = epidural space; yellow = subarachnoid space; red = spinal cord or cauda equina. The triangular blue epidural space is posterior. (Reprinted from Reina [8] with permission).

Note that the distances between the posterior aspects of the spinal cord and the posterior dura mater differ substantially at the different regions.

SURFACE ANATOMY

The spinous processes can be palpated in the midline as bony prominences running from the base of the skull to the gluteal cleft. A line joining the iliac crests approximates the position of the L4 spinous process. Similarly, a line joining the inferior poles of the scapula would indicate the level of T7 spine, whereas L2 approximates a line joining the lateral ends of the 12th rib. The most prominent bony point in the midline at the base of the neck is the spinous process of C7 (vertebra prominens) [1].

MICROANATOMY

To answer the questions "***Why are epidural blocks segmental?***" and do not block the entire spinal cord as does a subarachnoid (spinal) block, and "***Why is postdural puncture headache more prevalent in younger patients,***" we need to examine the microanatomy of the meninges [9]. We also have to briefly look at Fick's First Law of Diffusion (10), derived by Adolf Fick in 1855.

Diffusion over membranes and fascia barriers follows Fick's Law [10], simplified as $dQ/dt = P \times \Delta C$, where dQ/dt is the rate of diffusion (flux), P is the permeability constant of the drug and membrane conductance, and ΔC is the concentration gradient over the membrane. This is simplified, but the membrane conductance (P) will obviously change as the thickness and permeability of the membrane changes and the permeability constant of the drug changes (see also http://en.wikipedia.org/wiki/Fick's_laws_of_diffusion). Fick's Second Law of Diffusion is actually more applicable, as it deals with changing concentrations and volumes of regional anesthetic agents where the drug is constantly removed by the bloodstream. For the purposes of this chapter, it should be sufficient to understand that the diffusion of local anesthetic agents depends on the permeability of the drug (lipid solubility), the thickness and permeability of the membrane (dura and arachnoid in this case), and the difference of concentration of the drug on both sides of the membrane.

The article by Shantha and Evans (9), although relatively old, is a milestone paper and the reader is strongly encouraged to study this article in its entirety. The factual information of this article has not been disputed since its publication and it is largely beyond debate. The article explains why epidural blocks are segmental and why postdural puncture headache is more prevalent in younger patients than in older ones. These principles are summarized, together with Fig. (**6**), as follows:

1. To block the sodium channels of the nerve axons, the local anesthetic must diffuse to the axons.

2. Structurally, the dura is composed of thick collagen bundles mixed with elastic fibers and fibroblasts that run obliquely and longitudinally. It contains an abundant amount of polysaccharides. The thickness of the dura is greatest cephalad and is thinner in a caudad direction. The root dura is also thin compared to the spinal dura and becomes progressively much thinner toward the intervertebral foramen and continues as epi- and perineural connective tissue of peripheral nerves.

3. The spinal dura is relatively impermeable to local anesthetics. Studies have shown only very little radioactive lidocaine in the spinal dura itself [9].

4. The arachnoid mater is a membrane that covers the brain, the spinal cord, and the dorsal and ventral nerve roots and is situated between the dura and the pia maters. It consists of several layers of flat squamous cells laid one on top of the other with potential spaces (interarachnoid spaces) between the layers and a delicate network of collagen, elastic fibers, and blood vessels within.

5. The arachnoid covering the spinal roots has an important and remarkable histological feature. Proliferations of arachnoid cells lining villus structures have been consistently demonstrated in dogs, humans, primates, and rats. In humans and primates, arachnoid proliferations and villi have been demonstrated along both dorsal and ventral roots (Fig. **6**). These proliferations have been found in greater number and more extensively with advancing age see chapters 19 and 20), as observed in the sagittal sinus. Various types of arachnoid proliferations or villi have been described, and similar villus structures are in the optic nerve. There is no anatomic difference between the arachnoid villus structures of the spinal root, the sagittal sinus, or the optic nerve.

6. The endothelial lining of the arachnoid villi is a mosaic of lipid and pores, the latter occupying a larger part of the surface than in the blood-cerebrospinal fluid (CSF) barrier. Lipid-soluble substances can penetrate both lipids and pores, whereas water-soluble substances can escape and pass through the pores.

7. Between the dura and arachnoid maters is a potential space known as the subdural space.

8. There are five types of arachnoid villi: Types I through V (Fig. **6**). Type I protrudes into the subdural space; Type II partially protrudes the dura and reduces the thickness of the dura; Type III completely breaches the dura but does not protrude beyond it; Type IV protrudes out of the dura and lies in the epidural space, and Type V protrudes beyond the dura in proximity to epidural veins and partially protrudes into them. Types I, II, and II are found frequently, especially in young people, whereas Types IV and V are less frequently found, but are more prevalent in the older population group.

9. In young patients, epidural injections extend through the neural foramina around the spinal nerve roots, which explains the segmental nature of epidural anesthesia. The drug is effective if deposited in the subarachnoid space because the pia mater offers almost no resistance to diffusion. If the drug diffused through the spinal dura, the effect of the local anesthetic would occur on the spinal cord, similar to a subarachnoid block – non-segmental and blocking everything distal to the injection site.

10. In the older arteriosclerotic patient, however, there is lack of paravertebral spread, but because of the increase in number and size of arachnoid villi and the further penetration of the villi into the root dura, a decrease in the thickness of the root dura occurs, increasing the area of permeability and penetration into the spinal root.

11. Lack of paravertebral escape with the increased permeability area in the aged is most likely responsible for the faster onset and higher dermatomal levels of analgesia, even with smaller doses of local anesthetic. With little to no leakage into the paravertebral space through the intervertebral foramen, the result is a sharper rise in pressure and concentration in the epidural space, which facilitates increased penetration of the local anesthetic agent into the root subarachnoid space.

12. The phenomenon of *decreased* leakage of CSF into the paravertebral space is the most likely reason why the development of headache after lumbar puncture in the elderly compared to the younger is rare. In the aged, the leakage of CSF, thought to be at least partially responsible for postdural puncture headache, continues to leak into the epidural space but

cannot escape into the paravertebral space. This builds up enough pressure to cause partial or complete blockage of further CSF leakage. In young patients, CSF continues to escape from the subarachnoid space, to the epidural space, and to the paravertebral spaces. The result is low subarachnoid CSF pressure and its sequelae (spinal headache), dramatically relieved by pressure-equalizing measures such as epidural blood patch.

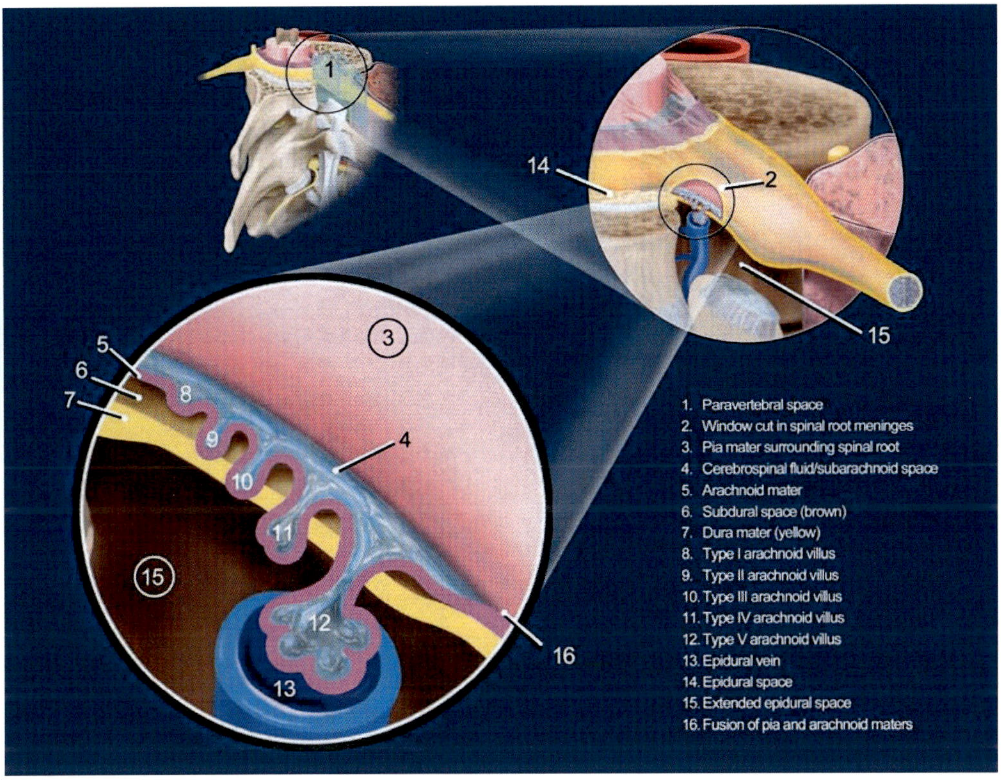

Figure 6: Arachnoid villi.

Type I: Simple arachnoid proliferations, consisting of several layers of arachnoid epithelial cells, are found along the root arachnoid. They are consistently found where the pia and arachnoid come together to obliterate the subarachnoid space. These proliferations come in many shapes and sizes and may protrude into adjacent subdural spaces.

Type II: Arachnoid villi partially protruding into the dural sheath without breaching the dural continuity, at the same time reducing the thickness of the dura at the site.

Type III: Villi that completely breach the dura but do not protrude beyond it.

Type IV: Villi protruding out of the dura lying in the epidural space.

Type V: Villi protruding beyond the dura in proximity to epidural veins and partially protruding into the veins, as commonly observed in the sagittal sinus.

(Types I through III are commonly found, especially in the young, whereas Types IV and V are less frequent, but their numbers increase with advancing age. See also Chapters 19 and 20).

SONOANATOMY

Although we describe the sonoanatomy of the neuraxium in this section, its value in an epidural block has not yet been fully described or appreciated. The basic principles of ultrasound technique apply [11], and in some patients, the clinical situation and the patient's body habitus dictates that we identify the correct lumbar spinal level. Ultrasound may be invaluable to find the midline if the patient is in the lateral position; to assess rotation of the vertebra if the patient has scoliosis and to measure the distance of the ligamentum flavum or laminae from the skin.

To obtain the images in this section we used a 6- to 13-MHz linear probe with a 38-cm footprint (HFL – 38, SonoSite Fujifilm, Bothell, WA, USA) for the thoracic region and a 2 to 5 MHz curvilinear ultrasound transducer probe with a 60 mm footprint (C-60, SonoSite Fujifilm, Bothell, WA, USA) for the lumbar region. The model was first placed in the prone position to prepare the images for the thoracic vertebrae (Figs. **7** and **8**).

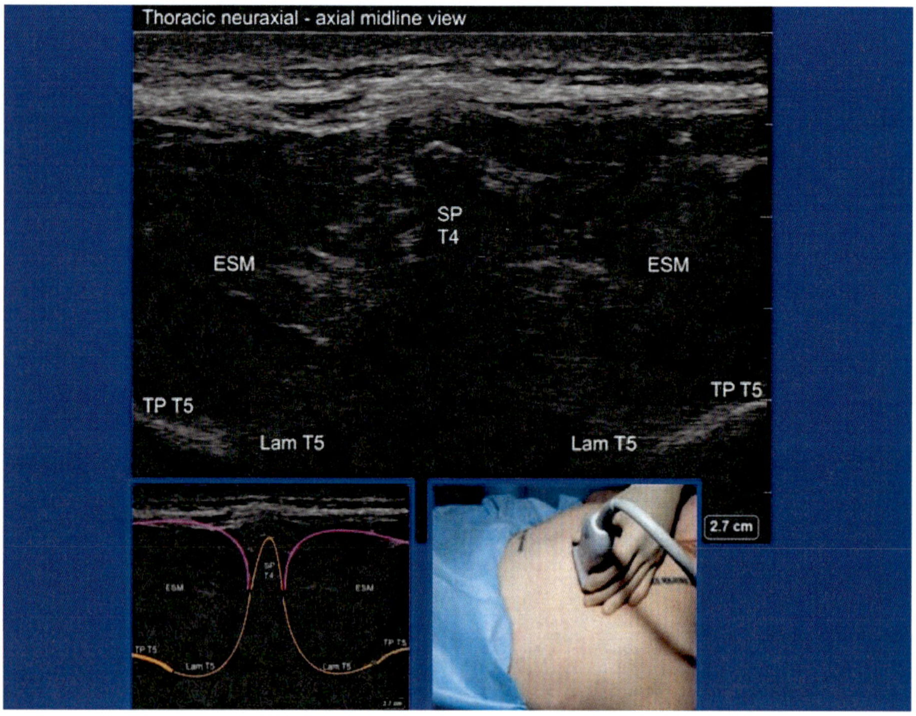

Figure 7: Sonoanatomy of the 5th thoracic vertebra as seen in the axial view. The left side of the image is the left side of the model.
ESM = erector spinae muscle; SP T4 = spinous process of the 4th thoracic vertebra; TP L5 = transverse process of the 5th thoracic vertebra; Lam L5 = lamina of the 5th thoracic vertebra.

Note that the spinous process of the 4th thoracic vertebra lies over parts of the vertebra of 5th thoracic vertebra. In the lumbar region, the spinous process would overlie the corresponding vertebra (L4 spinous process would lie over the L4 body and parts).

We turned the ultrasound transducer probe to the sagittal plane and moved it slightly off the midline with some medial tilt of the probe for the next image (Fig. **8**).

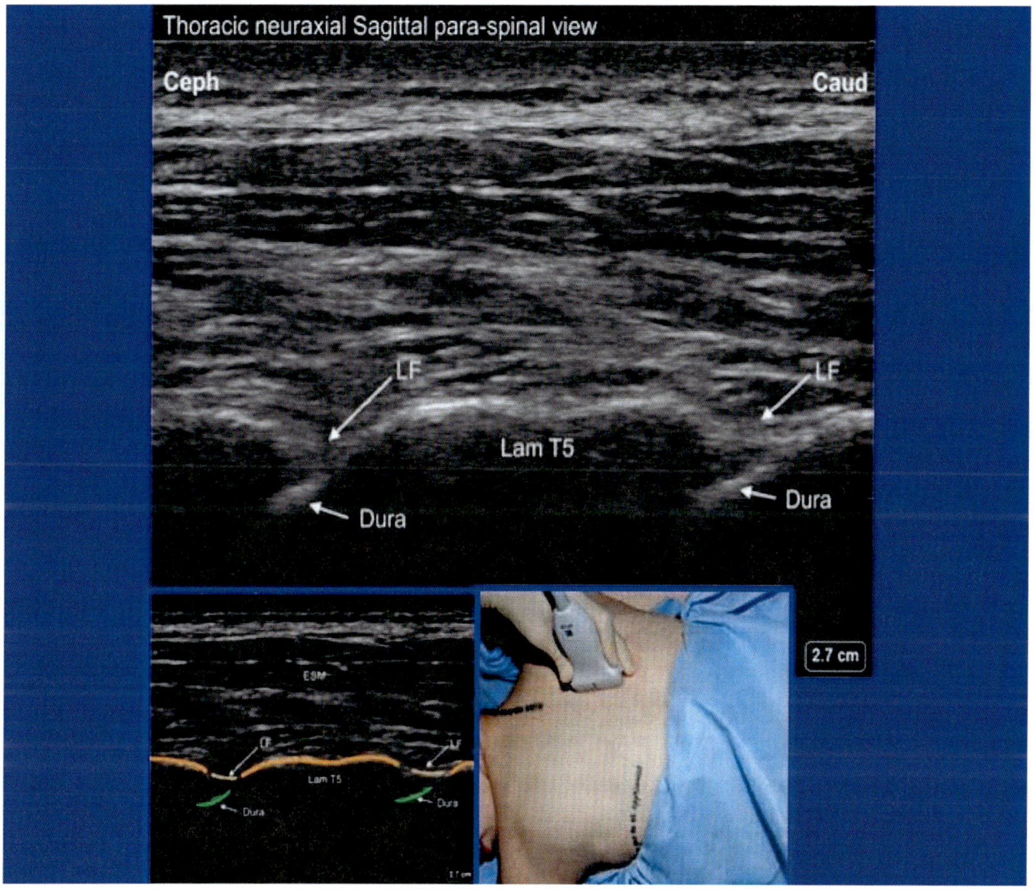

Figure 8: Sonoanatomy of the 5th thoracic vertebra as seen in the paramedian sagittal plane. *Ceph = cephalad; Caud = caudad; Lam T5 = lamina of the 5th thoracic vertebra; LF = ligamentum flavum; dura = dura mater.*

To obtain the images in the lumbar region, we placed the patient in the lateral position and set the probe in the axial plane at the level of the 4th lumbar vertebra. The sitting position, however, is similarly satisfactory for both of these regions.

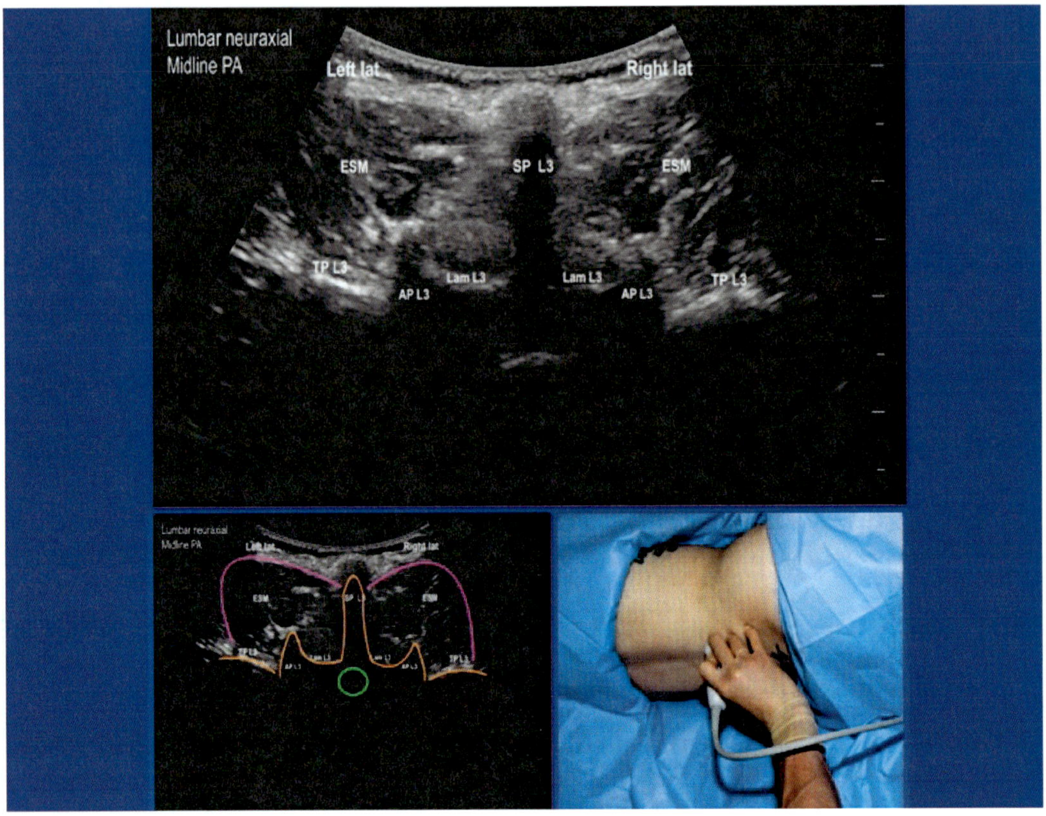

Figure 9: Sonoanatomy of the 4th lumbar vertebra as viewed in the axial plane.
Left lat = left lateral; Right lat = right lateral; ESM = erector spinae muscle; SP L3 = spinous process of the 3rd lumbar vertebra; TP L3 = transverse process of the 3rd lumbar vertebra; AP L3 = articular process of the 3rd lumbar vertebra; Lam L3 = lamina of the 3rd lumbar vertebra.

With the model still in the lateral position, the probe is turned into the sagittal plane and moved to a paramedian position with some medial tilt of the probe (Fig. **9**).

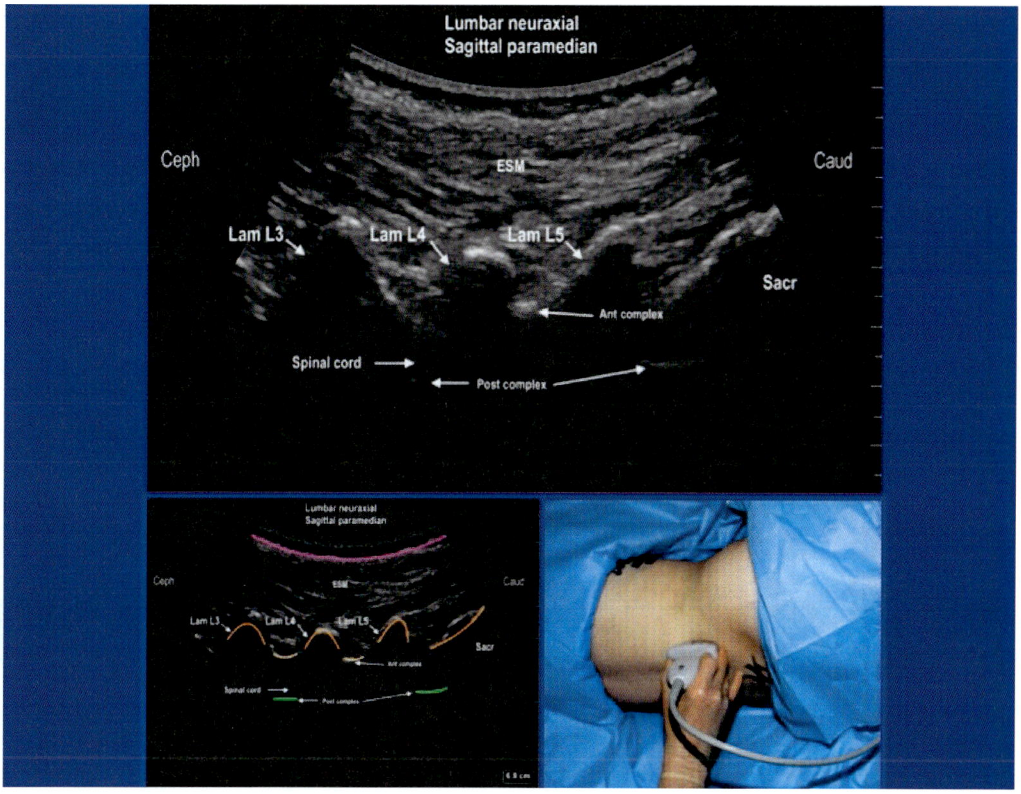

Figure 10: Sonoanatomy of the 3rd, 4th, and 5th lumbar vertebrae as viewed in the sagittal plane. *Ceph = cephalad; Caud = caudad; ESM = erector spinae muscle; Lam L3, L4, L5 = laminae of 3rd, 4th, and 5th lumbar vertebrae; Sac = sacrum.*

ACKNOWLEDGEMENTS

The author gratefully acknowledge the following people:

- The Head of the Department of Anesthesiology of the College of Medicine of the University of Florida, Dr. Tim Morey, and his department for their moral support and continuous encouragement.

- The faculty and fellows of the Division of Acute and Perioperative Pain Medicine of the above Department of Anesthesiology for affording the author the time to produce this work by covering his clinical duties.

- Drs. Anastacia Munro and Yury Zasimovich for their help with the preparation of the chapter and ultrasound images.

- Corey Astrom of the Department of Anesthesiology of the College of Medicine of the University of Florida for her professional and high quality text editing.

- Raeducation.com LLC for their financial support.

CONFLICT OF INTEREST

The authors confirm that this chapter contents have no conflict of Interest.

ABBREVIATIONS

Ao	=	abdominal aorta
AP L3	=	articular process of the 3rd lumbar vertebra
Caud	=	caudad
Ceph	=	cephalad
dura	=	dura mater
ESM	=	erector spinae muscle
L2	=	body of 2nd lumbar vertebra
Lam L3, L4, L5	=	laminae of 3rd, 4th, and 5th lumbar vertebrae
Lam T5	=	lamina of the 5th thoracic vertebra
Lamina	=	lamina of the 4th thoracic vertebra
Left lat	=	left lateral
LF	=	ligamentum flavum
LP	=	lumbar plexus
P Maj M	=	psoas major muscle
PVS	=	paravertebral space

Right lat	=	right lateral
Sac	=	sacrum.
SP L3	=	spinous process of the 3rd lumbar vertebra
SP T4	=	spinous process of the 4th thoracic vertebra
TP L3	=	transverse process of the 3rd lumbar vertebra
TP L5	=	transverse process of the 5th thoracic vertebra

REFERENCES

[1] Raff M. Continuous spinal and epidural anesthesia. In: Boezaart AP, Ed. Anesthesia and orthopaedic surgery. New York, McGraw-Hill, 2006; pp. 371–384.

[2] Masuda R Tanuma K. Subarachnoid (intrathecal) ligaments. In: Reina MA, Ed. Atlas of functional anatomy for regional anesthesia and pain medicine. New York, Springer, 2015; p. 652.

[3] Lirk P. The ligamentum flavum. In: Reina MA, Ed. Atlas of functional anatomy for regional anesthesia and pain medicine. New York, Springer, 2015; p. 640.

[4] Netter FH. The Ciba collection of medical illustrations, Volume 1: Nervous system. New York, NY: Ciba, 1967; p. 54.

[5] Lirk P. The ligamentum flavum. In: Reina MA, Ed. Atlas of functional anatomy for regional anesthesia and pain medicine. New York, Springer, 2015; p. 645.

[6] Boezaart AP. Computerized axial temo-epidurographic and radiologic documentation of unilateral epidural analgesia. Can J Anaesth 1989; 36: 697–700.

[7] Guo JJ, Luk KD, Karppinem J, Yang H, Cheung KM. Prevalence, distribution, and morphology of ossification of the ligamentum flavum: A population study 1736 magnetic resonance imaging scans. Spine 2010; 35:51–56.

[8] Lataster LMA, van Zundert AAJ. Anatomy of the thoracic spinal canal in different postures: An MRI investigation. In: Reina MA, Ed. Atlas of functional anatomy for regional anesthesia and pain medicine. New York, Springer 2015; p. 696.

[9] Shantha TR, Evans JA. The relationship of epidural anesthesia to neural membranes and arachnoid villi. Anesthesiology 1972: 37: 543-557.

[10] Mather LE, Tucker GT. Properties, absorption and disposition of local anesthetic agents. In: Cousins MJ, Horlocker TT, Car DB, Bridenbaugh PO, Eds. Neural Blockade in Clinical Anesthesia and Pain Medicine. Philadelphia: Wolter Kluwer/Lippencott Williams & Wilkins; 2009: p.53.

[11] Ihnatsenka BV, Boezaart AP. Ultrasound: Basic understanding and learning the language. Int J Shoulder Surg. 2010; 4:55–62.

Chapter 22:
The Applied Anatomy of the Abdominal and Pelvic Sympathetic Ganglia

CHAPTER 22

The Applied Anatomy of the Abdominal and Pelvic Sympathetic Ganglia

David A. Edwards[1] and André P. Boezaart[2,*]

[1]Vanderbilt University Medical Center, Department of Anesthesiology, Nashville, TN, USA; Assistant Professor, Vanderbilt University Medical Center, Department of Anesthesiology, Nashville Tennessee, South Africa and [2]Departments of Anesthesiology and Orthopaedic Surgery and Rehabilitation, Division of Acute and Perioperative Pain Medicine, University of Florida College of Medicine, Gainesville, Florida, USA

Abstract: The abdominal and pelvic sympathetic nervous system mediates visceral sensation and vasomotor tone to the abdominal organs and vessels, as well as sudomotor, vasomotor, and pilomotor function of the lower extremities. Pain sensation that is sympathetically maintained or mediated can be treated by a targeted block of the abdominal sympathetic ganglia or plexuses. A comprehensive understanding of the relevant physical anatomy and fluoroscopic or sonographic anatomy is a prerequisite for safely and effectively performing a sympathetic blockade.

Keywords: Abdominal aortic plexus, Cancer pain, Celiac ganglion, Celiac plexus, Chronic pain Ganglia, Ganglion impar Ganglion, Inferior hypogastric plexus, Intermesenteric plexus, Mesenteric plexus, Pancreas, Pelvis, Sacrum, Splanchnic nerves, Stomach, Superior hypogastric plexus, Sympathetic block, Sympathetic chain, Thoracolumbar spine.

MACROANATOMY FUNCTIONAL ANATOMY

The sympathetic innervation of the abdominopelvic organs (splanchnic) and the lower extremities arises from preganglionic neurons of the lateral horn of the 5th thoracic (T5) to the 2nd lumbar (L2) spinal cord levels. Preganglionic fibers exit the spinal cord with the somatic root and travel ventrally *via* white rami communicans to synapse within the paravertebral sympathetic ganglia. Postganglionic fibers exit the ganglia *via* gray rami communicans and branch along arteries to reach their target organs.

There are six major abdominal sympathetic plexuses: celiac, superior mesenteric, intermesenteric, inferior mesenteric, superior hypogastric, and inferior hypogastric

***Corresponding author André P. Boezaart:** Departments of Anesthesiology and Orthopaedic Surgery, Division of Acute and Peri-operative Pain Medicine, University of Florida College of Medicine, 1600 SW Archer Road, Gainesville, Florida 32610, USA; Tel: 352-846-0913 (Work); Fax: 352-392-7029;
E-mail: aboezaart@anest.ufl.edu

plexuses. These plexuses, along with the ganglion impar and sympathetic chain, constitute the most frequent targets for directed blockade for treatment of sympathetically maintained chronic pain conditions and abdominal and pelvic visceral pain conditions by pain physicians.

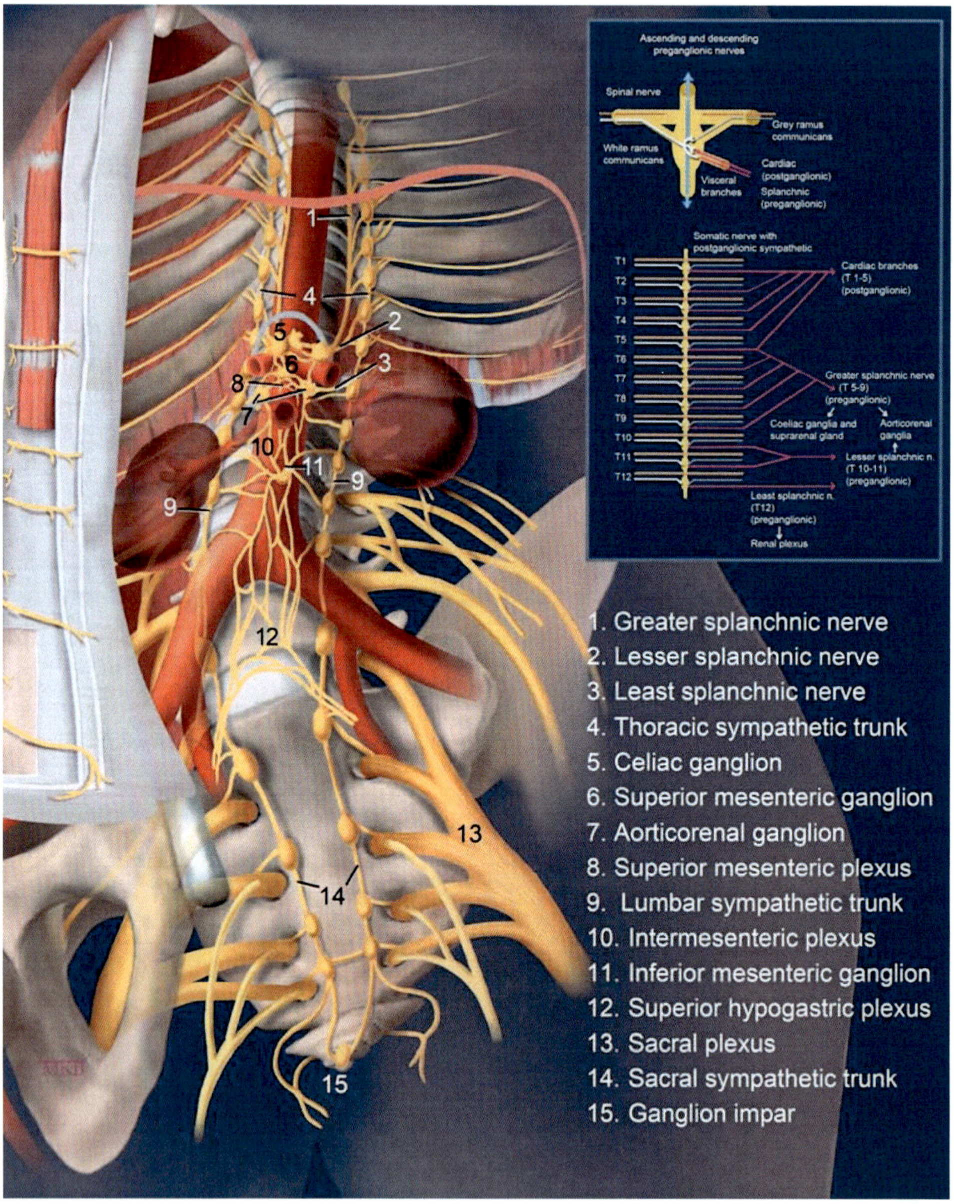

Figure 1: Antero-superior view of the abdominal and pelvic sympathetic chains, ganglia, and plexuses.

Celiac Plexus

The celiac ganglion consists of one to five ganglia situated anterior to the 12th thoracic (T12) or 1st lumbar (L1) vertebral bodies. The ganglia are situated anterior to the crura of the diaphragm bilaterally across the anterolateral surface of the aorta on the celiac trunk and are connected by the celiac plexus. The celiac plexus surrounds the celiac trunk and the superior mesenteric artery descends caudally to form the superior mesenteric ganglion and plexus and the left and right aorticorenal ganglia (Fig. **1**).

The celiac ganglion is formed by the coalescence of the preganglionic sympathetic fibers of the greater splanchnic nerve, which originate from the 5th (T5) to the 9th (T9) thoracic spinal nerves, the lesser splanchnic nerve originating from T10 to T11, and the least splanchnic nerve, originating from T12, that perforates the crura of the diaphragm carrying both efferent and afferent fibers. Postganglionic fibers exit the celiac ganglion to innervate the diaphragm, abdominal vessels, and abdominal visceral structures: the liver, biliary tract, pancreas, stomach, spleen, suprarenal glands, kidneys, ovaries, testes, small intestines, and colon to the splenic flexure. A celiac plexus block and neurolysis can be useful in the treatment of visceral organ cancer pain or chronic pancreatitis (Fig. **2**).

Superior, Inter-, and Inferior Mesenteric Plexuses

The mesenteric plexuses are caudal extensions of the celiac plexus fibers. They contain sympathetic fibers with inputs from the 1st and 2nd splanchnic nerves.

The **superior mesenteric ganglion and plexus** surround the superior mesenteric artery. The left and right aorticorenal ganglia sit laterally at the junction of the aorta and renal arteries. The caudal extension of the superior mesenteric plexus and the aorticorenal ganglia is the **intermesenteric plexus**, also called the **abdominal aortic plexus**. The **inferior mesenteric plexus** surrounds the inferior mesenteric artery and is the caudal extension of the intermesenteric plexus. It receives preganglionic inputs from the 2nd and 3rd lumbar splanchnic nerves (Fig. **1**).

Lumbar Sympathetic Chain

The lumbar sympathetic chain is a series of connected ganglia located antero-lateral to the 1st (L1) through the 4th (L4) lumbar vertebral bodies. Its axons exit the spinal cord through the ventral nerve roots and sympathetic fibers separate through the white rami communicans to form a chain of ganglia. Postganglionic fibers leave the ganglia *via* the gray rami communicans and regulate lower extremity vasomotor, sudomotor, and pilomotor tone. The largest portion of the lumbar sympathetic chain is situated along the 2nd and 3rd lumbar vertebral bodies, which is the reason a single-injection paravertebral sympathetic block at this level is usually sufficient for relieving sympathetic-mediated pain of the lower extremities (Fig. **3**).

Superior and Inferior Hypogastric Plexuses

The **superior hypogastric plexus** is a continuation of the inferior mesenteric plexus and it innervates the pelvic organs. It is retroperitoneal and lies caudad to the origin of the inferior mesenteric artery. It is situated anterior to the lower aorta, its bifurcation, and the sacral vessels, anterior to the 4th and 5th lumbar (L4 & L5) and 1st sacral (S1) vertebrae. The superior hypogastric plexus divides into left and right hypogastric nerves that travel on both sides lateral to the sigmoid colon and become the inferior hypogastric plexuses. It innervates the iliac vessels *via* the iliac plexuses and transmits pain sensation from the uterine cervix, proximal vagina, uterus, ovaries, testes, prostate distal colon, and rectum. It also contains sympathetic fibers from the pelvic splanchnic nerves on their way to innervate the left side of the transverse colon downward.

The **inferior hypogastric plexus** is a bilateral structure situated on both sides of the rectum, the lower portion of the bladder, the prostate, and seminal vessels in the male, or, the uterus, cervix, and vaginal fornices in the female. It is supplemented by preganglionic sympathetic fibers from the 1st and 2nd sacral splanchnic nerves. The inferior hypogastric plexus is responsible for vasomotor innervation and motor innervation to the vas deferens, seminal vesicles, prostate, and anal and bladder sphincters.

Ganglion Impar (or Ganglion of Walter)

The ganglion impar is the most inferior ganglion of the sympathetic nervous system and is a solitary midline structure situated anterior to the upper coccyx or lower sacrum and posterior to the rectum in the retrorectal space. It relays sympathetically maintained pain impulses that originate from the pelvic region. Blocking this ganglion with a local anesthetic agent by passing a needle through the anterior longitudinal ligament, also called the sacrococcygeal ligament, can be useful for the management of cancer-generated pain from the prostate, uterine cervix, rectum, and colon (Fig. **4**).

FLUOROSCOPIC ANATOMY

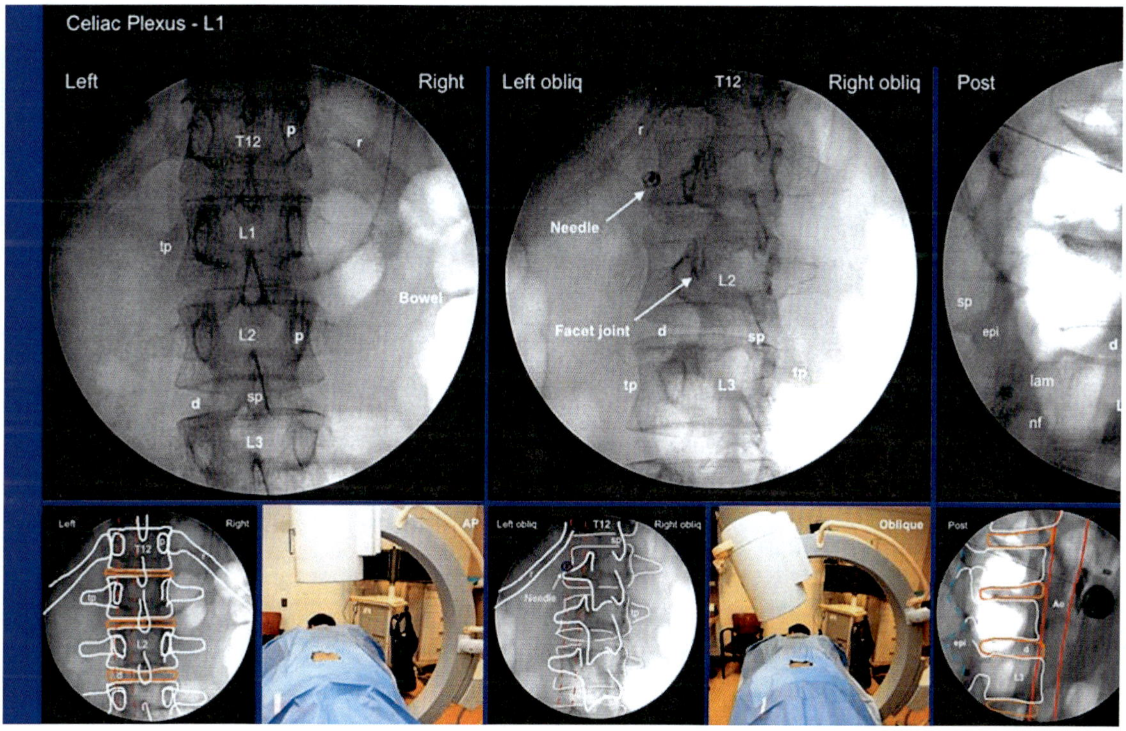

Figure 2: Fluoroscopic anatomy of antero-posterior, oblique, and transverse views showing needle placement a plexus.

Antero-posterior (AP) view showing T12-L3 vertebral bodies, spinous processes (sp), pedicles (p), transver discs (d), the T12 rib (r). The needle is viewed coaxial to the fluoroscopic image in the left oblique view. In th shows the tip of the needle anterior to the region of the aorta (Ao). The lamina (lam) and the zigzag pattern o identified in the lateral view.

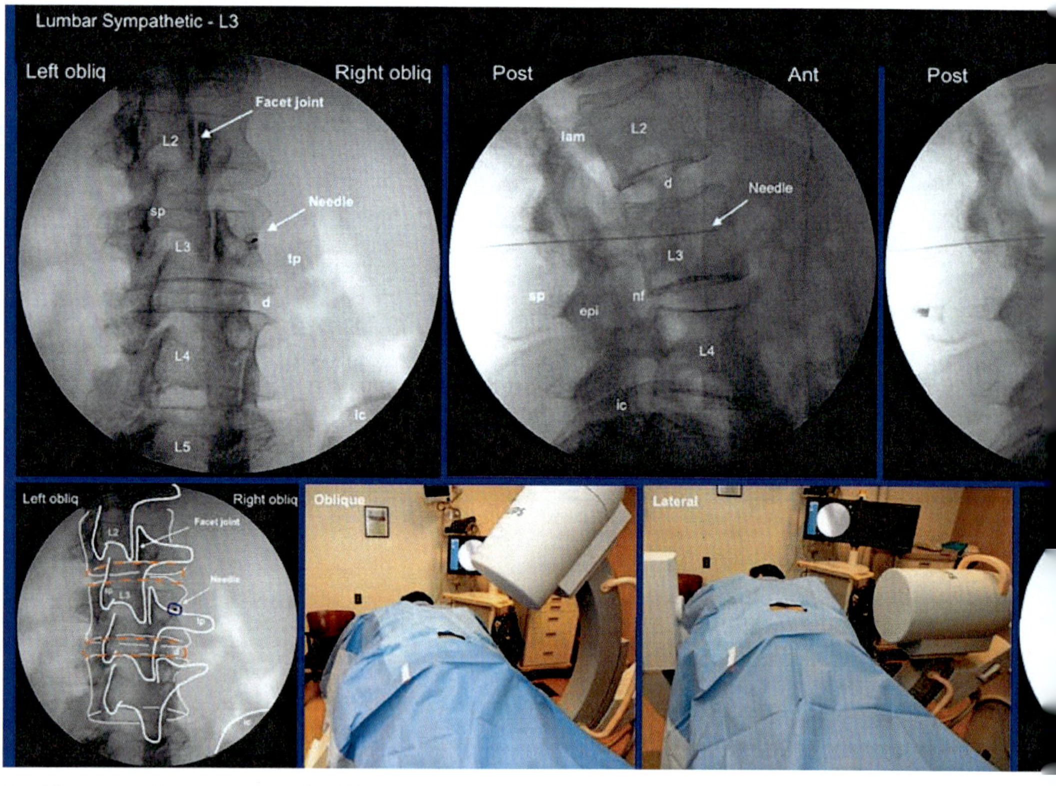

Figure 3: Fluoroscopic anatomy of oblique and transverse views showing placement of a needle an sympathetic chain.
In the right oblique view at the level of the lumbar vertebrae (L2-L5), the facet joints are seen coaxial to th viewed coaxial to the fluoroscopic image cranial to the right transverse process (tp) of L3. The interverteb (sp) are identified. In the lateral view the lamina (lam), zigzag pattern of the epidural space (epi), neurofo are identified. Radiocontrast dye can be seen spreading in a cranial-caudal direction along the anterolate which is the region of the sympathetic trunk (yellow line).

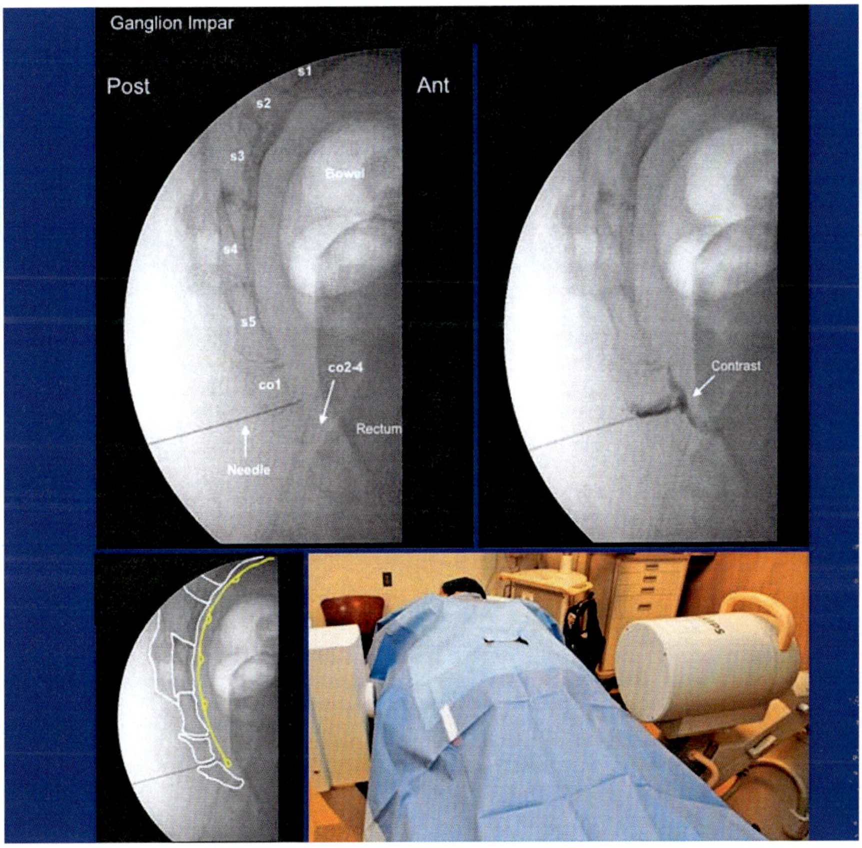

Figure 4: Fluoroscopic anatomy of the transverse view showing placement of a needle and dye extension onto
In the transverse view the sacral vertebrae (s1-s5) and coccygeal vertebrae (co1, co2-4) are identified intercoccygeal joint space between the first (co1) and 2nd (co2) coccygeal vertebrae, with radiocontrast d direction in the region of the ganglion impar (yellow line).

ACKNOWLEDGEMENTS

The authors gratefully acknowledge the following persons:

- The Head of the Department of Anesthesiology of the College of Medicine of the University of Florida, Dr. Tim Morey, and his department for their moral support and continuous encouragement.

- The faculty and fellows of the Division of acute and perioperative pain medicine for affording the author (APB) the time to produce this work by covering his clinical duties.

- George Hanna, Ravi Pathak, and Mihir Kamdar for providing the fluoroscopic images.

- Mary K. Bryson for her illustrations of Fig. (**1**).

- Corey Astrom of the Department of Anesthesiology of the College of Medicine of the University of Florida for her professional and high quality text editing.

- Raeducation.com LLC for their financial support.

CONFLICT OF INTEREST

The authors confirm that this chapter contents have no conflict of interest.

ABBREVIATIONS

Ao = aorta

Co1 = first coccygeal ligament

Co2 = second coccygeal ligament

Epi = epidural space

Ic = iliac crest

Lam = lamina

Nf = neuroforamen

Sp = spinous process

Tp = transverse process

SUGGESTED FURTHER READING

[1] Netter FH. Atlas of Human Anatomy. 2nd Ed. Teterboro, NJ: ICON Learning Systems; 2001.
[2] Whitaker RH, Borley NR. Instant Anatomy. 4th Ed. West Sussex, United Kingdom: Wiley-Blackwell: 2010.

Chapter 23:
Applied Macroanatomy and Sonoanatomy of the Nerves of the Head and Neck

CHAPTER 23

Applied Macroanatomy and Sonoanatomy of the Nerves of the Head and Neck

Johan P. Reyneke[1] and André P. Boezaart[2,*]

[1]*Center for Orthognathic Surgery, Cape Town Mediclinic, Department of Maxillofacial and Oral Surgery, University of the Western Cape, South Africa and* [2]*Departments of Anesthesiology and Orthopaedic Surgery and Rehabilitation, Division of Acute and Perioperative Pain Medicine, University of Florida College of Medicine, Gainesville, Florida, USA*

Abstract: The trigeminal ganglion gives off three branches. One of them is the ophthalmic nerve, which again splits into three branches: the lacrimal, the frontal, and the nasociliary nerves. The other two branches are the maxillary and mandibular nerves. In this chapter the authors discuss all the branches of these nerves as well as the nerves of the cervical plexus. The innervation of the skin of the head, the eye, nose, mouth, teeth, tongue, ear and larynx are discussed in detail. Finally the authors outline the sonoanatomy of infraorbital and greater occipital nerves, the superficial cervical plexus and that of the eye and orbit.

Keywords: Cutaneous innervation, External nasal nerve, Facial muscles, Fifth cranial nerve, Greater auricular nerve, Greater occipital nerve, Infratrochlear nerve, Innervation of the teeth, Laryngeal nerve, Larynx, Lingual nerve, Mandibular division, Mandibular nerve, Maxillary division, Ophthalmic division, Optic nerve, Orbit,Sonoanatomy, Superior trochlear nerve, Supraorbital nerve, Tongue, Trigeminal ganglion, Trigeminal nerve, Vestibular sulcus, Zygomatic facial nerve, Zygomatic temporal nerve.

CUTANEOUS (SENSORY) INNERVATION OF THE FACE

The trigeminal nerve is the fifth and the largest of the cranial nerves (CN V) and is the principle sensory nerve of the face and head. The skin of the face is innervated in three zones by the branches of the three divisions of the trigeminal nerve (Fig. **1**). The trigeminal nerve is mostly a sensory nerve but supplies motor innervation to the muscles of mastication and also the mylohyoid, anterior belly of the digastric, tensor palati, and tensor tympani. The motor root arises in the pons and joins the mandibular nerve in the foramen ovale. The muscles of facial expression receive their motor innervation from the facial nerve (seventh cranial

***Corresponding author André P. Boezaart:** Departments of Anesthesiology and Orthopaedic Surgery, Division of Acute and Peri-operative Pain Medicine, University of Florida College of Medicine, 1600 SW Archer Road, Gainesville, Florida 32610, USA; Tel: 352-846-0913 (Work); Fax: 352-392-7029; E-mail: aboezaart@anest.ufl.edu

nerve). The same nerves that supply sensory innervation to the skin over the muscles carry the proprioceptive impulses from the facial muscles.

The fifth cranial nerve has three divisions: the ophthalmic, the maxillary, and the mandibular divisions, and the numbers of terminal branches from each division are five, three, and three respectively.

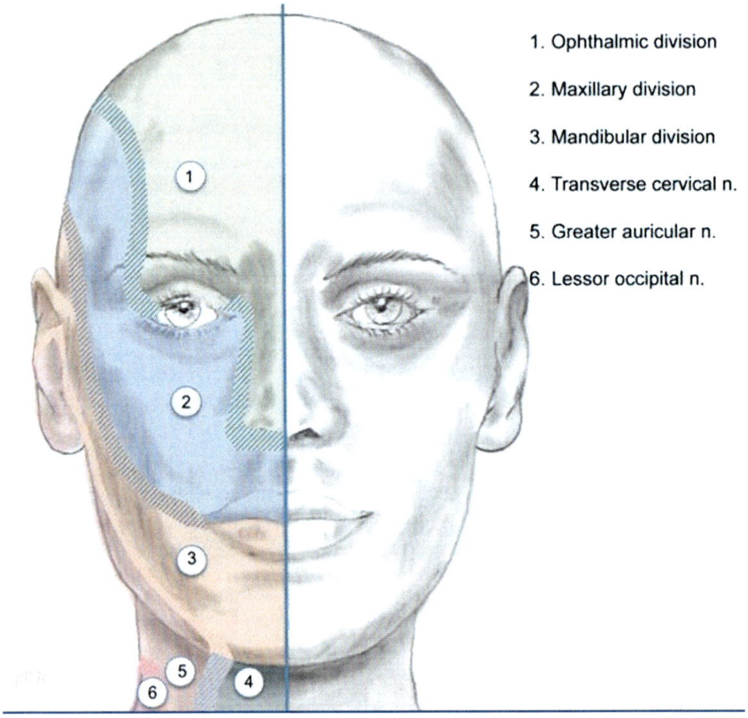

Figure 1: A schematic presentation of the sensory innervation of the face – a frontal view. *The fifth cranial nerve (CN V) is responsible for the cutaneous nerve supply of the face through its three divisions: ophthalmic (1), maxillary (2), and mandibular (3)divisions.*

Cutaneous Branches of the Ophthalmic Division (CN V_1)

The ophthalmic division leaves the upper part of the trigeminal ganglion and runs forward in the lateral wall of the cavernous sinus below the trochlear nerve (CN IV). At the anterior end of the cavernous sinus, it gives off meningeal branches, the tentoreal nerves, which supply all the supra tentoreal dura mater except in the bony floor of the middle cranial fossa. The ophthalmic nerve finally divides into a frontal, a lacrimal, and a nasociliary nerve. The frontal nerve runs in the roof of the orbit where it divides into a medial and lateral and the supraorbital nerves.

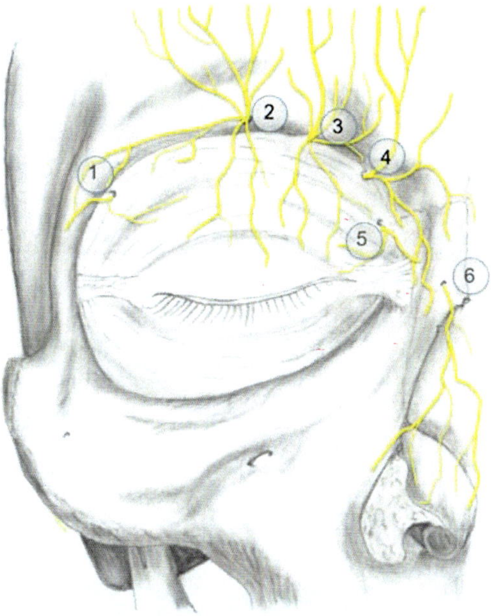

Figure 2: The superior orbit, upper eyelid, and frontal area of the head and superior aspect of the nose are supplied by the five branches of the ophthalmic division of trigeminal nerve.
(1) lacrimal nerve, (2) lateral supraorbital nerve, (3) medial supraorbital nerve, (4) superior trochlear nerve, (5) infratrochlear nerve, and (6) the external nasal nerve.

- Lacrimal nerve (1, Fig. **2**): innervates a small area of skin and conjunctiva over the lateral part of the upper eyelid and the lacrimal gland.

- Supraorbital nerves (2,3, Fig. **2**): The medial (2) and lateral (3) supraorbital nerves enter the face toward the medial end of the orbit through a notch, the supraorbital notch or foramen. They break up into several branches and pass superiorly. They innervate the forehead and scalp up to the vertex, however, they have substantial overlap with cervical nerves from the second (C2) and third (C3) cervical nerves beyond the vertex. The nerves also reach the conjunctiva of the upper eyelid and the mucosa of the frontal sinus.

- Supratrochlear nerve (4, Fig. **2**): This nerve passes upward and medial to the supraorbital nerves, divides into several branches, emerges through the medial canthus, and innervates the middle of the forehead up to the hairline as well as the conjunctiva of the eye and skin of the nose.

- Infratrochlear nerve (5, Fig. **2**): Passes above the palpebral ligament and innervates the medial part of the upper eyelid and the bridge of the nose.

- External nasal nerve (6, Fig. **2**): This nerve passes through the ethmiod sinuses and emerges between the nasal bone and upper lateral cartilage of the nose. It supplies sensory innervation to the lateral nose down to the tip.

Cutaneous Branches of the Maxillary Division (CN V_2)

The maxillary division is the second of the three divisions of the trigeminal nerve. It arises from the trigeminal ganglion and passes through the foramen rotundum, enters the pterygo-palatine fossa, and curves laterally through the pterygo-palatine fissure to the infratemporal fossa. It enters the infraorbital groove as the infraorbital nerve (Fig. **3**).

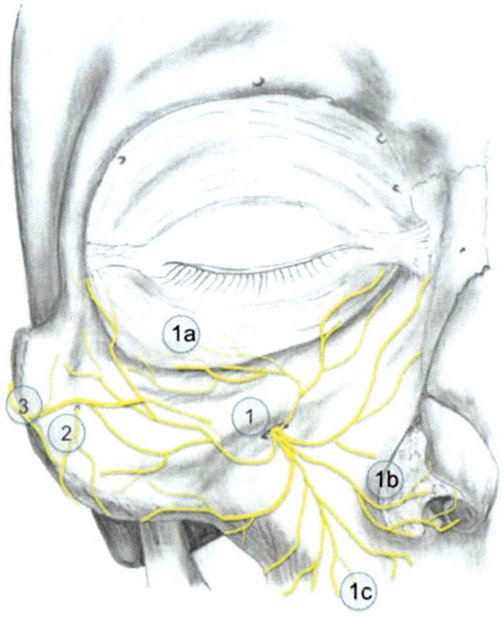

Figure 3a: The lower eyelid, skin over the nostril, cheek, lower lip, gingiva from the premolars to the centerline, skin over the hairless part of the temple, and lateral canthus of the eye are innervated by the three branches of the maxillary division of the trigeminal nerve.
The infraorbital nerve (1), has three branches: (1a) a palpebral branch, (1b) a nasal branch, and (1c) a labial branch. (2) Zygomatic facial nerve and (3) zygomatic temporal nerve.

- Infraorbital nerve (1, Fig. **3a**): This nerve runs in the floor of the orbit and exits through the infraorbital foramen. It breaks up into several branches, the palpebral branch (1a), the nasal branch (1b) and the labial branch (1c) that radiate away from the foramen.

- Palpebral branches (1a, Fig. **3a**) supply sensory innervation to the lower eyelid and cheek.

- Nasal branches (1b, Fig. **3a**) innervate the skin over the lower lateral cartilages of the nose (nostril).

- Labial branches (1c, Fig. **3a**) innervate the upper lip and labial gingiva from the midline to the second premolar.

- Zygomatico facial nerve (2, Fig. **3a**): Emerges from one or two foramina in the zygomatic bone and its branches supply sensory innervation to the overlying skin and lateral canthus of the orbit.

- Zygomatico temporal nerve (3, Fig. **3a**): Emerges in the temporal fossa through a foramen on the temporal (posterior) surface of the zygomatic bone. The nerve innervates a small area of skin over the front of the temple (the "hairless" part of the temple).

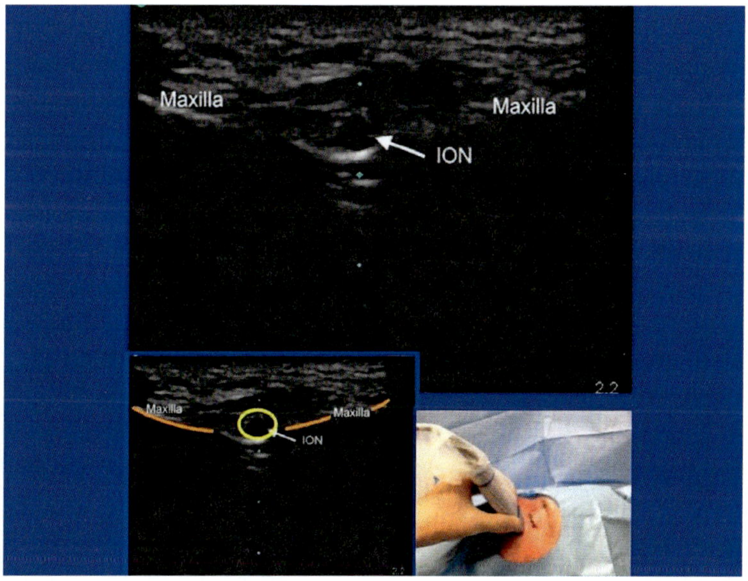

Figure 3b: Sonoanatomy of the infraorbital nerve.
ION = infraorbital nerve.

The ultrasound probe that was used was a 6 - 13-MHz linear probe with a 25 mm footprint (HFL – 25, SonoSite Fujifilm, Bothell, WA, USA).

Cutaneous Branches of the Mandibular Division (CN V_3)

The mandibular division is the third division of the trigeminal nerve and arises from the trigeminal ganglion in the cranium and enters the infratemporal fossa through the foramen ovale. Immediately below the skull, the trunk of the trigeminal nerve gives off a twig to the meninges and a branch to the medial pterygoid muscle. It then divides into an anterior (predominantly motor) and a posterior division (predominantly sensory).

Branches of the Trunk of the Trigeminal Nerve (CN V)

1. A meningeal branch.

2. The motor nerve to the medial pterygoid and tensor palati muscles.

Branches of the Anterior Division of the Mandibular Nerve

- The long buccal nerve (2, Fig. **4**): This sensory nerve arises from the mandibular nerve medial to the mandibular ramus and innervates the oral mucosa posterior to the lower bicuspid teeth. It gives off a few cutaneous twigs before it perforates the buccinators muscle and innervates a "thumb print" area of skin over the cheek between the areas of the infraorbital nerve and the greater auricular nerve. (Note: The greater auricular nerve, which originates from C2 supplies sensory innervation to an area of skin over the angle of the mandible and the parotid gland).

- Nerve to lateral pterygoid (not depicted): It arises with the long buccal nerve (2, Fig. **4**) and supplies motor fibers to the muscle as it passes over it.

- Deep anterior and posterior temporal nerves (not depicted): These nerves enter the temporal fossa between the skull and the lateral pterygoid muscle and supply motor fibers to the temporal muscle.

- Nerve (3, Fig. **4**) to the masseter muscle (10, Fig. **4**): The masseteric nerve (3, Fig. **4**) arises from the posterior deep temporal nerve, runs anterior to the temporomandibular joint, and enters the masseter muscle on its deep surface by passing through the coronoid notch. It also gives two twigs to the temporomandibular joint.

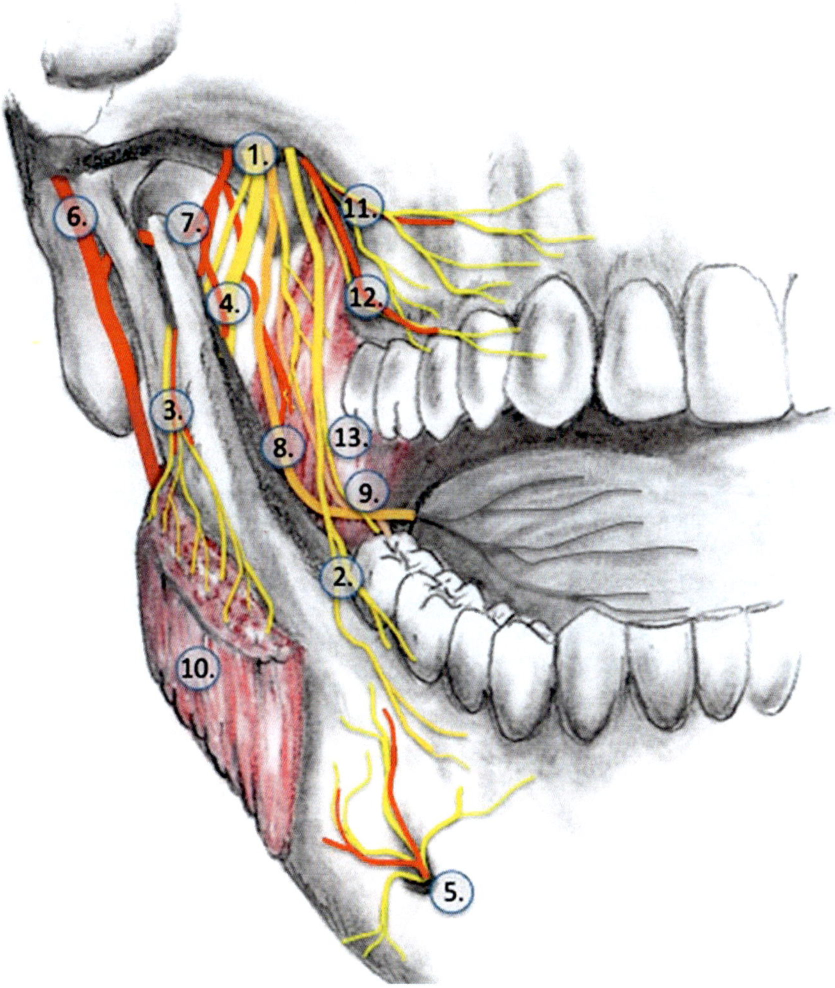

Figure 4: Nerves and vessels medial and lateral to the mandibular ramus Part of the masseter muscle is removed.
(1) Mandibular nerve, (2) long buccal nerve, (3) massetric nerve, (4) inferior alveolar nerve, (5) mental nerve, (6) superficial temporal artery, (7) maxillary artery, (8) lingual nerve, (9) nerve to mylohyoid muscle (10), masseter muscle, (11) medial superior alveolar nerve, (12) posterior superior alveolar nerve, and (13) medial pterygoid muscle.

Branches of the Posterior Division of the Mandibular Nerve

- Auriculotemporal nerve (not depicted): The nerve arises from the mandibular nerve (1, Fig. **4**), runs laterally tightly underneath the oval foramen and medially from the mandibular ramus. It continues dorsally dorsally, penetrates the parotid gland, and then passes around the neck of the mandibular condyle behind the superficial temporal vessels. The auricular part supplies sensory innervation to the external acoustic meatus and the surface of the eardrum and skin above this level (see "Innervation of the ear"). The temporal part of this nerve supplies the hairy skin over the temple (that part where gray hair appears first).

- Inferior alveolar nerve (4, Fig. **4**): It runs vertically downward with the inferior alveolar artery, enters the mandibular foramen, and runs in the inferior alveolar canal. It supplies sensory innervation to the teeth and gingiva of the lower dental arch.

- Mental nerve (5, Fig. **4**): This is the terminal branch of the inferior alveolar nerve and it exits from the mandible through the mental foramen. The nerve breaks up into tufts of branches and supplies the skin and mucous membrane of the lower lip and gingiva from the midline to the bicuspid teeth.

- Mylohyoid nerve (9, Fig. **4**): This is the only motor fiber of the posterior division of the mandibular nerve and it leaves the inferior alveolar nerve near the mandibular foramen. The nerve divides into a number of branches to innervate the mylohyoid muscle and the anterior belly of the digastric muscle.

- Lingual nerve (8, Fig. **4**): This is an entirely sensory nerve and it innervates the mucosa of the anterior two-thirds of the tongue and adjacent floor of the mouth. It emerges from beneath the lateral pterygoid muscle and runs anteriorly between the mandible and the medial pterygoid muscle, inferior and medial to the last molar tooth, above the posterior border of the mylohyoid muscle.

MOTOR INNERVATION OF THE FACIAL MUSCLES

The seventh cranial nerve (CN VII) contains no sensory fibers on the face and the proprioceptive impulses from the facial muscles are conveyed centrally by the trigeminal nerve.

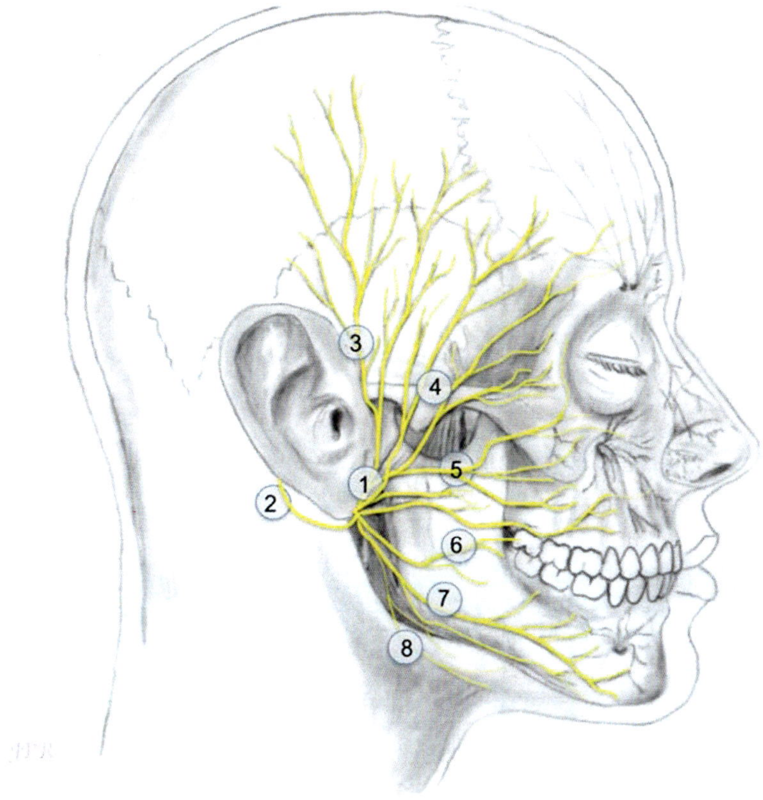

Figure 5: Lateral view of the face indicating the extra cranial course of the facial nerve (CN VII). The soft tissue and parotid gland have been removed.
(1) Facial nerve, (2) posterior auricular nerve, (3) auriculotemporal nerve (CN V_3), (4) temporal branches of CN VII, (5) zygomatic branches (CN VII), (6) buccal branches (CN VII), (7) mandibular branches (CN VII), and the (8) cervical branches (CN VII).

Extra Cranial Course of the Facial Nerve

The facial nerve (1, Fig. **5**) exits the cranium through the stylomastoid foramen and immediately provides the posterior auricular branch (2, Fig. **5** of chapter 13) that passes behind the ear to supply motor innervation to the occipitofrontalis muscle. It also provides a branch to the posterior belly of the digastric and stylohyoid muscles.

It then enters the parotid gland on its posteromedial surface and divides into two branches, the temporozygomatic and cervicofacial nerves. These nerves divide, rejoin, and divide again to exit the parotid gland in five main groups of branches.

1. Temporal branches (4, Fig. **5**)
2. Zygomatic branches (5, Fig. **5**)
3. Buccal branches (6, Fig. **5**)
4. Mandibular branches (7, Fig. **5**)
5. Cervical branches (8, Fig. **5**)

THE INNERVATION OF THE ORAL CAVITY

Nerve supply to the palate: The maxillary nerve and pterygo-palatine ganglion occupy the pterygo-palatine fossa. The maxillary nerve through the ganglion sends branches into the nose and down into the palate (Fig. **6**).

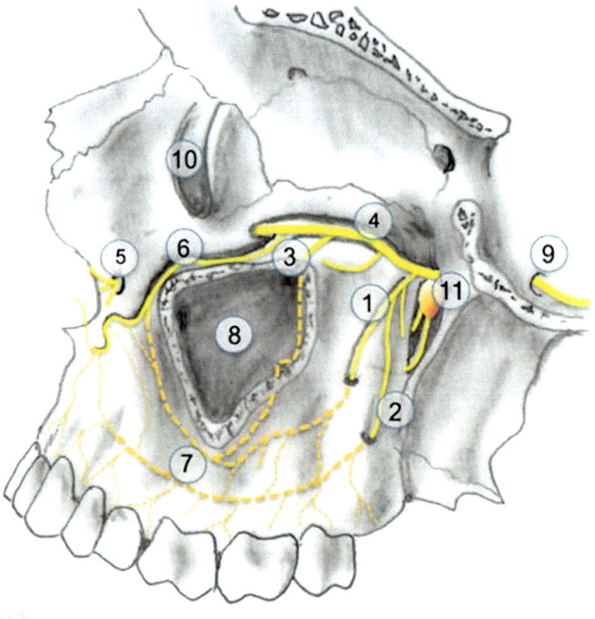

Figure 6: A diagram of the maxillary nerve and related structures.
(1) The upper branch of the superior posterior alveolar nerve, (2) the lower superior posterior alveolar nerve, (3) superior medial alveolar nerve, (4) the maxillary nerve, (5) infraorbital nerve, (6) anterior superior alveolar nerve, (7) branches to the gingiva, periostium, premolar, and molar teeth, (8) maxillary sinus, (9) the maxillary nerve exits from the foramen rotundum, the (10) lacrimal duct and the (11) pterygo-palatine ganglion.

- The lessor palatine nerve: The soft tissue of the soft palate receives sensory innervation from the lesser palatine nerve as a branch of the maxillary nerve *via* the pterygo-palatine ganglion. The nerve enters the posterior hard palate through the lessor palatine foramen.

- The greater palatine nerve: The nerve enters the hard palate through the greater palatine foramen and gives sensory innervation to the hard palate and palatal gingiva as far forward as the incisor teeth.

- The nasopalatine nerve: This nerve is the terminal branch of the anterior superior alveolar nerve, which runs along the nasal septum and enters the oral cavity through the incisive canal. The nerve has anastomoses with the greater palatine nerve and supplies the gingiva just posterior of the maxillary incisor teeth.

Innervation of the Vestibular Sulcus of the Maxilla and Cheek

1. Superior posterior alveolar branches of the maxillary nerve (1, 2, Fig. **6**) (CN V_2) supply the posterior maxillary sulcus and then pierce the posterior wall of the maxilla and pass forward in the bone above the molar teeth, which they supply. It also supplies the mucosa of the maxillary sinus.

2. The superior medial alveolar (3, Fig. **6**) branches off the infraorbital nerve on the floor of the orbit and runs down in the lateral wall of the maxilla to innervate the premolar teeth and mucosa of the maxillary sinus.

3. The infraorbital nerve (5, Fig. **6**) (CN V_2) innervates the maxillary vestibule anterior to the second bicuspid teeth and its innervation extends to the midline of the maxilla to supply the upper lip. There is substantial overlap with the above nerves.

Innervation of the Teeth

The Maxillary Teeth

1. The posterior superior alveolar nerves (1,2, Fig. **6**) only supply the posterior maxillary gingiva and molar teeth.

2. The middle posterior alveolar nerve (7, Fig. **6**) supplies the anterior buccal root of the first molar, as well as the two bicuspid teeth.

3. The anterior superior alveolar nerve (a branch of the infraorbital nerve (5, Fig. **6**)) gives sensory innervation to the upper canine and incisor teeth.

The Mandibular Teeth

1. The main trunk of the inferior alveolar nerve (4, Fig. **4**) innervates the three lower molars and two bicuspids.

2. The terminal branch of the inferior alveolar nerve (4, Fig. **4**) innervates the lower canine and lower incisor teeth.

Innervation of the Mandibular Vestibular Sulcus and Cheek

1. The long buccal nerve (CN V_3) (2, Fig. **4**) is a branch of the mandibular nerve (1, Fig. **4**) and enters the oral cavity through the buccinator muscle. It supplies the mandibular vestibule and gingiva through overlap with the mental nerve anteriorly.

2. The mental nerve (CN V_3) (5, Fig. **4**) is the terminal sensory branch of the inferior alveolar nerve and it enters the oral cavity through the mental foramen. This nerve innervates the mandibular vestibule and gingiva anterior to the second mandibular bicuspid teeth and reaches the midline of the mandible.

Innervation of the Floor of the Mouth and Tongue

- The lingual nerve (8, Fig. **4**) (CN V_3) runs on the lingual side of the mandibular ramus over the medial pterygoid muscle. It then runs anteriorly and medial to the internal oblique ridge on the bone medial to the second molar tooth, turns medial, runs over the posterior border of the mylohiod muscle and enters the tongue. The anterior two-thirds of the lingual nerve, whose trigeminal component mediates common sensibility (cell bodies in the trigeminal ganglion). The chorda tympani component mediates taste (cell bodies in the geniculate ganglion of VII). The parasympathetic secretomotor fibers to the anterior lingual salivary gland run in the chorda tympani from the superior salivatory nucleus.

- The glossopharyngeal nerve supplies the posterior one-third of the tongue (2, Fig. **7**), including the papilla vallate. The nerve carries fibers of sensibility and taste as well as parasympathetic secretomotor fibers to the glands.

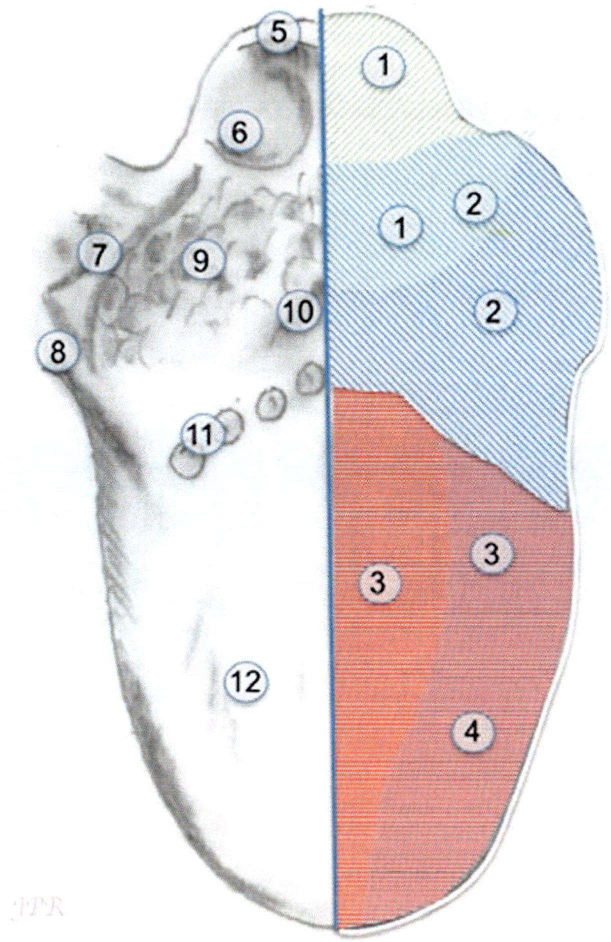

Figure 7: A schematic representation of the nerve supply of the tongue and related structures. *(1) Vagus nerve, (2) glossopharyngeal nerve, (3) trigeminal nerve, (4) facial nerve, (5) epiglottis, (6) vallecula of the epiglottis, (7) palatine tonsil, (8) palatoglossal fold, (9) lymphoid nodules, (10) foramen cecum, (11) papillae cicumvelata, and (12) papillae fungiform and viliform.*

INNERVATION OF THE NOSE

The nerves of sensation all arise as branches of the maxillary nerve (CN V_2) except the anterior ethmoidal nerves, which are branches of the nasociliary nerve in the orbit (10, Fig. **14b**). The nerves reach the nasal cavity through the anterior ethmoidal foramen and the cribriform plate of the ethmoid bone through branches of the pterygo-palatine ganglion, the anterior superior alveolar, and the greater palatine nerves.

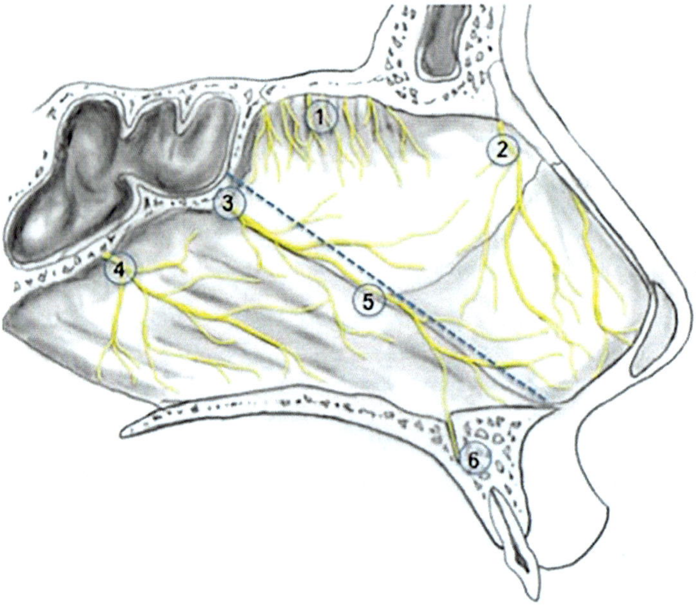

Figure 8: Innervation of the nasal septum.
(1) olfactory nerve, (2) anterior ethmoidal nerve, (3) sphenopalatine fossa, (4), posterior branches of the sphenopalatine nerve, (5) nasopalatine nerve, (6) nasopalatine nerve in the incisive canal.

- The nasal septum: Note that the septum is innervated in halves (antero-superior and postero-inferior).
  - The antero-superior section is supplied by the anterior ethmoidal nerve (2, Fig. **8**).
  - The postero-inferior section is supplied be the nasopalatine nerve (5, Fig. **8**).
- The lateral wall of the nose: Note that the lateral wall is innervated in quadrants by branches of the ophthalmic (CN V_1) and maxillary (CN V_2) nerves.
  - The postero-superior lateral nasal branches (CN V_1) (1, Fig. **9**) innervate the postero-superior area through the pterygo-palatine

ganglion and enter the nasal cavity through the sphenopalatine foramen.

- The postero-inferior branches of the greater palatine nerve (2, Fig. **9**) innervate the postero-inferior area.

- The anterior ethmoidal nerve (3, Fig. **9**) innervates the antero-superior area. It passes out of the nasal cavity between the nasal bones and the upper lateral cartilages and becomes the external nasal nerve.

- The anterior inferior quadrant of the lateral wall of the nose receives sensory innervation from the anterior superior alveolar nerve (4, Fig. **9**). The nerve terminates as a tiny septal branch.

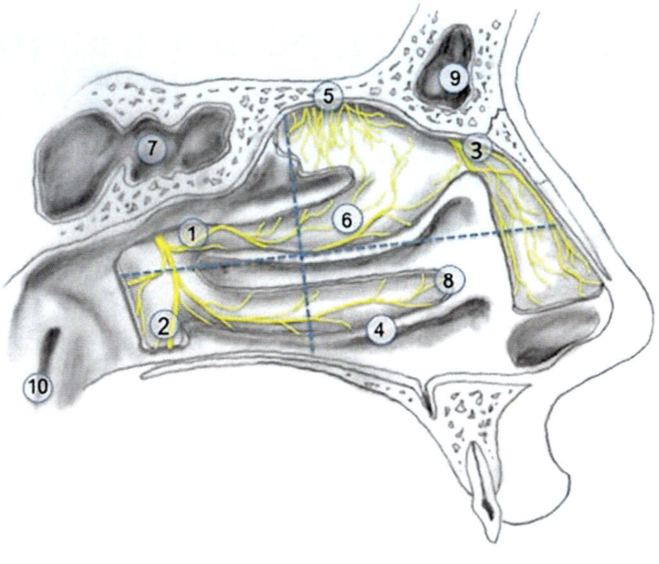

Figure 9: Innervation of the lateral wall of the nose.
(1) lateral posterior nasal branches, (2) greater palatine nerve, (3) anterior ethmoidal nerve (CN V1), (4) anterior superior alveolar nerve, (5) olfactory nerve (CN I), (6) superior turbinate, (7) sphenoid sinus, (8) inferior turbinate, (9) frontal sinus, (10) Auditory (Eustachian) tube.

- The olfactory nerves (5, Fig. **9**) (CN1) are formed as processes of the olfactory cells in the epithelium in the olfactory area of the brain and supply an individual with a sense of smell. They pass through the cribriform plate of the ethmoid bone into the roof of the nasal cavity.

- The external nasal nerve exits the nasal cavity between the nasal bone and upper lateral cartilage and runs down on the lower lateral cartilage to the tip of the nose (6, Fig. **2**).

- The infratrochlear nerve supplies sensory innervation to the skin over the nasal bones (the bridge of the nose) above the exit of the external nasal nerve (5, Fig. **2**).

- The nasal branches of the infraorbital nerve (CN V_2) innervate the skin around the nostrils (1b, Fig. **3a**).

CUTANEOUS INNERVATION OF THE EAR

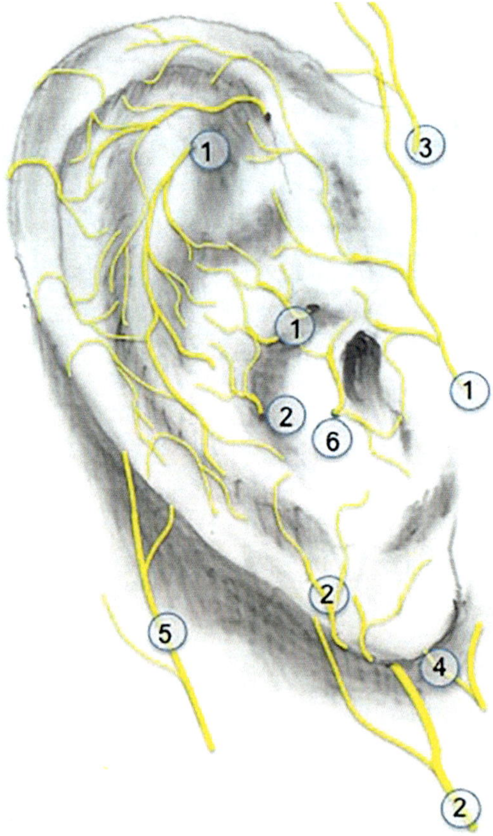

Figure 10: Innervation of the external ear.
(1) auriculo-temporal nerve, (2) greater auricular nerve, (3) temporal branches of CN VII, (4) posterior auricular branch of CN VII, (5) lessor occipital nerve, (6) auricular branch of CN X, CN VII and CN IX via Arnold's nerve.

Several sensory nerves innervate the external ear.

- Auriculotemporal nerve (1, Fig. **10**) (CN V_3): This nerve enters the auricular region running dorsally from the mandibular condyle. It innervates the anterior portion of the auricle (anterior part of the helix and the tragus), the skin over the temporomandibular joint, and the temporal region. This nerve also innervates the outer surface of the eardrum and the external acoustic meatus.

- Greater auricular nerve (2, Fig. **10**) (C2, C3) runs dorsally and innervates the skin on the cranial-dorsal aspect of the helix. The anterior branch of the greater auricular nerve innervates the lower lateral one-third of the helix with fibers from the second cervical nerve (C2).

- Facial nerve (Fig. **5**) (CN VII): This nerve passes through the stylomastoid foramen and then a branch from this nerve, the posterior auricular nerve (4, Fig. **10**), provides motor innervation to the muscles on the cranial aspect of the ear. The auricular branch of vagus conducts sensory impulses from the skin behind the auricle through the posterior auricular nerve (4, Fig. **10** of chapter 13) to the auricular branch of the vagus nerve (CN X) (6, Fig. **10**).

- Lesser occipital nerve (5, Fig. **10**) (C3) overlaps the greater auricular nerve (3, Fig. **10**) and supplies the upper, cranial one-third, and the lower lateral one-third of the helix of the ear with sensory innervation.

- Vagus nerve (CN X): The concha and the cymba conchae of the ear are innervated by the auricular branch of this nerve.

CUTANEOUS INNERVATION OF THE HEAD

The sensory innervation of the scalp is derived from the trigeminal nerve and the second (C2) and third (C3) cervical spinal nerves. There is substantial overlap between areas of sensory innervation of the scalp that can be summarized as follows (Fig. **11**):

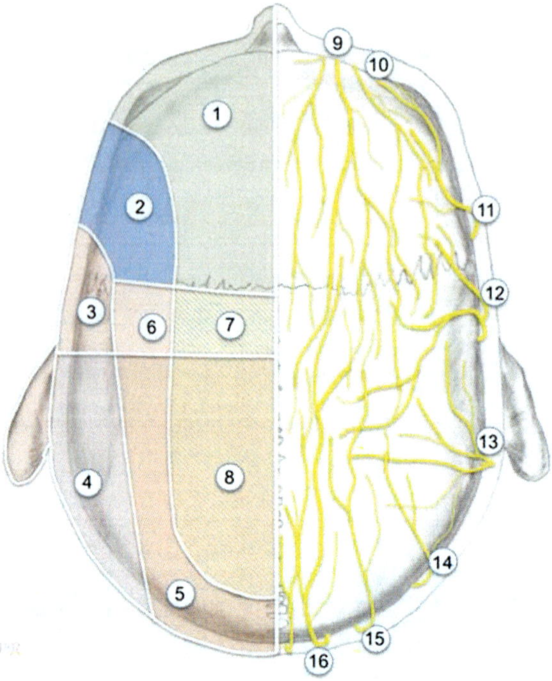

Figure 11a: Regions of sensory innervation and nerves of the head in a schematic representation. A vertical view of the head.
(1) Ophthalmic nerve (CN V_1), (2) maxillary nerve (CN V_2), (3) mandibular nerve (CN V_3), (4) lessor occipital nerve (C2), (5) greater occipital nerve (C3), (6) C2 and CN V_2, (7) C3 and CN V_1, (8) C2, C3, and CN V_1, (9) supraorbital nerve (medial branch), (10) supraorbital nerve (lateral branch), (11) temporal branches of CN V_3, (12) auriculotemporal nerve branches (CN V_3), (13) posterior auricular nerve, (14) lessor occipital nerve (C3), (15) greater occipital nerve (C2), and (16) the third occipital nerve.

Anterior to a line extending from the ear to the vertex of the head, the sensory innervation is provided by the trigeminal nerve, except for the skin over the lower one-half of the ramus of the mandible and the lower one-half of the auricle, which are innervated by the ventral rami of the second and the third cervical nerves through the greater auricular nerve. Posterior to that line, the sensory innervation is entirely provided by the cervical nerves; the antero-inferior part from the ventral rami (C2, C3) through the auricular nerve and lesser occipital branches of the cervical plexus. The postero-superior part is supplied of sensory innervation by the dorsal rami of the second and, to a lesser extent, the third cervical nerves, through the greater and third occipital nerves, respectively.

The branches of the three divisions of the trigeminal nerve supply the frontal one-half and lateral part of the head (Fig. **11**).

1. Medial supraorbital and lateral supraorbital nerves (9,10, Fig. **11**) (CN V_1) enter the face at the superior orbital rim through a notch or foramen and run superiorly and posteriorly. The antero-medial area of the scalp to the forehead and the scalp receive their sensory innervation from these nerves. There is substantial overlap with the lesser and greater occipital nerves and the third occipital nerve (14, 15, 16, Fig. **11**) (C2 and C3) that may extend to the posterior one-half of the head.

3. The pre-auricular area is innervated by branches of the maxillary division of the trigeminal nerve (CN V_2) through the auriculotemporal nerve (12, Fig. **11**).

The occipital region and the dorsal part of the neck receive sensory innervation from the dorsal branches of the spinal nerves (Fig. **11**):

1. The greater occipital (C2) dorsal branch of the fourth spinal nerve (15, Fig. **11**)

2. Third occipital nerve (C3) (16, Fig. **11**)

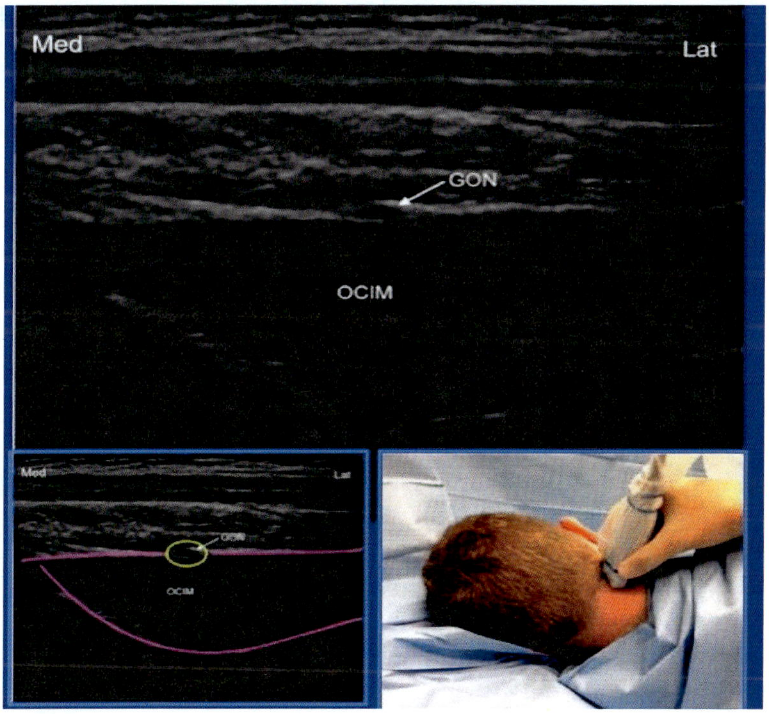

Figure 11b: Sonoanatomy of the greater occipital nerve.

3. The medial branch of the dorsal branch of the fourth spinal nerve (C4)

4. Lessor occipital nerve (C3) from the cervical plexus (14, Fig. **11**)

GON = greater occipital nerve; OCIM = obliquus capitis inferior muscle.

The ultrasound probe that was used was a 6 - 13-MHz linear probe with a 25 mm footprint (HFL – 25, SonoSite Fujifilm, Bothell, WA, USA).

CUTANEOUS INNERVATION OF THE NECK

The Anterior Neck

Transverse cervical nerve: The anterior portion of the neck is supplied by the transverse cervical nerve (C3), while the mandibular angle and lateral area of the neck is supplied by the greater auricular nerve. The skin behind the auricle of the ear, the lower part of the helix, and the lateral part of the neck is supplied by the lesser occipital nerve (C3) (4,5,6, Fig. **1**).

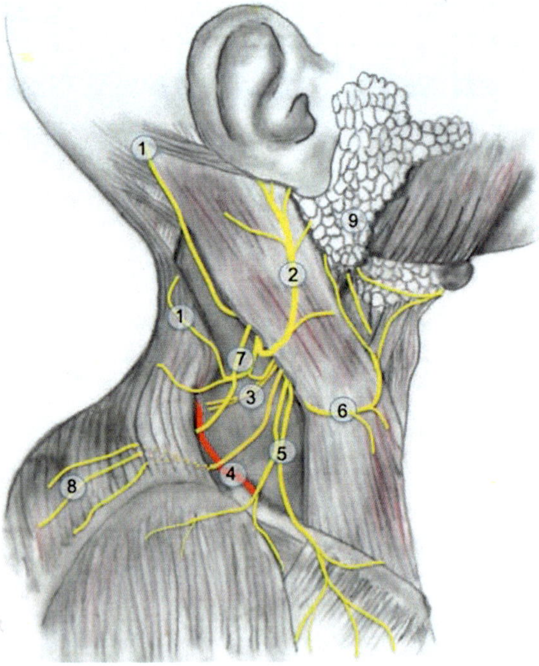

Figure 12a: Superficial nerve supply to the neck.
(1) Lessor occipital nerve (C2), (2) greater auricular nerve (C2, 3), (3) C2 and C3 to trapezius muscle, (4) transverse cervical artery, (5) supraclavicular nerve, (6) transverse cervical nerve, (7) accessory nerve, (8) supra-acromion nerve, and (9) the parotid gland.

The Posterior Neck

The dorsal part of the neck receives sensory innervation from the dorsal branches of the spinal nerves (Fig. **12**).

- Greater auricular nerve (2, Fig. **12**) (C2, C3): This nerve originates from the cervical plexus and innervates the skin over the sternocleidomastoid muscle through its posterior branch.

- Lesser occipital nerve (1, Fig. **12**) (C3): The lower one-half of the neck behind the ear and the skin that covers the lateral aspect of the neck is innervated by this nerve.

- Supraclavicular nerve (5, Fig. **12**) innervate the lower part of the neck the skin covering the clavicle, the pectoral area and skin overlying the shoulder.

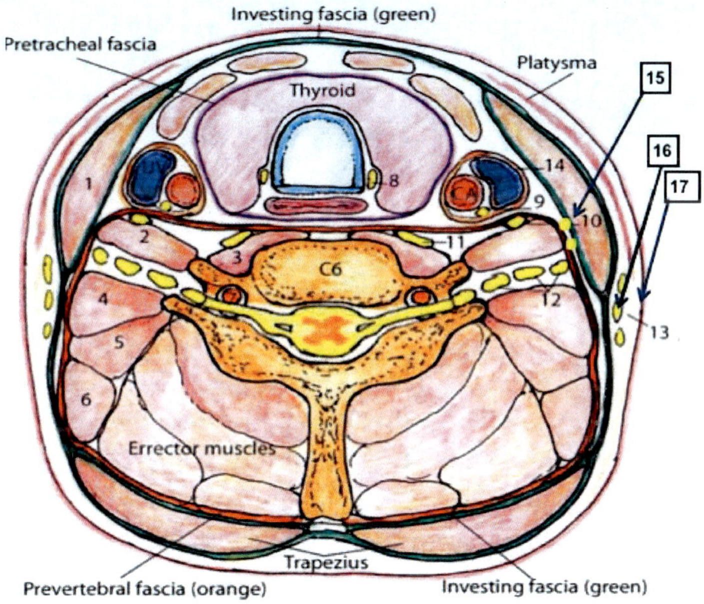

Figure 12b: Schematic trans sectional anatomy of the neck through the region of the 6th cervical vertebra showing the superficial cervical plexus.
(1) sternocleidomastoid muscle, (2) anterior scalene muscle, (3) longus colli muscle, (4) middle scalene muscle, (5) posterior scalene muscle, (6) levator scapulae muscle, (7) vertebral artery, (8) recurrent laryngeal nerve, (9) vagus nerve, (10) phrenic nerve, (11) middle cervical sympathetic ganglion, (12) brachial plexus (13) superficial cervical plexus, (14) carotid sheath, (15) supraclavicular nerves under sternocleidomastoid muscle, (16) supraclavicular nerves under the skin, (17) punctum nervosum.

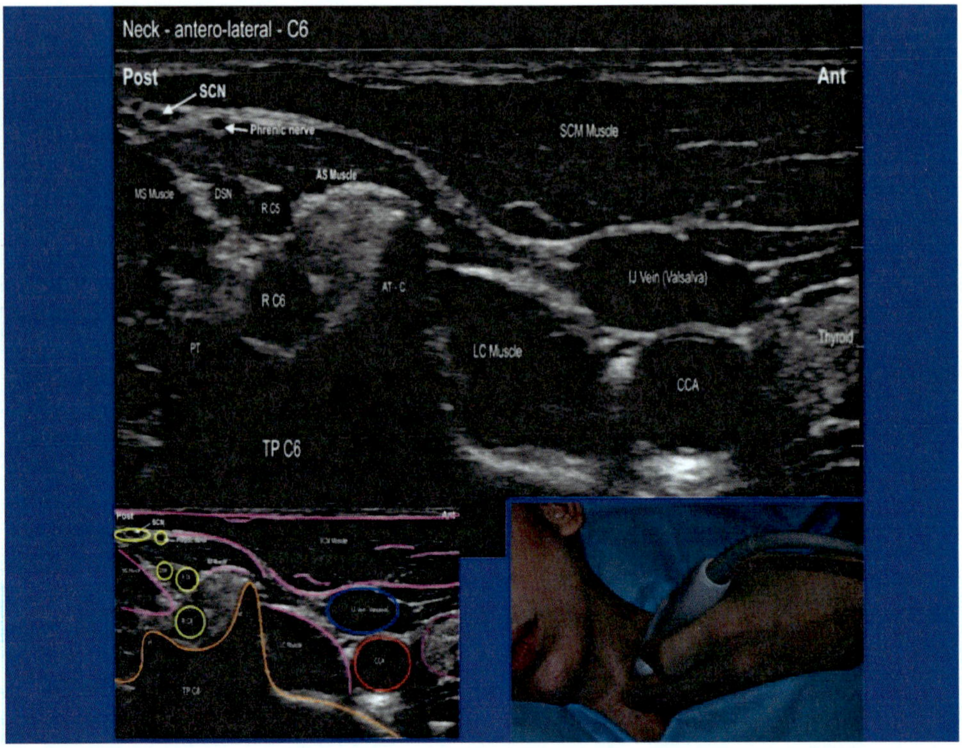

Figure 12c: Sonoanatomy of the superficial cervical plexus at the level of the 6th cervical vertebra – anterolateral view.

Post = posterior, Ant = anterior, CCA = common carotid artery, IJV = internal jugular vein (Valsalva maneuver applied), R C5 = 5th cervical spinal nerve root (C5), R C6 = 6th cervical spinal nerve root (C6), DSN = dorsal scapular nerve originating from the C5 spinal root, TP C6 = transverse process of the 6th cervical vertebra (C6), PT = Posterior tubercle of the transverse process of C6, AT C = large anterior tubercle of the transverse process of C6 (also known as the Carotid tubercle or Chassaignac's tubercle), AS Muscle = anterior scalene muscle, MS Muscle = middle scalene muscle, LC muscle = longus colli muscle (longus capitis muscle is not present at this level), SCM muscle = sternocleidomastoid muscle, SCN = supraclavicular nerves.*

The ultrasound probe that was used was a 6- to 13-MHz linear probe with a 38 mm footprint (HFL – 38, SonoSite Fujifilm, Bothell, WA, USA)

INNERVATION OF THE LARYNX

The Upper one-Half of the Larynx

- The superior laryngeal nerve (1, Fig. **13a**): This nerve is a branch off of the vagus nerve and it divides into internal (1a) and external branches (1b). The internal branch pierces the thyroid membrane, divides into several branches, and innervates the larynx and the aryepiglottic fold to the base of the tongue, epiglottis, and mucus membrane as far as the vocal folds with sensory and secretomotor fibers.

- The muscles are innervated by the recurrent laryngeal nerve (8, Fig. **13a**) by fibers derived from the accessory nerve (cell bodies lie in the nucleus ambiguous).

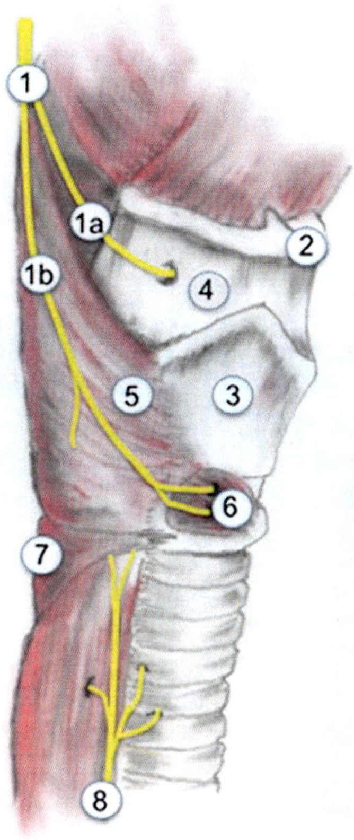

Figure 13a: Nerves of the larynx – right external view.
(1) Superior laryngeal nerve (branches of vagus nerve (CN X)), (1a) internal branch, (1b) external branch, (2) hyoid cartilage, (3) thyroid cartilage, (4) thyrohyoid membrane, (5) inferior pharyngeal constrictor muscle, (6) cricothyroid muscle, (7) cricopharyngeus muscle, and (8) recurrent laryngeal nerve.

The Lower One-Half of the Larynx

- The recurrent laryngeal nerve (8, Fig. **13a**) ascends in the groove between the trachea and the esophagus and enters the larynx deep to the lower border of the inferior pharyngeal constrictor muscle (5, Fig. **13a**).

- The lower part of the larynx receives sensory and secretomotor innervation by the recurrent laryngeal branch of the cricothyroid nerve.

- The recurrent laryngeal nerve innervates all the intrinsic muscles of the larynx except the cricothyroid muscle.

- The cricothyroid muscle receives its motor innervation from the external branch of the superior laryngeal nerve (1, Fig. **13a** and **13b**).

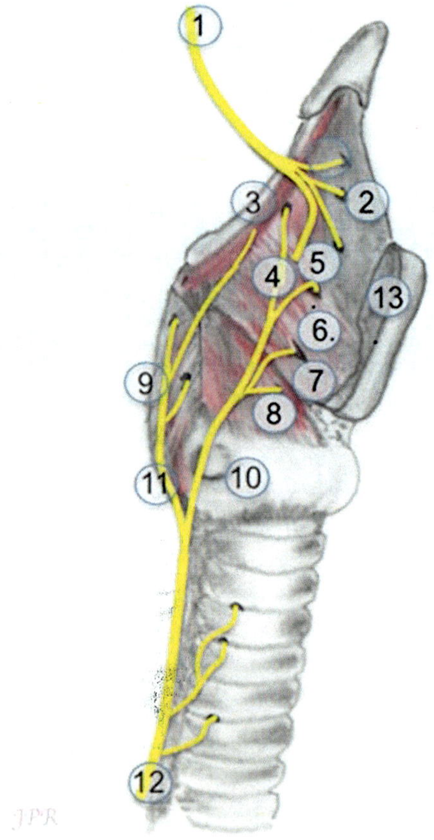

Figure 13b: Nerves of the larynx – right internal view – thyroid cartilage lamina removed.
(1) Lateral branch of the superior laryngeal nerve, (2) sensory branches of the superior laryngeal nerve to the larynx, (3) aryepiglottic muscle, (4) anastomosis between the nerves, (5) thyroepiglottic muscle, (6) transverse and oblique aryarytenoid muscles, (7) vocalis muscle, (8) lateral cricoarytenoid muscle, (9) posterior cricoarytenoid muscle, (10) cricothyroid articular facet, (11) anterior and posterior branches of the inferior laryngeal nerve, (12) recurrent laryngeal nerve, and (13) the thyroid cartilage lamina removed.

INNERVATION OF THE ORBIT

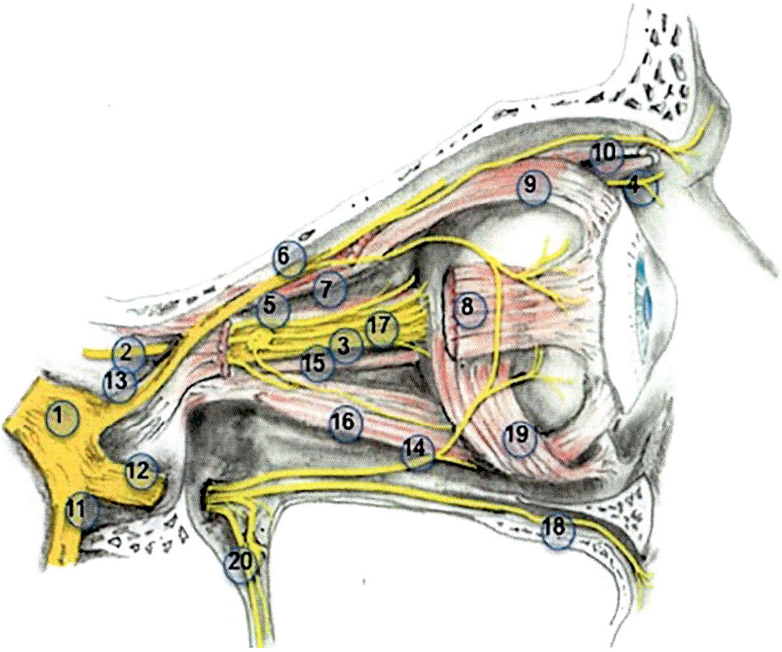

Figure 14a: Nerves of the orbit – A lateral view of the right orbit with part of the lateral rectus muscle removed.
(1) Trigeminal nerve and ganglion, (2) oculomotor nerve, (3) optic nerve (CN II), (4) lacrimal nerve, (5) ciliary ganglion, (6) frontal nerve, (7) levator palpebrae superior muscle, (8) lateral rectus muscle, (9) superior rectus muscle, (10) superior oblique muscle, (11) mandibular nerve (CN V V3), (12) maxillary nerve (CN V V2), (13) ophthalmic nerve (CN V V1), (14) zygomatic nerve, (15) medial rectus muscle., (16) inferior rectus muscle, (17) long and short ciliary nerves, (18) infraorbital nerve, (19) inferior oblique muscle, and (20) pterygopalatine ganglion.

- Optic nerve (3, Fig. **14a**) (C1): The optic nerve is, in fact, an outdrawn cord of white matter of the brain, lies loose within a tube of arachnoid and dura mater, and is surfaced by pia, arachnoid and dura mater similar to all spinal roots.

- Infraorbital nerve (18, Fig. **14a**) enters the infraorbital canal and proceeds to the skin of the face, innervating the antrum and upper central incisors.

- Zygomatic nerve (14, Fig. **14a**) passes along the lower side of the lateral wall and enters the zygoma. It then divides into the zygomatic-facial and zygomatic-temporal nerves, innervating the skin of the face.

- Frontal nerve (7, Fig. **24a** of chapter 13): This is a direct continuation of the ophthalmic nerve (13, Fig. **24a** of chapter 13). It enters the orbit through the superior orbital fissure and runs above all the orbital muscles on the levator palpebrae superior muscle (10, Fig. **24a** of chapter 13) to divide into the supraorbital (4) and supratrochlear (6) branches.

- Abducent nerve (not depicted) (C VI): This nerve passes forward and then diverges away from the optic nerve and innervates the lateral rectus muscle.

- Oculomotor nerve (2, Fig. **14a**) (C III): The superior division of this nerve runs forward above the optic nerve and supplies motor innervation to the overlying superior rectus and levator palpebrae muscles. It carries sympathetic fibers from the cavernous plexus to the smooth muscle part of the levator palpebrae muscle (10, Fig. **14a**).

- Supraorbital nerve (4, Fig. **14a**) passes through the notch or foramen and turns upward into the forehead.

- Supratrochlear nerve (6, Fig. **14a**): This medial and smaller branch leaves the orbit and runs upward into the forehead.

- Lacrimal nerve (9, Fig. **14b**): This smallest branch of the ophthalmic nerve passes through the lateral part of the superior fissure and runs forward above the lateral rectus muscle. It receives postganglionic parasympathetic fibers from the zygomatic nerve and innervates the lacrimal gland. It also gives a twig to the upper eyelid, the palpebral nerve.

- Trochlear nerve (C IV): The fourth cranial nerve is a motor nerve and innervates only the superior oblique muscle. It enters the orbit through the superior orbital fissure, passes medially above the other structures, and then enters the superior oblique muscle.

- Nasociliary nerve (7, Fig. **14b**) originates from the ophthalmic nerve and passes through the superior orbital fissure between the heads of the lateral rectus muscle. It runs antero-medially above the optic nerve to the medial wall of the orbit and ends by dividing into the infratrochlear (1, Fig. **14b**) and anterior ethmoidal (10, Fig. **14b**) nerves. It also gives off three branches: 1. A branch to the ciliary ganglion (11, Fig. **14a & b**), which runs on the lateral side of the optic nerve to reach the ganglion, 2. The posterior ethmoidal branch (not depicted) passes through the posterior ethmoidal foramen and supplies the mucous membrane of the ethmoid and sphenoid sinuses, and 3. Two long ciliary branches (5, Fig. **14b**) pass along the medial side of the optic nerve and then pierce the sclera. The nerve fibers supply sensory innervation to the eyeball except for the retina. These nerves also transmit postganglionic sympathetic fibers, which enter the nasociliary nerve from the internal carotid plexus and innervate the dilator of the pupil.

- Infratrochlear nerve (1, Fig. **14b**): The smaller of the two branches of the nasociliary nerve leaves the orbit below the trochlea. It supplies the skin of the eyelids and upper one-half of the external nose.

- Anterior ethmoidal nerve (10, Fig. **14b**) is a terminal branch of the nasociliary nerve and leaves the orbit through the anterior ethmoidal foramen and crosses above the ethmoidal sinuses. It descends into the nasal cavity through a slit-like aperture at the side of the crista galli and supplies the nasal mucosa. It then enters the deep surface of the nasal bone and emerges between the nasal bones and the upper lateral nasal cartilage as the external nasal nerve to supply the skin of the lower one-half of the nose.

- Ciliary ganglion (11, Fig. **14b**): The ciliary ganglion is a small body (2 mm in diameter) and lies in the adipose tissue between the lateral rectus muscle and the optic nerve in front of the ophthalmic artery as the artery spirals around the nerve. Three roots enter the ganglion: (1) a sensory branch of the nasociliary nerve that passes through the ganglion without relay to innervate the cornea, iris, and ciliary body, (2) the sympathetic root, and (3) the motor root.

- Short ciliary nerves (6, Fig. **14b**): These branches of the ciliary ganglion usually number 12 or more. Each nerve contains fibers of all three roots of the ganglion (motor, sensory, and sympathetic). The nerves pierce the back of the sclera and pass to their respective destinations in the eyeball.

- Long ciliary nerves (5, Fig. **14b**) pierce the posterior part of the sclera medial to the short ciliary nerves. These nerves also carry sympathetic fibers and are the motor innervation to the dilator pupillae muscle, while a few sensory fibers supply the cornea.

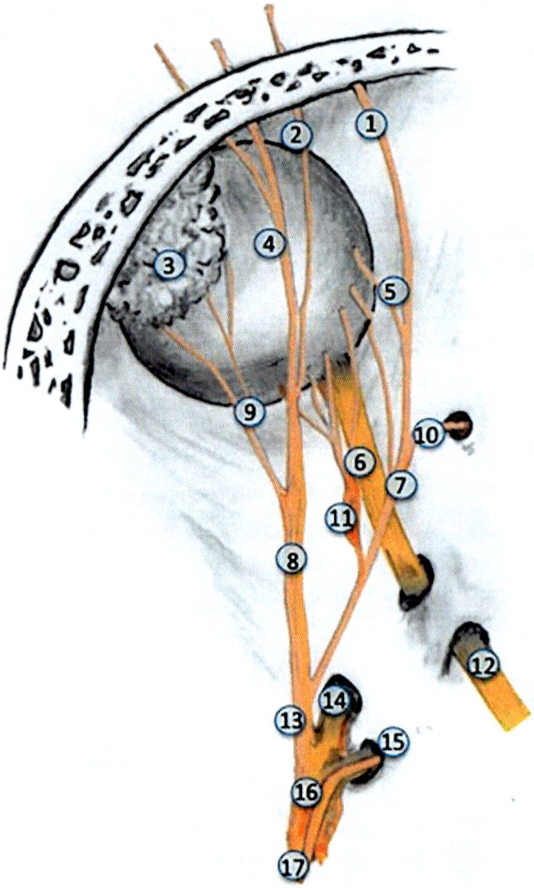

Figure 14b: Schematic representation of the nerves of the eye and orbit.
(1) Infratrochlear nerve, (2) supratrochlear nerve, (3) lacrimal gland, (4) supraorbital nerve, (5) long ciliary nerve, (6) short ciliary nerve, (7) nasociliary nerve, (8) lacrimal nerve, (10) anterior ethmoidal nerve, (11) ciliary ganglion, (12) optic nerve, (13) ophthalmic nerve, (14) maxillary nerve, (15) mandibular nerve, (16) trigeminal ganglion, (17) motor root of trigeminal nerve.

The ultrasound probe that was used was a 6 - 13-MHz linear probe with a 25 mm footprint (HFL – 25, SonoSite Fujifilm, Bothell, WA, USA) *(Ophthalmic ultrasound are done with the thermal index (TI) and mechanical index (MI) limits of <1.0 and <0.23 respectively).*

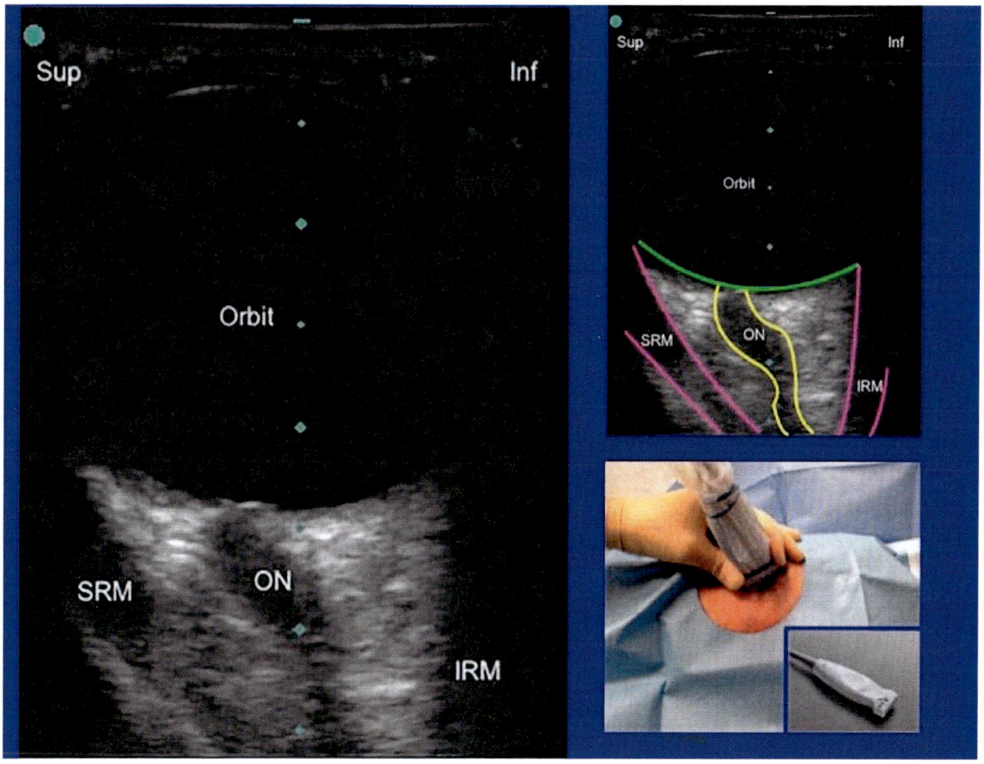

Figure 14c: Sagittal sonoanatomy of the eye.
SRM = superior rectus muscle; IRM = inferior rectus muscle; ON = optic nerve.

ACKNOWLEDGEMENTS

- The Head of the Department of Anesthesiology of the College of Medicine of the University of Florida, Dr. Tim Morey, and his department for their moral support and continuous encouragement.
- The faculty and fellows of the Division of acute and perioperative pain medicine for affording the author (APB) the time to produce this work by covering his clinical duties.
- Drs. Barys Ihnatsenka and Yury Zasimovich for their help in the preparation of the ultrasound images for this chapter.
- Corey Astrom of the Department of Anesthesiology of the College of Medicine of the University of Florida for her professional and high quality text editing.

- Raeducation.com LLC for their financial support.

- The senior author (JPR) produced the illustrations and Dr. Barys V. Ihnatsenka provided Fig. (**12b**).

CONFLICT OF INTEREST

Prof. JP Reyneke declares the following potential conflicts of interest:

1) Consultant for Biomet Microfixation, Tradeport avenue, Jacksonville, Fl. USA.

2) Speakers' Bureau: Present international courses on Orthognathic Surgery for Biomet Microfixation, Jacksonville, FL, USA.

3) Speakers' Bureau: Present international courses on Orthognathic Surgery for Osteomet, Dallas, TX, USA.

Prof. AP Boezaart declare no conflict of interest.

ABBREVIATIONS

Ant	=	anterior
AS Muscle	=	anterior scalene muscle
AT C	=	large anterior tubercle of the transverse process of C6
CCA	=	common carotid artery
CN	=	cranial nerve
DSN	=	dorsal scapular nerve originating from the C5 spinal root
GON	=	greater occipital nerve
IJV	=	internal jugular vein
ION	=	infraorbital nerve
IRM	=	inferior rectus muscle

LC muscle	=	longus colli muscle
MS Muscle	=	middle scalene muscle
OCIM	=	obliquus capitis inferior muscle.
ON	=	optic nerve.
Post	=	posterior
PT	=	Posterior tubercle of the transverse process of C6
R C5	=	5th cervical spinal nerve root (C5)
R C6	=	6th cervical spinal nerve root (C6)
SCM muscle	=	sternocleidomastoid muscle
SCN	=	supraclavicular nerves.
SRM	=	superior rectus muscle
TP C6	=	transverse process of the 6th cervical vertebra (C6)

SUGGESTED FURTHER READING

[1] Last RJ. ANATOMY Regional and Applied. Fifth ed. 1973, Edinburgh & London, Churchill Livingstone.

[2] Romanes GJ, revised; Cunningham's Manual of Practical Anatomy, Vol 3. Thirteenth ed. 1966, London, Oxford University Press.

[3] Radlanski RJ, Wesker KH. The Face Pictorial Atlas of Clinical Anatomy. 2012, London, Quintessence Publishing.

[4] Netter FH, Atlas of Human Anatomy, Ed. Colacino S. Fifth print, 1906-1991. Ciba-Geigy Collection of Medical Illustrations.

[5] Janfaza P, Nadol JB, Galla RL, Montgomery WW, Surgical Anatomy of the Head and Neck. 2001, Philadelelphia, Lippencott Williams & Williams

Subject Index

Subject Index

A

B

C

D

E

F

G

H

I

L

P

V

Z

Made in United States
North Haven, CT
04 November 2026

21727465R10221